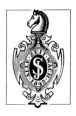

Michael Strobel
Hans-Werner Stedtfeld

Diagnostic Evaluation of the Knee

With a Foreword by John A. Feagin

Translation by Terry C. Telger

With 369 Figures (Mostly in Color)
Containing 541 Separate Illustrations
and 109 Tables

Springer-Verlag Berlin Heidelberg New York
London Paris Tokyo Hong Kong

Dr. Michael Strobel
Klinik und Poliklinik für Unfall- und Handchirurgie
Westfälische Wilhelms-Universität, Jungeblodtplatz 1
D-4400 Münster

PD Dr. Hans-Werner Stedtfeld
Städtisches Klinikum, Zentrum Chirurgie
Fachabteilung Unfallchirurgie, Flurstraße 17
D-8500 Nürnberg

Translator
Terry C. Telger
6112 Waco Way, Ft. Worth, TX 76133, USA

ISBN 3-540-50710-8 Springer-Verlag Berlin Heidelberg New York
ISBN 0-387-50710-8 Springer-Verlag New York Berlin Heidelberg

Library of Congress Cataloging-in-Publication Data
Strobel, Michael. [Diagnostik des Kniegelenkes. English]
Diagnostic evaluation of the knee / Michael Strobel, Hans-Werner Stedtfeld :
with a foreword by John A. Feagin : translation by Terry C. Telger. p. cm.
Translation of: Diagnostik des Kniegelenkes.
Includes bibliographical references. Includes index.
ISBN 3-540-50710-8 (alk. paper). – ISBN 0-387-50710-8 (alk. paper)
1. Knee-Wounds and injuries-Diagnosis. 2. Knee-Mechanical properties. 3. Arthroscopy. I. Stedtfeld,
Hans-Werner, 1944-II. Title. [DNLM: 1. Arthroscopy. 2. Knee Injuries-diagnosis. 3. Knee Joint.
WE 870 S919d]   RD561.S7713   1990   617.5'8207545-dc20   DNLM/DNLC
for Library of Congress   90-10232 CIP

© Springer-Verlag Berlin Heidelberg 1990
Printed in Germany

Typesetting, printing and binding: Appl, Wemding
2124/3145-543210 – Printed on acid-free paper

To our wives

Foreword

Knee surgeons world wide have been aware that a beautifully illustrated book on diagnostic evaluation of the knee existed. What we in the English-speaking world did not appreciate was the superb quality of the text that accompanied these splendid illustrations. Now, Dr. Michael Strobel and Dr. Hans-Werner Stedtfeld's work, *Diagnostic Evaluation of the Knee,* has been translated by Mr. Terry Telger into an English text that is clear and cogent. The authors' message is comprehensive and straight forward. They show how diagnosis of knee disorders lends itself to a disciplined, orderly thought process based on a substantial body of scientific knowledge. This book, through effective illustrations, clarity of text and thought, and subject organization, leads the reader through the diagnostic evaluation of the knee in an enjoyable and unforgettable way.

Some may think the diagnostic process is dead with the advent of magnetic resonance imaging. They are wrong: the diagnostic process has never been more alive, and M. Strobel and H.-W. Stedtfeld capture the excitement of modern day diagnosis through the integration of many disciplines – anatomy, pathophysiology, general examination, special examinations, and special studies. This is the unique character of this book and why it will be a text appreciated by all who care for the knee-injured patient.

Diagnostic Evaluation of the Knee is a timely work: it fills a needed void, and yet is also an in-depth reference companion. This scientific text is truly deserving of the broad dissemination that will be gained through translation. We appreciate having *Diagnostic Evaluation of the Knee* available in English.

August 1990

JOHN A. FEAGIN, M. D.
Durham, North Carolina

Preface

The knee joint, like no other joint in the human body, forms a focal point for diagnostic evaluations by the traumatologist and orthopaedist as well as by the sports physician and general practitioner. This is because of the exceptional vulnerability of the knee joint and its extremely complex anatomic and biomechanical structure.

New scientific discoveries in anatomy, biomechanics, pathophysiology, and diagnostics have led to a significant evolution and reframing of traditional views. This accounts both for the vast body of literature and for the frequent contradictory reports on the diagnosis, classifications, and treatment of knee injuries and their sequelae. Our knowledge of anatomy, too, has been greatly expanded, leading to new functional descriptions for a number of anatomic structures.

While many different tests and procedures are available for examinations of the knee, there is much diversity of opinion as to their appropriate use and value.

Injuries and diseases of the knee deserve special attention because, though very common, they are complex in terms of their detection and differential diagnosis. Examiners must cope with a frustrating lack of consensus in the classification of these lesions and in the evaluation of diagnostic test procedures. This diagnostic "tentativeness" leads to errors that can result in chronic, refractory, and at times irreversible damage to the entire joint. What is true in the diagnostic realm is even more true in treatment, as evidenced by the fact that, to date, more than 300 different surgical procedures have been described for repairs and reconstructions of the ACL, yet there is still no generally accepted "procedure of choice."

Similar problems exist with regard to evaluations of the menisci and patella. By contrast, fractures about the knee joint (femoral condyles, proximal tibia, patella) pose few diagnostic problems because they are so accessible to visualization and evaluation by a variety of radiologic techniques.

This book is intended as a reference work and "diagnostic companion" that will guide the examiner in the conduct of clinical examination procedures, both general and specialized, as well as in the various radiologic studies, machine evaluations, and diagnostic arthroscopy.

We express particular thanks to Dr. A. Menschik of Vienna for his generous help, his many useful comments, and for proofreading the chapter on biomechanics and biometry.

We thank Prof. Dr. M. Reiser (Institute of Clinical Radiology, Westphalian Wilhelm University, Münster) for his kind and energetic support in compiling the chapters on X-ray examinations and magnetic resonance imaging. Prof. Dr. P. E. Peters, Director of the Department of Clinical Radiology of the Westphalian Wilhelm University of Münster, furnished the many X-ray films that are reproduced in this text, and his assistance is gratefully acknowledged.

We thank Prof. Dr. E. Brug (Director, Clinic of Traumatology and Hand Surgery, Westphalian Wilhelm University of Münster) and Prof. Dr. H. Bünte (Director, Clinic of General Surgery, Westphalian Wilhelm University of Münster) for the generous help, which proved to be essential in the planning of this book.

We are also indebted to Dr. Sciuk for proofreading the chapter on scintigraphy. We thank our friend Dr. Hans Pässler (Bopfingen) for his support and for supplying several of the illustrations.

We thank Dr. H. Neumann, Dr. U. Sulkowski, and Mrs. U. Strobel for their extensive help with proofreading, Mrs. C. Werfs and Mrs. M. Wiewer for typing the manuscript, and Mr. Eschkötter for his outstanding photographic documentation of the clinical examination and numerous findings.

It was a pleasure working with the publishing staff at Springer Verlag, whom we thank for their excellent work in the production of this book. Finally, we give special recognition and our sincere thanks to Mr. Terry C. Telger (Ft. Worth, TX) for undertaking the English translation.

Münster, July 1990   MICHAEL STROBEL
                                                 HANS-WERNER STEDTFELD

Contents

Anatomy, Proprioception, and Biomechanics

General Clinical Diagnosis

Special Clinical Diagnosis

Special Diagnostic Procedures

Terminology and Definitions

Anatomy, Proprioception, and Biomechanics

1
Anatomy, Proprioception, and Biomechanics

An understanding of normal and pathologic anatomy is of fundamental importance in diagnosing conditions of the knee joint and in performing optimum anatomic repairs on injured capsuloligamentous structures [34, 77, 235, 285, 313, 321, 451, 452, 466, 470].

Our anatomic depictions of the knee stabilizers should not lead the reader to view these structures in isolation, for even putatively "simple" injuries rarely involve isolated portions of the capsule or ligaments. Rather, we wish to encourage a comprehensive view that appreciates the close functional and anatomic ties among the ligamentous structures of the knee. In the diagnosis and treatment of ligamentous knee injuries, we have found it very helpful to distinguish between anatomic complexes and functional units. It must be realized that chronic instabilities are based not just on a deficiency of the ligaments affected by the primary injury but also on an abnormal laxity of the entire functional unit that is responsible for stabilizing the joint in the given direction or plane [470, 491, 492].

This chapter presents an overview of the functional anatomy of the knee joint. Our presentation is highlighted and clarified by photographs showing a series of anatomic preparations obtained from cadaveric limbs. All photographs pertain to the *right* knee.

1.1
Introduction

The knee joint, the largest articulation in the human body, unites the two bones with the longest lever arms, the tibia and femur. There is a remarkable lack of congruity between the bony articular surfaces of the tibia and femur (see Sect. 1.9 for more details). Lacking the primary bony constraint of the hip joint [67, 466], for example, the knee must rely essentially on ligamentous and muscular elements for its stability (Fig. 1-1). We distinguish the "active" ("dynamic") stabilizers of the knee, such as the musculotendinous units, from "passive" ("static") stabilizers such as the ligaments, menisci, and osseous structures [296, 466].

The most widely used classification of the knee stabilizers was introduced by Nicholas [479] (Table 1-1). More detailed classifications have been proposed by James [321] and by Wagner and Schabus [680].

In addition to the bony structures of the knee (Sect. 1.2), we recognize five different complexes about the knee joint, designated by their location as anterior, central, medial, lateral, and posterior (Sects. 1.3 through 1.7).

1.2
Bony Structures

1.2.1
Femur

The condyles forming the distal end of the femur resemble two adjacent wheels that converge anteriorly (Fig. 1-2). Between them is the intercondylar notch, whose roof forms a 40° angle posteriorly with the axis of the femoral shaft. During extension the ACL engages with the vault of the intercondylar notch in a way that limits the range of knee extension [355, 470, 487, 488] (see Fig. 1-10a).

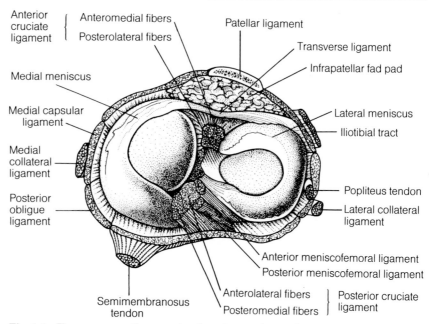

Fig. 1-1. Transverse section proximal to the meniscus plane

Table 1-1. Classification of the knee stabilizers. (After Nicholas [281])

Medial complex:
    Medial collateral ligament
    Posteromedial capsule
    Semimembranosus muscle
    Pes anserinus
Lateral complex:
    Iliotibial tract
    Lateral collateral ligamentü
    Popliteus muscle
    Biceps femoris muscle
Central complex:
    Anterior cruciate ligament
    Posterior cruciate ligament
    Medial meniscus
    Lateral meniscus

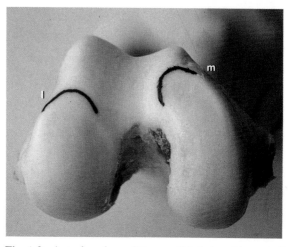

Fig. 1-2. Anterior view of the medial (m) and lateral (l) femoral condyles, showing the condylopatellar sulci (limiting grooves; *marked in black*)

The tibial surfaces of the femur merge anterosuperiorly with the femoral patellar surface, from which they are separated by the "limiting grooves" (condylopatellar grooves; Figs. 1-2 and 1-3). The medial limiting groove appears as an irregularly marked concavity on the superior third of the medial condyle, and the lateral groove as a constant, better marked impression on the middle third of the articular surface [536]. The development of the medial and lateral grooves and their different degrees or prominence can be explained in biomechanical terms. When the knee is extended, the lateral condyle engages with the lateral meniscus at the start of terminal (automatic) rotation, whereas the medial condyle glides past the medial meniscus until full extension is reached [470]. This explains why the medial

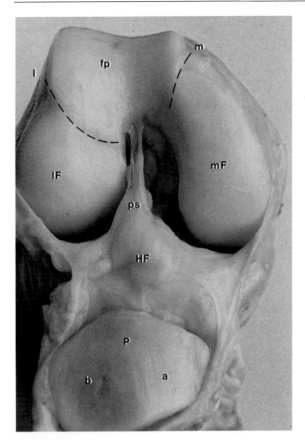

Fig. 1-3. Anterior view of the knee joint in 90° flexion. The quadriceps tendon has been divided, and the patella and patellar ligament have been reflected forward to expose the joint cavity.
Medial femoral condyle *(mF)*, lateral femoral condyle *(lF)*, femoral patellar surface *(fp)*, limiting groove *(broken lines)*, impression of the limiting groove in the medial *(m)* and lateral *(l)* portions of the condyles, infrapatellar fat pad *(HF)*, infrapatellar plica *(ps)*, crest of patella *(P)*, medial facet *(a)*, lateral facet *(b)*

the patella. The remaining fibers pass over the anterior surface of the bone and blend with the patellar ligament [264]. The posterior surface of the patella is covered with cartilage as far as the apex and articulates up to 90° flexion with the femoral patellar surface. The posterior surface of the patella presents a smaller, usually convex medial facet and a larger, concave lateral facet, which apposes to the lateral femoral condyle (Fig. 1-3) [167, 348]. The facets are separated from each other by a vertical ridge, the median retropatellar crest. In about 70% of the population the medial facet itself presents a ridge (secondary median retropatellar crest) that is better marked inferiorly than superiorly [675]. This ridge divides the facet into two more or less well-defined areas, the more medial of which is called the "Odd" facet [26, 217, 264, 703] and reaches the proximal portion of the patella in 70% of cases [675].

Active and passive tension are exerted upon the patella by the quadriceps femoris muscle and the medial and lateral longitudinal retinacula in the vertical direction, and in the transverse direction by the variably marked structures of the vastus medialis obliquus, by the vastus lateralis with its inconstant distal portion, and by the medial and lateral transverse retinacula (Figs. 1-4 and 1-5) [658]. Thus, the complicated gliding path of the patella is defined and delimited on virtually all planes by longitudinal and transverse musculotendinous units.

impression is considerably less constant. Identification of the limiting grooves on the lateral radiograph is helpful in differentiating between the medial and lateral femoral condyles [307, 536] (see Figs. 1-45 and 1-46).

1.2.2
Patella

The patella, the largest sesamoid bone in the human body, is embedded in the tendon of the quadriceps femoris muscle, about 50% of which inserts on the superior border (base) of

1.2.3
Tibia

The tibial plateau is inclined posteriorly at an angle of 3°–8° (retroversion), and it is also displaced posteriorly relative to the axis of the tibial shaft (retroposition) [42, 67]. The intercondylar eminence functions as a fixed central pivot allowing rotation of the femur upon the tibia. Accordingly, its sides are covered by a very strong and thick cartilage layer. The eminence subdivides the upper tibial surface into the anterior and posterior intercondylar areas and the medial and lateral tibial plateaus. The medial plateau is concave in sagittal section,

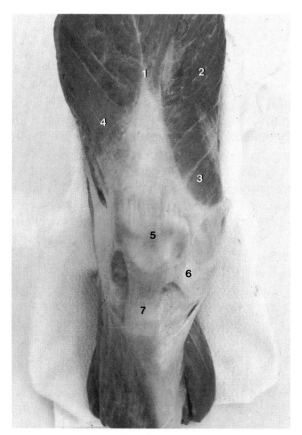

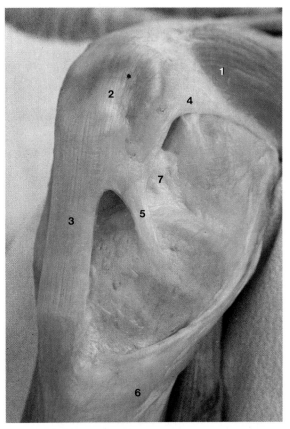

Fig. 1-4. Anterior view of the knee joint in 80° flexion, with fascia lata removed. Rectus femoris *(1)*, vastus medialis *(2)*, vastus medialis obliquus *(3)*, vastus lateralis *(4)*, patella *(5)*, medial patellotibial ligament (medial transverse retinaculum) *(6)*, patellar ligament *(7)*

Fig. 1-5. Anteromedial view in 80° flexion, with fascia lata and medial longitudinal retinaculum removed. Vastus medialis obliquus *(1)*, patella *(2)*, patellar ligament *(3)*, medial patellofemoral ligament *(4)*, medial patellotibial ligament *(5)*, pes anserinus *(6)*, infrapatellar fat pad *(7)*

whereas the lateral plateau is convex and shorter [167, 255, 341, 444]. Another difference is that the medial plateau has a sharp-edged posterior border, while that of the lateral plateau is rounded and blends smoothly with the posterior tibial surface [307].

1.3
Anterior Complex (Table 1-2)

1.3.1
Quadriceps Femoris Muscle

The development of the quadriceps femoris muscle in man paralleled his assumption of an erect gait and is credited with enabling that form of locomotion [167, 173]. With its five constituent muscles, the quadriceps femoris is the most powerful active stabilizer of the knee (Fig. 1-4). Only one of the muscles, the rectus femoris, is biarticular, since it arises from the anterior inferior iliac spine. The rest are monoarticular and arise at various levels on the fem-

Table 1-2. Structures of the anterior complex

Quadriceps femoris muscle
   Vastus lateralis muscle
   Vastus intermedius muscle
   Rectus femoris muscle
   Vastus medialis muscle
   Vastus medialis obliquus muscle
Patellar ligament
Infrapatellar fat pad
Medial retinaculum
Lateral retinaculum

oral shaft [42, 67]. The most distal portion of the vastus medialis muscle and fibers arising from the adductor magnus tendon insert on the patella at a sharp angle, forming a separate expansion called the vastus medialis obliquus muscle (Fig. 1-4) [680].

The distal part of the vastus medialis differs functionally and anatomically from its more proximal portion. The differences consist in the orientation of the muscle fibers relative to the femoral shaft axis (about 17° for the vastus medialis vs 50° for the vastus medialis obliquus) and in the different muscular origins and insertions [572]. In approximately two-thirds of cases there is even an anatomic boundary formed by a superficial branch of the femoral nerve or by a distinct fascial plane [572].

The major portion of the vastus lateralis is situated more proximally and unites with its tendon of insertion about 5–6 cm above the superior border of the patella. The most distal portions, highly variable in their prominence, arise from the posterior surface of the iliotibial tract and send a short tendon to the lateral patellar border [658]. In women, the distal portion of the vastus lateralis inserts on the superolateral point of the patella, while in men the insertion is more evenly distributed proximal and distal to the superolateral part of the patella [243].

Because of its very oblique course, this portion of the muscle is called the vastus lateralis obliquus, analogous to the vastus medialis obliquus on the medial side [243, 573]. When the medial muscles are deficient, the vastus lateralis obliquus fibers predispose to patellar dislo-

cation or may exacerbate disturbances of patellar gliding [243].

In addition to its primary function as the extensor of the knee, the quadriceps femoris functions as the dynamic partner of the PCL. In that capacity it helps to stabilize the knee joint on the sagittal plane [296, 466, 470, 572]. By their anatomic arrangement, the vasti medialis and lateralis exert a restraining effect that stabilizes the knee in rotation, as electromyographic studies have confirmed [579]. In addition, the quadriceps, through its attachments with the retinacula, can impart a primary tension to the knee ligaments that protects them from the potentially damaging effects of abrupt forces [470, 579].

Because athletes in particular require effective rotatory stabilization and rely heavily on the protective effect of primary muscular tension on the ligaments, the vasti medialis and lateralis muscles are powerfully developed in most athletes. Atrophy of the vastus medialis is seen in patients with ACL insufficiency or an old meniscus tear [33, 470], and there are many other knee lesions in which vastus medialis atrophy is a suggestive sign of serious damage [610] (see Sect. 2.2.3).

The quadriceps muscle is linked to adjacent structures by numerous proprioceptive reflexes (see Sect. 1.8). Even a varus or valgus displacement of the knee joint will affect the tonus of the vasti muscles [513]. When a valgus- or varus-producing stress is applied to the slightly flexed knee, valgus displacement causes a medial pull to be exerted on the patella, while varus displacement causes the patella to be pulled laterally [470]. The stretching of the vasti by the imposed stress causes the vastus on the affected side to contract, exerting a pull that tends to recenter the patella. Since valgus-producing stresses are common, patellar dislocation would be more prevalent were it not for the reflex medial "checkrein." The changing contractions of the vasti also benefit the knee by raising the pressure in the medial or lateral part of the femoropatellar joint [470], thereby assisting cartilage nutrition ("cartilage massage"). As a result, muscular imbalances like those associated with angular deformities or certain major knee operations (extensive arthrotomy that disrupts the proprioception between the patella and vasti) lead to a unilateral retropatellar pressure rise with resultant cartilage damage (see Sect. 1.8 for more details).

1.3.2
Medial and Lateral Retinacula

The medial and lateral longitudinal retinacula are fibrous tracts that originate from the vasti medialis and lateralis muscles and extend to the tibia, running parallel to the patellar ligament. These structures, which comprise the "reserve extensor apparatus," course between the patellar ligament and medial collateral ligament on the medial side, and between the iliotibial tract and patellar ligament on the lateral side. Deep to the superficial longitudinal fibers on each side is a separate, transverse layer, the medial and lateral transverse retinacula. The transverse layer provides passive anterior tension and contains distinct fibrous tracts that can be demonstrated in isolation as the medial and lateral patellofemoral ligaments and the medial and lateral patellotibial ligaments [658] (Figs. 1-5 and 1-6).

1.3.3
Infrapatellar Fat Pad

Between the patellar ligament and anterior joint capsule lies the infrapatellar fat pad (Fig. 1-3). Though most authors ascribe no special functional significance to the fat pad, Müller [467, 470] states that it acts as a shock-absorbing element for peak loads during contraction of the quadriceps muscle.

Because the infrapatellar fat pad contributes to the blood supply of the ACL, it plays an important role in revascularization following a repair or autologous reconstruction of the ligament [18, 470]. The middle third of the patellar tendon with a fat-pad pedicle is sometimes used as a vascularized ligament replacement [39].

1.4
Central Complex (Table 1-3)

The ACL and PCL are the central passive guide elements of the knee joint (the "central pivot") and are fundamental to preserving the physiologic rolling-gliding motion of the femur on the tibia [278]. Lesions of the ACL result in an experimentally confirmed disintegration of this rolling-gliding process [707] with consequent damage to the joint, especially to

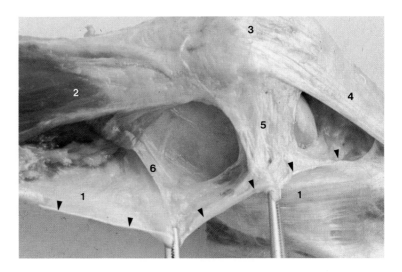

Fig. 1-6. Lateral view in 30° flexion, with the iliotibial tract released at its anterior border *(arrowheads)* and retracted laterally. Iliotibial tract *(1)*, vastus lateralis muscle *(2)*, patella *(3)*, patellar ligament *(4)*, lateral patellofemoral ligament *(5)*, Kaplan fibers (distal superficial portion) *(6)*

Table 1-3. Structures of the central complex

Anterior cruciate ligament (ACL)
Posterior cruciate ligament (PCL)
Anterior meniscofemoral ligament (of Humphrey)
Posterior meniscofemoral ligament (of Wrisberg)
Medial meniscus
Lateral meniscus

the posterior meniscus horns and the articular cartilage with associated radiographic changes (see Fig. 6-10 b) [10, 22, 29, 33, 73, 105, 235, 306, 318, 491, 492, 494].

The cruciate ligaments, whose function can be modeled by a crossed four-bar linkage, form the basic kinematic mechanism of the knee joint [448, 450, 470] (Fig. 1-7). It should be noted, however, that the crossed four-bar linkage is a simplified model which takes into account only the cruciate ligaments and does not fully portray the complex biomechanics of the knee joint. This led Menschik, in 1974 [450], to describe the Burmester curve, which takes into account the kinematics of the cruciate as well as the collateral ligaments of the knee (Fig. 1-8) (see Sect. 1.9) and illustrates how the courses of the ligaments are interdependent.

The suggestion of Müller [470] that the ACL, with its complicated fiber pattern, may itself be structured along the lines of a crossed four-bar linkage illustrates the complexity of the biomechanics.

Ontogenetically the cruciate ligaments (Fig. 1-9) migrated into the knee joint from the posterior side, so they are covered only anteriorly by synovial membrane. Thus they are intra-articular but extrasynovial. In front of the ACL is a synovial fold (infrapatellar plica) of variable prominence which, if hypertrophied, may be mistaken for the ACL on arthroscopic inspection (see Fig. 11-50).

1.4.1
Anterior Cruciate Ligament

The anterior cruciate ligament (ACL) originates from an elliptical area approximately 15–20 mm long on the posteromedial surface of the lateral femoral condyle. It passes forward, downward, and medially to the anterior intercondylar area of the tibia, where it inserts between the anterior attachments of the menisci (Fig. 1-10 a).

Two functional subdivisions of the ligament are recognized:

1. Anteromedial fibers
2. Posterolateral fibers

In their approximately 3-cm course, the fibers intertwine in a way that results in a triangular

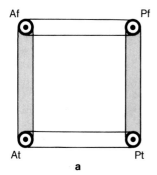
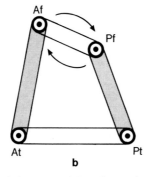
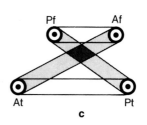

Fig. 1-7 a–c. Kinematic model of the crossed four-bar linkage, which takes into account only the anterior *(AfAt)* and posterior *(PfPt)* cruciate ligaments. We can understand the principle of the "crossed" four-bar linkage by taking the model in its uncrossed state (**a**), matching the lengths of the side bars to the relative lengths of the cruciate ligaments (**b**), and then crossing the bars *(arrows)* to obtain the crossed four-bar linkage (**c**). AtPt represents the distance between the attachment sites of the cruciate ligaments on the tibial plateau, PfAf the distance between the femoral insertion areas

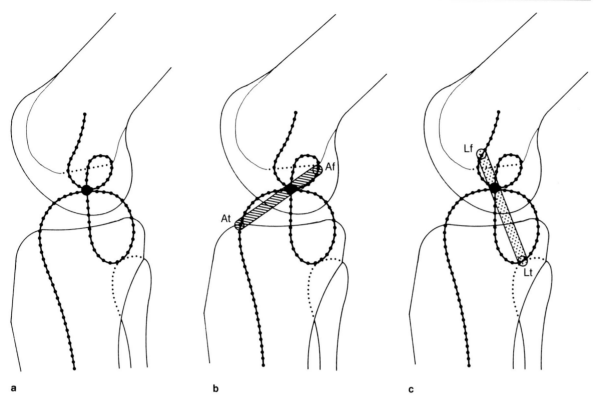

Fig. 1-8a-c. Construction of the Burmester curve (**a**), which takes into account the course of the cruciate ligaments (e.g., the ACL, AfAt) (**b**) and that of the collateral ligaments (e.g., the lateral collateral ligament, LfLt) (**c**). All the sites of origin and insertion lie on the Burmester curve. The cruciate and collateral ligaments pass through the instant center of the motion system (●)

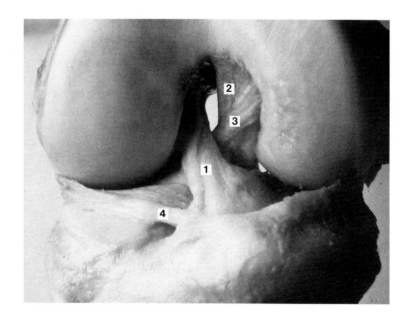

Fig. 1-9. Anterior view in slight flexion (left knee). The anterior capsule, retinacula, patella, and synovial investment of the cruciates have been removed. ACL *(1)*, PCL *(2)*, anterior meniscofemoral ligament *(of Humphrey) (3)*, transverse ligament of the knee (inconstant) *(4)*

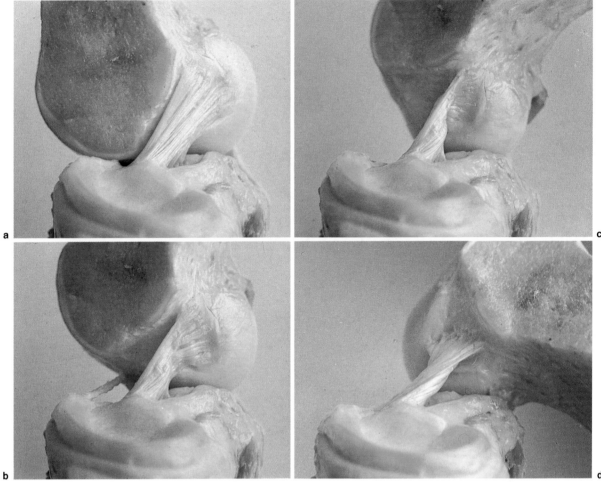

Fig. 1-10 a-d. Medial view with the medial femoral condyle removed, showing the behavior of the ACL with increasing flexion of the joint: extension (**a**), 30° flexion (**b**), 60° flexion (**c**), 120° flexion (**d**)

area of insertion in the anterior intercondylar area. At that site the longer anteromedial fibers are situated anteriorly and the shorter posterolateral fibers posteriorly. In the extended knee the anteromedial fibers originate from the most superior part of the femoral insertion area of the ACL, while the posterolateral fibers originate from the most inferior part [680]. Identification of separate fiber bundles by dissection is somewhat controversial, and several authors [16, 355, 500] found no microscopic or macroscopic evidence of an anatomic subdivision of the ligament into different bundles.

More recent studies suggest that the fibers of the ACL are arranged more along the lines of a scissor lattice [14], which is a more effi-cient arrangement in terms of coping with changing fiber tensions. If the fiber arrangement were strictly parallel, potentially disruptive tension differences could develop within the ligament.

During extension the ACL engages against the roof of the intercondylar notch in a way that limits further extension (Fig. 1-10 a). With increasing flexion the ligament bundles twist around each other, the posterolateral fibers rotating beneath the anteromedial fibers [191, 487] (Fig. 1-10 b-d). The ligament loses its proximal fan shape as flexion increases, assuming more the shape of a rounded cord. Van Dijk [674] showed that the fibers of the ACL are not parallel in extension, as one might assume, but show external torsion of 46°. When the knee is flexed to 90°, the torsion angle increases to 105°, as manifested by an increased overall twisting of the ligament (Fig. 1-10 d).

If we consider the individual fibers as separate biomechanical structures, we find that the fibers mimic the pattern of an uncrossed four-bar linkage in extension (fibers are uncrossed, Fig. 1-10 a) but adopt the form of a crossed four-bar linkage with increasing flexion (crossing of the fibers, Fig. 1-10 d). However, this analogy is subject to the same limitations cited by Menschik [448, 450] with regard to transfering the mechanism of the four-bar linkage directly to ligamentous (biologic) structures. The four-bar model allows motion only on one plane, and a rigid connection must exist between the hinge points (the origin and insertion of the cruciate ligaments). But these conditions are not fully satisfied in the knee joint, which allows motion on more than one plane. The tension on different fibers changes with the angle of knee flexion.

There is diversity of opinion as to which fibers are tight in flexion and which are tight in extension [42, 167, 209, 279, 311, 467]. As with the anteromedial fibers, opinions differ on how tension is developed in the posterolateral fibers [167, 279, 311, 466, 488]. The discrepant and in some cases contradictory results of different in vitro stress tests presumably relate to differences in experimental conditions (joint position, applied force, measuring apparatus). The clinical relevance of studies on the tension and fiber orientation of the ACL is based on the fact that the structures provide their greatest stabilizing effect in joint positions where their state of tension is maximal.

The anatomic course of the ligament is a fundamental consideration in ACL reconstructions. The anatomic position of the tibial insertion site and especially the choice of the femoral insertion site (drill channel) are critical in terms of the functional behavior of the selected cruciate ligament replacement [254, 500]. It has been shown that the "extra-anatomic" over-the-top position for the femoral insertion leads to an average of 10 mm of elongation with a tension up to 200 N exerted on the reconstructed ligament. This compares with an elongation of only 1–3 mm and a tension up to 45 N when the ligament is given a transosseous, strictly anatomic area of insertion. The goal in every such procedure, then, is to achieve an isometric tension in the reconstructed ligament. That is the only way to ensure adequate stability while maintaining a full range of joint motion and protecting the reconstruction from excessive elongation and peak stresses [500].

It can be especially difficult to determine the optimum tibial and femoral attachments for the cruciate ligament reconstruction in knees with chronic instability. Frequently the ligament stumps are atrophied or have been previously removed by surgery. The key to success is to make certain that the reconstructed ligament remains isometric during function. This is done by identifying the optimum sites of attachment, whose determination has been the object of numerous investigations [15, 64, 185, 218, 223, 226, 261, 497].

It is important to consider that the ACL is not a simple "thin cord" but a complex anatomic structure. Accordingly, there exists (at least in theory) a set of isometric points, which might be more accurately described as an isometric area [64].

An isometric ligament placement is defined as one in which the distance between the tibial and femoral insertion points does not change by more than 1.5–2 mm when the knee is flexed from 0° to 90° [64, 218, 226, 261]. Special devices for determining the most favorable isometric points have already been developed [218].

The isometric points for the ACL are located approximately 5 mm posterosuperior to the center of the normal anatomic insertion [218], or at the site of attachment of the anterosuperior fibers [497]. An over-the-top position is also possible. In this case the isometric point can be approximated by attaching the ligament to a 2- to 4-mm-deep notch prepared in the posterosuperior aspect of the lateral femoral condyle [497].

A comparison of the effect of the femoral and tibial insertion sites on isometry shows that the femoral insertion is of greater importance than the tibial insertion [64, 223]. However, the tibial insertion has a major bearing on the length of the substitute ligament and its orientation in the joint [223]. Above all, one should avoid placing the tibial drill hole too far anteriorly, as this can result in limitation of extension.

The following conclusions may be drawn from the results of the many experimental studies to determine the optimum isometric points for the attachment of a reconstructed ACL:

1. There is no single, absolute isometric point. The discrepancies in published findings are due not just to differences in experimental conditions but also to the fact that each knee joint has its own isometric points. Individual knees also differ markedly in their bony dimensions and in the strength and thickness of their cruciate ligaments.
2. The position of the femoral insertion is critical for an isometric reconstruction of the ACL as well as the PCL.
3. An isometric ligament placement is essential for a good surgical outcome and for the long-term survival and stability of the graft.

The major practical implication is that the surgeon should drill the femoral channel for a cruciate ligament replacement only after identifying the most favorable individual isometric point or area, defined as the site where there is less than a 2-mm change in the distance between the tibial and femoral insertions when the knee moves from extension to 90° flexion.

1.4.2
Posterior Cruciate Ligament

The posterior cruciate ligament (PCL) arises from the inner surface of the medial femoral condyle [209, 296]. Its course is opposite to that of the ACL, which it crosses at a 90° angle in passing to the posterior intercondylar area and posterior tibial surface (Figs. 1-11 and 1-12). The area of attachment on the medial femoral condyle is horizontal in extension and thus differs from the vertical femoral attach-

ment of the ACL (Figs. 1-12a and 1-15a) [209, 680].

The ligament consists of a long, thick anterolateral fiber system and a shorter posteromedial fiber system [42, 167, 209, 311, 470, 569, 680].

Like the ACL, the PCL twists upon itself with increasing flexion (Fig. 1-12), so again the kinematic principle of the four-bar linkage is observed. Thus, the fiber systems form an uncrossed four-bar linkage in extension (fibers parallel, Fig. 1-12a) and a crossed four-bar linkage in flexion (fiber crossed, Fig. 1-12c). In contrast to the ACL, the fibers of the PCL twist from 51° of external rotation in extension to 30° of internal rotation as the knee flexes [674]. This is a further illustration of the opposite functional behaviors of the cruciate ligaments, which, however, work jointly in the service of knee-joint kinematics (Fig. 1-13).

Because the PCL is the most powerful ligamentous structure of the knee joint, it is viewed as the "central stabilizer" of the knee

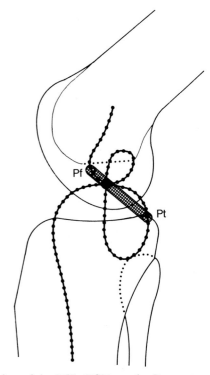

Fig. 1-11. Position of the PCL (PfPt) on the Burmester curve

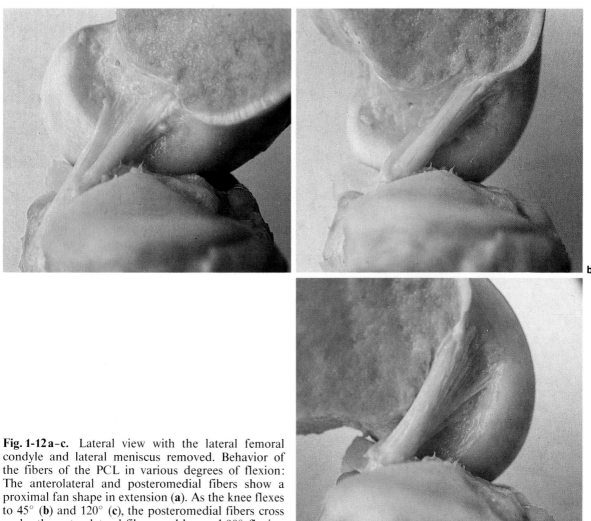

Fig. 1-12 a-c. Lateral view with the lateral femoral condyle and lateral meniscus removed. Behavior of the fibers of the PCL in various degrees of flexion: The anterolateral and posteromedial fibers show a proximal fan shape in extension (**a**). As the knee flexes to 45° (**b**) and 120° (**c**), the posteromedial fibers cross under the anterolateral fibers and beyond 90° flexion occupies the more anterior position

[278, 294, 296]. Hughston [296] calls it the "key to the knee joint" and makes it the basis for his classification of instabilities.

As with the ACL, the goal in PCL reconstructions is to achieve an isometric placement of the graft. The femoral isometric area lies posterosuperiorly in the normal area of attachment of the PCL. Studies by Grood et al. [226] show that there is no absolute isometric point for this ligament. The tibial isometric insertion site is located at the attachment of the posterolateral fibers. An isometric placement can also be achieved with a modified over-the-back position. However, this requires making about a 5-mm-deep notch to advance the liga-

ment substitute into the more anterior, isometric area [185]. As with the ACL, placement of the femoral insertion is critical to achieving an isometric reconstruction.

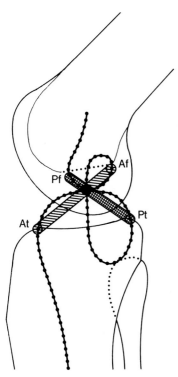

Fig. 1-13. The origins *(PfAf)* and insertions *(PtAt)* of the cruciate ligaments lie on the Burmester curve. Their point of intersection coincides with the instant center of the motion system *(●)*

1.4.3
Anterior and Posterior Meniscofemoral Ligaments

The PCL may be accompanied by two ligaments which, if present, both originate from the inner surface of the medial femoral condyle. The anterior meniscofemoral ligament (of Humphrey) passes over the front of the PCL and was identifiable in many of our specimens as a well-defined, separate band (Fig. 1-14). Heller [268], however, describes it as being fused to the surface of the PCL and present in 35% of his specimens. He could identify both ligaments in only 6% [268]. In our material the anterior meniscofemoral ligament was present in 72% of knees, the posterior meniscofemoral ligament in 78%.

Behind the PCL, the posterior meniscofemoral ligament (of Wrisberg) descends to the posterior horn of the lateral meniscus [268].

The variable and at times very marked prominence of this ligament led Robert [554] in 1855 to describe it as the "posterior crossed ligament," as opposed to the anatomic PCL, which he called the "middle crossed ligament." When both meniscofemoral bands are present, which we noted in 61% of our material, they form a looplike structure that wraps around the insertion of the PCL (Fig. 1-15).

The anterior meniscofemoral ligament is tight in flexion (Fig. 1-15 b), while the posterior meniscofemoral ligament is tight in extension (Fig. 1-15 a). Both ligaments tighten with internal rotation of the tibia. Their function is to stabilize the posterior horn of the lateral meniscus and prevent its entrapment [268, 680] (Fig. 1-15 b).

1.4.4
Menisci

The small area of contact between the femoral condyles and tibial plateau is partially corrected by the interposition of the fibrocartilage menisci. These C-shaped or crescent-shaped cartilages rest on the medial and lateral tibial plateau, have a wedge-shaped cross section, and are vascularized from their base, which is adherent to the capsule [167, 168, 311, 680] (Fig. 1-16).

The medial meniscus is supplied by the articular branch of the descending genicular artery and medial superior genicular artery, and the lateral meniscus by the lateral inferior genicular artery. The posterior portions of the menisci derive their blood supply from direct branches of the popliteal artery and middle genicular artery. Numerous studies show that the anterior and posterior horns have a copious blood supply, while the supply of the intermediate portion is restricted to the basal zone [17, 40, 46]. This is consistent with the results of laser Doppler flowmetry, which registers the highest blood flow rates in the anterior and posterior horns and basal region [641].

Bird [46] demonstrated the presence of small canals in the menisci by electron microscopy. Reportedly, these canals run between two col-

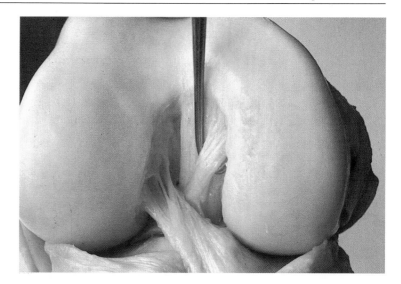

Fig. 1-14. Anterior view of the left knee with the synovial investment removed. The hook has been passed beneath the anterior meniscofemoral ligament (of Humphrey)

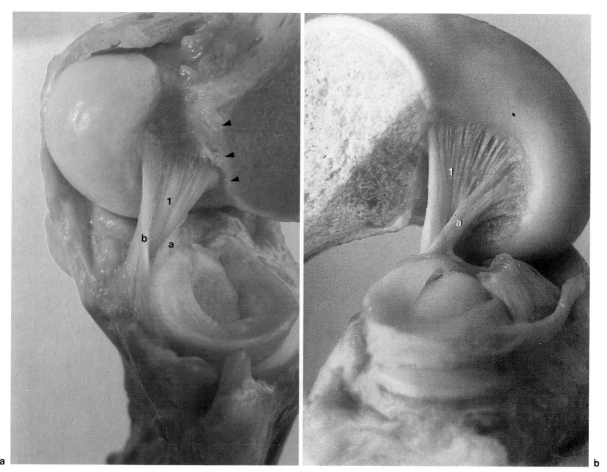

Fig. 1-15a, b. Posterolateral view of the knee joint in extension (**a**) and lateral view in flexion (**b**) with the lateral capsule, lateral ligaments, and lateral femoral condyle removed. Roof of the intercondylar notch *(arrowheads)*, PCL *(1)*, anterior meniscofemoral ligament (of Humphrey) (**a**), posterior meniscofemoral ligament (of Wrisberg) (**b**)

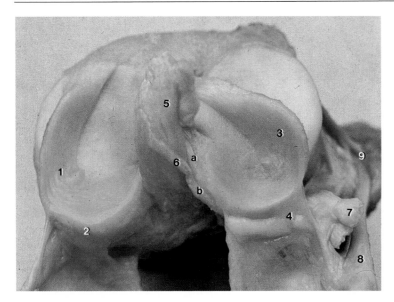

Fig. 1-16. Superior view with the femoral condyles removed, showing the medial meniscus *(1)* and its attachments to the posteromedial capsule *(2)*, the lateral meniscus *(3)* and its attachments to the posterolateral capsule *(4)*, the PCL *(5)*, anterior meniscofemoral ligament *(6a)*, posterior meniscofemoral ligament *(6b)*, popliteus tendon *(7)*, lateral collateral ligament *(8)*, fibular head *(9)*

lagenous bundles which in turn surround the vascular structures within the meniscus. Their function may be to collect transsudated fluid from the vessels and carry it to the fibrocartilage cells of the meniscus. It is conceivable that this intrameniscal fluid flow from fenestrated arteries through the sinusoidal canal system to the meniscal surface performs a nutritive function for the meniscus. It may also perform a shock-absorbing function as a "water cushion" [46]. Further studies are needed to clarify these issues.

1.4.4.1
Medial Meniscus

The larger medial meniscus extends from the anterior intercondylar area of the tibia (anterior horn region) to the posterior intercondylar area (posterior horn region). In the middle third the base of the meniscus is firmly attached to the thickened medial capsule layer, which in turn is separated from the medial collateral ligament by an interposed bursa. The posterior third of the meniscus has strong fibrous attachments to the posterior oblique ligament [295] and semimembranosus tendon [680] (Fig. 1-16). This firm attachment accounts for the relatively low mobility of the medial

meniscus and its consequent proneness to injury.

1.4.4.2
Lateral Meniscus

Viewed from above, the lateral meniscus presents a more circular shape than the medial meniscus. Its anterior horn arises just lateral to the insertion of the ACL, to which it is sometimes united by fiberlike attachments [168, 311]. In its further course it has isolated attachments with lateral capsuloligamentous structures. Thus, the lateral capsule sends fibers to the base of the meniscus in the area where the tendon passes upward and forward between the meniscus and the lateral collateral ligament (popliteal hiatus). The fibers of the PCL that insert into the posterior horn of the lateral meniscus were described previously (Fig. 1-15); attention must be given to these fibers in a lateral meniscectomy, especially when dealing with a discoid meniscus.

The two anterior horns of the menisci are interconnected by the transverse ligament of the knee (Fig. 1-9), which is inconstant and of variable prominence. This ligament is believed to have little functional significance.

Both the medial and lateral menisci are essential stabilizers of the knee joint, bearing approximately 45% of the body weight (Table 1-4) [311]. They move posteriorly during flexion and anteriorly during extension [1, 42, 65, 67, 168, 311, 680] (Fig. 1-17). They serve to distribute the synovial fluid while helping to check rotational movements and absorb peak loads [279, 467].

Table 1-4. Functions of the menisci

1. Buffer between the femur and tibia
2. Relieve pressure on the articular cartilage
3. Transform compressive and tensile stresses
4. Enlarge area of femorotibial contact
5. Stabilization
6. Aid nutrition of cartilage surfaces
7. Reinforce medial collateral ligament
8. Proprioception
9. Limitation of hyperflexion and hyperextension

1.5
Medial Complex (Table 1-5)

Both medial and lateral structures show a three-layer arrangement consisting of a superficial (fascia lata), intermediate (collateral ligaments), and deep layer (capsular ligaments). In addition, the capsuloligamentous structures of the medial and lateral complex are envisioned as consisting of an anterior, middle, and posterior third (Fig. 1-18) [173, 321, 466, 680, 689].

1.5.1
Medial Collateral Ligament

The medial (tibial) collateral ligament is the dominant ligamentous structure of the medial side. It arises from the medial femoral epicon-

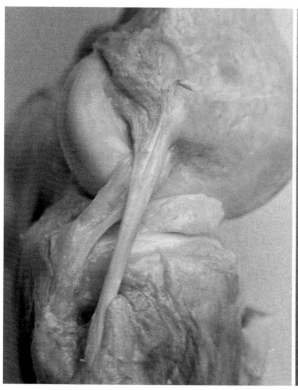
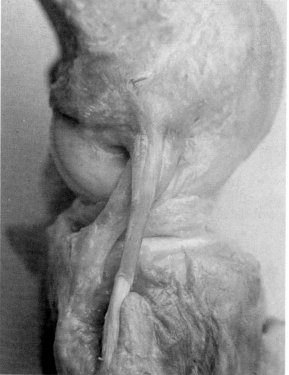

Fig. 1-17a, b. Lateral view in extension (**a**) and 45° flexion (**b**). From its anterior position in extension (**a**), the lateral meniscus moves posteriorly with increasing flexion

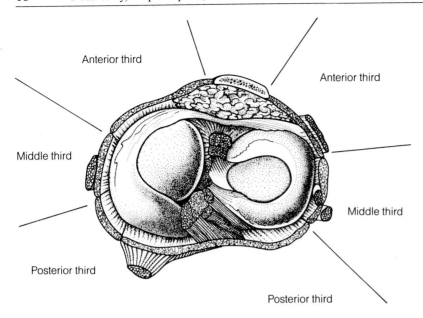

Anterior third

Anterior third

Middle third

Middle third

Posterior third

Posterior third

Fig. 1-18. Transverse section proximal to the meniscus plane, showing the subdivision of the medial and lateral sides of the joint into thirds (see also Fig. 1-1)

Table 1-5. Structures of the medial complex

Medial retinaculum
Medial collateral ligament
Medial capsular ligament
Posterior oblique ligament
Semimembranosus muscle
Pes anserinus
   Semitendinosus muscle
   Gracilis muscle
   Sartorius muscle

dyle, anterior to the adductor tubercle, and descends for 9–11 cm before inserting on the medial tibial border, overlapped by the muscle group of the pes anserinus (Fig. 1-19) [1, 42, 66, 67, 167, 680, 688]. It is attached anteriorly to the medial retinaculum, and its posterior fibers blend with the posterior oblique ligament and posteromedial capsule [174] (Fig. 1-20).

The medial collateral ligament sends posterosuperior and posteroinferior expansions to the posterior oblique ligament, the posteroinferior fibers first passing over the semimembranosus tendon before blending with the ligament (Fig. 1-20). These fibers insert on the posterior tibial border and the posterior horn of the medial meniscus.

During flexion the posterior expansions lose little of their tension, because all the medial ligaments including the posterior oblique ligament are "self-tightening" (Fig. 1-21). This is made possible by their elliptical area of attachment on the medial epicondyle [311], their attachment to the medial meniscus, and their common flexion axis with the ACL and PCL. This relationship is a logical consequence of the Burmester curve (Fig. 1-22) [449, 470].

A bursa separates the medial collateral ligament from the underlying capsular ligament, visible only after removal of the medial collateral ligament, and from the medial meniscus (Fig. 1-23). The interposed bursa enables the ligament to glide backward over the medial capsular layer with little friction as the knee is flexed.

The function of the medial collateral ligament is to stabilize the knee against valgus forces in extension and especially in flexion, and also to stabilize against forces producing external rotation. That is why the competency of the medial collateral ligament is tested clinically by applying a valgus stress with the knee slightly flexed (about 20°) and the tibia externally rotated. The external rotation relaxes the cruciate ligaments so that they will contribute less to primary medial stabilization.

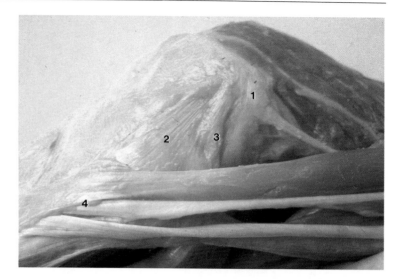

Fig. 1-19. Medial view in 90° flexion with the fascia lata removed. Adductor tubercle *(1)*, triangular form of the medial collateral ligament *(2)* continuous posteriorly with the posterior oblique ligament *(3)*, pes anserinus *(4)*

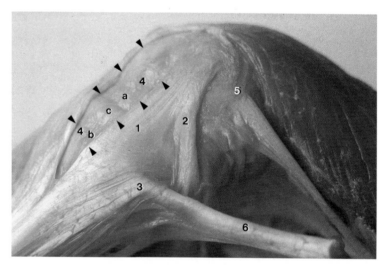

Fig. 1-20. Medial view in 90° flexion with the pes anserinus removed. Medial collateral ligament *(1)*, split in line with its fibers (arrowheads), with posterosuperior expansion to the posterior oblique ligament *(2)* and posteroinferior expansion to the posterior tibial obli-que ligament *(3)*. Medial capsular ligament *(4)* with meniscofemoral ligament *(a)* and meniscotibial ligament *(b)*, bulge of medial meniscus *(c)*, adductor tubercle *(5)*, tendon of semimembranosus muscle *(6)*

1.5.2
Medial Capsular Ligament

In contrast to the anterior third of the capsule, which has little functional significance, and the posterior third of the capsule, which is fused with the posterior femoral oblique ligament (see below), the thick middle third of the capsule is of major importance (Figs. 1-20 and 1-23). This accounts for its designation as the "medial capsular ligament." Its attachments to the base of the meniscus subdivide the ligament anatomically into a meniscofemoral and a meniscotibial component [279, 295]. The fiber orientation corresponds to that of the medial collateral ligament.

Tight in extension [354], the medial capsular ligament loses tension as the knee begins to flex but tightens again with greater flexion due to the increasing separation of its origin and

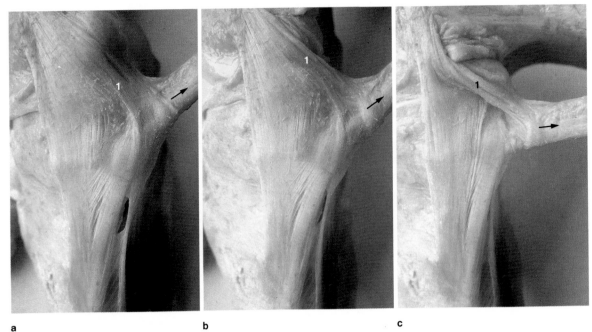

a   b   c

Fig. 1-21 a–c. Medial view with the pes anserinus removed, in extension (**a**), 30° flexion (**b**), and approximately 100° flexion (**c**). Tendon of semimembranosus muscle *(arrow)* is retracted posteriorly. Note the "winding" of the posteromedial capsule *(1)* and posterior oblique ligament with increasing flexion

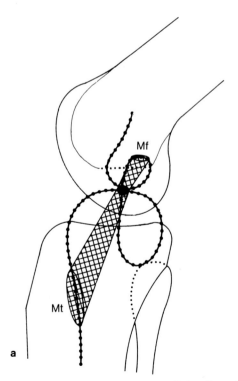

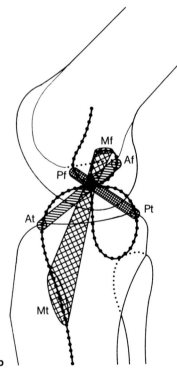

a   b

Fig. 1-22 a, b. Course of the medial collateral ligament *(MfMt)*, whose areas of origin and insertion lie on the Burmester curve (**a**). Anterior *(AfAt)* and posterior *(PfPt)* cruciate ligaments and medial collateral ligament *(MfMt)* on the Burmester curve (**b**) with a common point of intersection at the instant center *(●)* of the motion system *(schematic)*

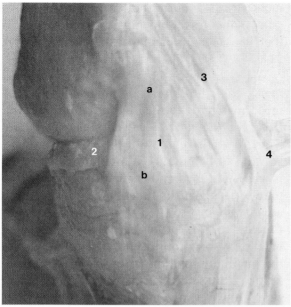

a   b

Fig. 1-23 a, b. Medial view after removal of the medial collateral ligament, in extension (**a**) and 90° flexion (**b**). The medial capsular ligament *(1)*, with its menisco-femoral (**a**) and meniscotibial components (**b**), is at-tached both to the medial meniscus *(2)* and to the pos-teromedial capsule *(3)*, which is made tense by the semimembranosus muscle *(4)*

insertion. This results from the shape of the condyle and the physiologic recession of the medial meniscus (Fig. 1-23).

Thus, the medial capsular ligament stabilizes the knee against valgus-producing and externally rotating forces in extension and also at higher angles of flexion [311, 416].

Opinions differ as to the functional importance of the medial capsular ligament. While Kennedy and Fowler [354] assign it an important role in medial stabilization of the knee, Warren et al. [688, 689] and Hertel [279] believe that it performs only a minor stabilizing function. Our own studies indicate no increase of valgus laxity or anterior displacement following isolated division of the medial capsular ligament.

1.5.3
Posterior Oblique Ligament

The posterior oblique ligament, whose functional importance was first described by Hughston and Eilers [295], forms the connecting link between the medial and posterior structures (Fig. 1-24). It should not be confused with the oblique popliteal ligament.

The posterior oblique ligament (known also as the posterior medial collateral ligament or posteromedial ligament) originates from the adductor tubercle and runs distally with three arms [420] (Fig. 1-24).

1. The main, central arm passes to the posterior tibial border and medial meniscus [295, 311].

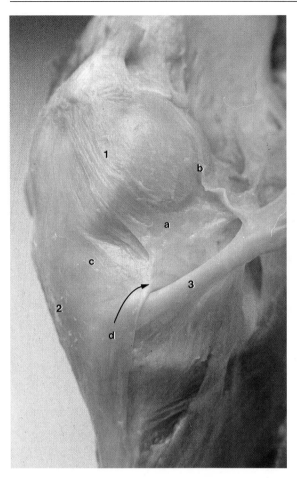

Fig. 1-24. Posteromedial view in extension. Posterior oblique ligament *(1)* with its main arm *(a)* and lateral fibers *(b)*, medial collateral ligament *(2)* with its posterosuperior arm *(c)*, posterior tibial oblique ligament *(d)*, which winds over *(arrow)* the semimembranosus tendon *(3)* and inserts with the posterior oblique ligament on the posterior tibial border

meniscus to stabilize the knee joint on the sagittal plane. It is frequently involved in injuries that cause anteromedial instability [285, 296, 311, 354, 409, 479].

We distinguish the posterior oblique ligament from the "posterior tibial oblique ligament," which is formed by the posteroinferior fibers of the medial collateral ligament and winds over the tendon of the semimembranosus muscle (Fig. 1-24). Although this structure is well developed and is identifiable in all anatomic specimens, its function has not yet been adequately investigated or described. A major function of the posterior tibial oblique ligament may be proprioception and to support the internally rotating action of the semimembranosus muscle when the joint is near extension. However, no studies have yet been done on the postulated proprioceptive feedback mechanism for this action.

1.5.4
Semimembranosus Muscle

The biarticular semimembranosus muscle is part of the ischiocrural muscle group (hamstrings), originates from the ischial tuberosity, and has five attachments with the posteromedial ligamentous structures of the knee (Fig. 1-25):

1. A main insertion on the medial tibial condyle, below the medial collateral ligament.
2. A medial expansion to the posterior capsule, posterior oblique ligament, and posterior horn of the medial meniscus [295, 321]. The meniscal attachment prevents entrapment of the meniscus by drawing it posteriorly during flexion (Fig. 1-26). The fibers to the posterior capsule reinforce the capsule and make it tense (Fig. 1-27).
3. A lateral expansion to the oblique popliteal ligament (Figs. 1-27 and 1-28).
4. Fibers to the posterior aspect of the medial tibial condyle.
5. Distal expansions to the fascia of the popliteus muscle, the periosteum, and the posterior and posteromedial tibial surface.

2. The medial arm passes to the semimembranosus tendon.
3. The lateral arm joins with the semimembranosus tendon to help form the oblique popliteal ligament.

The posterior oblique ligament acts with the medial collateral ligament to stabilize the knee against valgus-producing and externally rotating forces in extension and also in flexion, where it is "dynamized" (made tense) by the semimembranosus muscle [174, 295, 420, 680]. It works with the ACL, the medial collateral ligament, and the posterior horn of the medial

The semimembranosus muscle, with its complex pattern of insertion, is the prime stabilizer of the posteromedial corner of the joint. Its tendinous fibers connect with, or are involved in the formation of, numerous posterior and posteromedial ligamentous structures. Dynamically tensed in this way, these ligamentous structures cannot be regarded as purely "passive" stabilizers of the knee (Figs. 1-27 and 1-28).

1.5.5
Pes Anserinus

The sartorius muscle, semitendinosus muscle, and gracilis muscle comprise the pes anserinus, a multi-layer muscle group that inserts on the medial aspect of the tibia, distal to the tibial tuberosity (see Fig. 1-19). Together with the semimembranosus, these muscles are responsible for medial stabilization of the knee joint and internal rotation of the tibia [42, 67, 167, 467].

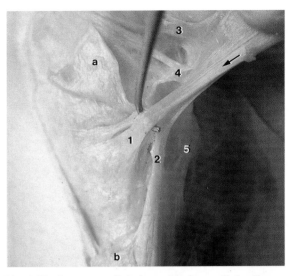

Fig. 1-25. Posteromedial view with the medial collateral ligament divided and its stumps reflected upward *(a)* and downward *(b)*. Insertions of the semimembranosus muscle *(arrow)* on the medial side (*1*, over hook) and posterior side *(2)* of the medial tibial condyle, on the oblique popliteal ligament *(3)*, the posterior capsule and posterior oblique ligament *(4)*, and the popliteal aponeurosis and posterior tibial surface *(5)*

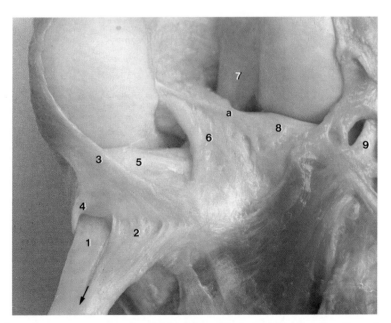

Fig. 1-26. Posterior view with the semimembranosus muscle reflected downward *(arrow)* to show its insertion on the posterior border of the medial tibial condyle *(1)*, in the direction of the medial meniscus *(2)*. Expansions of the posterior oblique ligament *(3)* and posterior tibial oblique ligament *(4)* in the direction of the medial meniscus *(5)*. PCL *(6)* with posterior meniscofemoral ligament *(a)* and attachment to posterior horn of lateral meniscus *(8)*, ACL *(7)*, popliteus tendon *(9)*

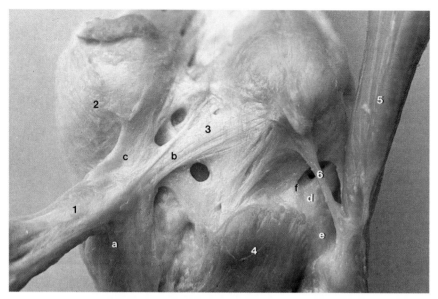

Fig. 1-27. Posterior view in extension, with gastrocnemius muscle removed. Semimembranosus muscle *(1)* with its attachments to the medial and posterior aspect *(a)* of the medial tibial condyle, oblique popliteal ligament *(b)*, and posterior oblique ligament *(c)*. The posterior oblique ligament *(2)* and oblique popliteal ligament *(3)*, which represents a prolongation of the main semimembranosus muscle fibers *(b)*, function with the arcuate popliteal ligament *(6)* to enhance posteromedial and posterolateral stability. Slips from the tendon *(d)* of the popliteus muscle *(4)* attach to the head of the fibula *(e)*, the posterolateral capsuloligamentous structures *(f)*, and the lateral meniscus. Biceps femoris muscle *(5)*

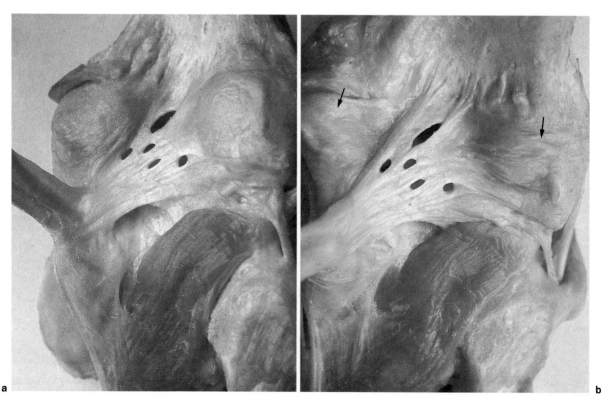

Fig. 1-28a, b. Posterior view with the gastrocnemius muscle removed. The posterior capsuloligamentous structures *(arrows)*, which have close attachments to the semimembranosus muscle, become lax as the joint moves from extension **(a)** to slight flexion **(b)**

1.6
Posterior Complex (Table 1-6)

1.6.1
Posterior Capsule

For convenience the posterior capsule is sub-divided into three parts consisting of a medial, a lateral, and a middle third. The medial and lateral thirds form caplike coverings over the posterior aspect of the femoral condyles and are the sites of origin for the two heads of the gastrocnemius muscle. Since the posterior capsule is tight in extension, it stabilizes against valgus, varus, hyperextension, and rotatory forces in that position [173, 279, 321] (Figs. 1-27 and 1-28a). As the knee is flexed, the capsule becomes lax, and the medial and lateral collateral ligament become the primary stabilizers (Fig. 1-28).

1.6.2
Oblique Popliteal Ligament

In its course between the lateral attachment of the semimembranosus muscle and the femoral condyles, the oblique popliteal ligament reinforces the posterior capsule. Numerous openings in the ligament and posterior capsule, visible from behind, are present for the passage of nerves and blood vessels (Fig. 1-28).

The powerfully developed oblique popliteal ligament contributes greatly to the strength of the posterior capsule. It is tight in extension and lax in flexion (Fig. 1-28). In extension it acts to prevent medial or lateral opening of the joint space. Though lax in flexion, the ligament can still contribute to joint stability in that position owing to the dynamizing action of the semimembranosus muscle.

Table 1-6. Structures of the posterior complex

Posterior capsule
  Oblique popliteal ligament
  Arcuate popliteal ligament
Semimembranosus muscle
Popliteus muscle
Gastrocnemius muscle
Biceps femoris muscle

1.6.3
Arcuate Popliteal Ligament

The arcuate popliteal ligament is a fan-shaped band of variable prominence which spans the posterolateral joint region [1, 42, 167, 343] (Fig. 1-29). It continues distally in a course that parallels the lateral collateral ligament.

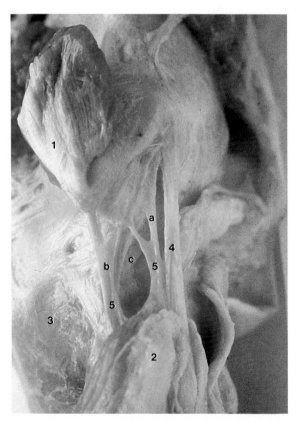

Fig. 1-29. Lateral view with the lateral head of the gastrocnemius muscle *(1)* reflected upward and the biceps femoris *(2)* reflected downward. Popliteus muscle *(3)*. Posterior to the lateral collateral ligament *(4)* is the variable arcuate popliteal ligament *(5)* with its lateral *(a)* and posterior *(b)* expansions. The popliteus tendon *(c)* passes beneath the arcuate popliteal ligament and lateral collateral ligament

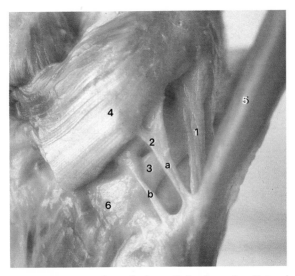

Fig. 1-30. Posterolateral view of the lateral collateral ligament *(1)*, the arcuate popliteal ligament *(2)* with its lateral *(a)* and posterior *(b)* expansions, tendon of popliteus muscle *(3)*, lateral head of gastrocnemius *(4)*, biceps femoris muscle *(5)*, junction of popliteus tendon and muscle belly *(6)*

The arcuate ligament consists of a lateral and a posterior portion. The latter extends from the fibular head to the capsular structures below the lateral head of gastrocnemius [173, 321], passing directly over the popliteus tendon to the posterior tibial border and posterior capsule [167, 621] (Fig. 1-30). Variable slips connect the arcuate popliteal ligament with the lateral meniscus, the popliteus tendon, and the posterior capsule (Fig. 1-31).

Although the arcuate popliteal ligament can be demonstrated in isolation by dissection, it belongs functionally to the arcuate complex along with the lateral collateral ligament, the popliteus tendon, and the posterior third of the lateral capsule. The arcuate complex stabilizes the posterolateral corner of the knee against varus-producing and externally rotating forces [296, 321, 621].

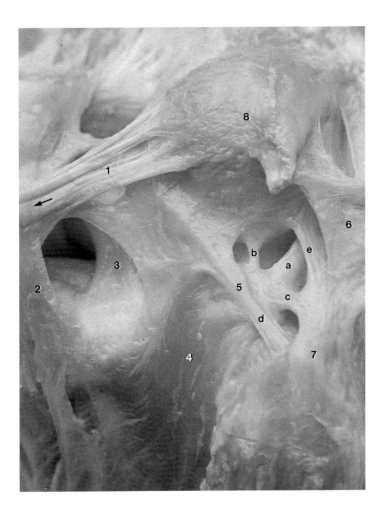

Fig. 1-31. Posterior view in extension, with the gastrocnemius muscle cut away. Semimembranosus muscle *(arrow)* with its extensions to the oblique popliteal ligament *(1)* and posteromedial part of the upper tibia *(2)*. Insertion of the PCL *(3)*. The popliteus muscle *(4)* sends its main tendon *(a)* to the lateral femoral condyle but also distributes slips to the posterolateral capsule *(b)* and fibular head *(c, 7)*. Arcuate popliteal ligament *(5)* with its posterior *(d)* and lateral *(e)* fibers. The biceps femoris muscle *(6)*, here retracted laterally, inserts on the fibular head *(7)*. An expansion toward the lateral origin of gastrocnemius *(8)* connects the biceps femoris with the lateral femoral condyle

1.6.4
Popliteus Muscle

The popliteus muscle arises by a tendon that attaches anterior and distal to the femoral origin of the lateral collateral ligament. The tendon runs posteriorly through a groove on the lateral femoral epicondyle, medial to the collateral ligament (Figs. 1-17, 1-27, 1-31, 1-32, 1-33) [42, 67, 95, 616]. At the level of the lateral meniscus the tendon passes through the "popliteal hiatus" bounded anteroinferiorly by the inferior fasciculus and posterosuperiorly by the superior fasciculus. The popliteus tendon is attached to the lateral meniscus by both fasciculi (Figs. 1-34 and 1-35). The tendon is not intra-articular, however, but is covered by synovial membrane on the medial side [95]. Shortly after traversing the popliteal hiatus, which averages 1.3 cm in length, the femoral tendon of origin is reinforced by fibers from the fibular head, from posterolateral joint structures (arcuate popliteal ligament), and from the lateral meniscus [32, 95, 278, 384] (Figs. 1-31 and 1-33).

In addition to its function as an internal rotator, the popliteus muscle plays a significant role in the automatic rotation of the knee. Because of its anatomic position, it can impart an internal rotating action to the knee when flexion is initiated from the terminal position of extension [321, 384, 466]. Through its attachment to the lateral meniscus, the popliteus can actively move the meniscus and prevent its entrapment as the knee flexes [32, 95, 384] (Figs. 1-34 and 1-35). It contributes to posterolateral joint stability by its connection with the arcuate popliteal ligament, to which it likewise can impart tension (Fig. 1-31) [152, 383]. Experimental studies demonstrate its significant stabilizing action against varus stress in the range from 0° to 90° flexion. Indeed, significant posterolateral instability cannot exist when the popliteus tendon is intact [483]. Electromyographic studies by Peterson et al. [523] indicate that the popliteus muscle is involved in the mechanism of the active pivot-shift sign (see Fig. 3-54). Functionally, the popliteus muscle belongs to the arcuate complex mentioned above. Its femoral insertion lies on the

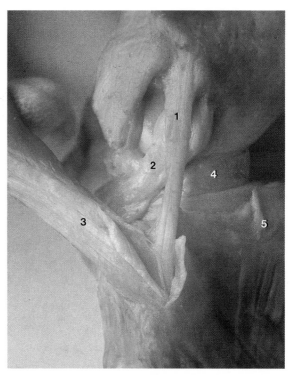

Fig. 1-32. Lateral view. The popliteus tendon *(2)* passes beneath the lateral collateral ligament *(1)* in its proximal third and is overlapped by the biceps femoris muscle *(split) (3)* in its distal third. Lateral meniscus *(4)*. Attachment of the iliotibial tract *(5)*

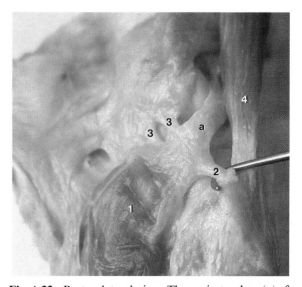

Fig. 1-33. Posterolateral view. The main tendon *(a)* of the popliteus muscle *(1)* passes to the lateral femoral condyle. Other slips attach to the fibular head *(2, over hook)* and posterolateral capsuloligamentous structures *(3)*. Biceps femoris muscle *(4)*

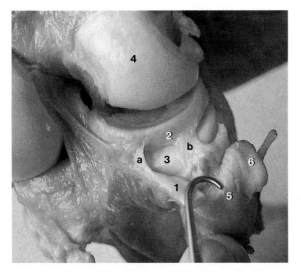

Fig. 1-34. Posterolateral view with the posterolateral capsule removed. Popliteus tendon *(1, under probe)* with its superior fasciculus *(a)* and inferior fasciculus *(b)*, lateral meniscus *(2)*, lateral tibial plateau *(3)*, femoral condyle *(4)*, fibular head *(5)*, biceps femoris muscle *(6)*

Burmester curve (Fig. 1-36), and this circumstance should be considered in the repair and reconstruction of posterolateral injuries.

Clearly, the functional significance of the popliteus muscle has been overlooked for many years [152]. But when we consider its manifold functions and the problems that are associated with its reconstruction, especially in chronic lesions, its importance for knee-joint stability becomes apparent. It is not surprising that posterolateral instabilities involving injury to the popliteus muscle and the PCL are among the most difficult-to-treat of all ligamentous knee injuries.

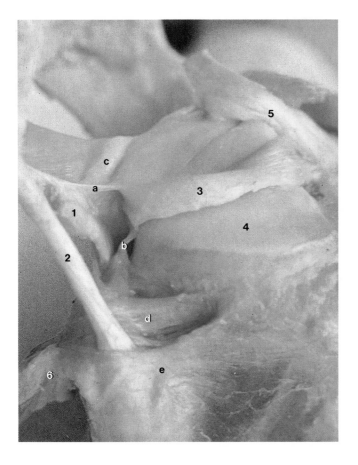

Fig. 1-35. Lateral view with lateral femoral condyle removed. The popliteus tendon *(1)* runs below the lateral collateral ligament *(2)*. Note the attachments of the superior fasciculus *(a)* and inferior fasciculus *(b)* to the lateral meniscus *(3)*, which in turn has close contact with the posterolateral capsule *(c)*. Lateral tibial plateau *(4)*, ACL *(5)*, insertion of biceps femoris muscle *(6)* on fibular head with both a deep *(d)* and superficial *(e)* attachment

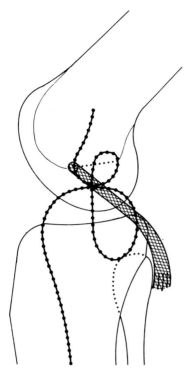

Fig. 1-36. Position of the popliteus muscle on the Burmester curve

Table 1-7. Structures of the lateral complex

Lateral retinaculum
Lateral collateral ligament
Lateral capsular ligament
Iliotibial tract
   Tractotibial ligament
   Kaplan fibers
Arcuate complex
Biceps femoris muscle

1.7
Lateral Complex (Table 1-7)

As on the medial side, the lateral capsuloligamentous structures are arranged in three layers [173]. The superficial layer contains the fascia lata, iliotibial tract, and biceps femoris muscle; the middle layer contains the lateral collateral ligament; and the deep layer contains the lateral capsular ligament and joint capsule.

1.7.1
Lateral Capsule, Lateral Capsular Ligament

The lateral capsule is weaker and thinner than the medial capsule, but like the latter it is firmly attached to the ipsilateral meniscus.

The anterior third of the capsule extends between the lateral margin of the patellar ligament and the anterior border of the iliotibial tract [173]. It is reinforced by the lateral longitudinal retinaculum and by fibers that diverge from the iliotibial tract.

The middle third of the capsule extends from the iliotibial tract to the level of the lateral collateral ligament. It consists of meniscofemoral and meniscotibial components. This part of the capsule contains more fibers than the anterior third and, following the nomenclature on the medial side, is termed the "lateral capsular ligament."

1.6.5
Gastrocnemius Muscle

The gastrocnemius muscle arises by two heads attached to the posterosuperior portions of the femoral condyles. It bounds the popliteal fossa distally and unites with the soleus muscle to form the triceps surae muscle. It inserts on the tuber calcanei along with the tendon of the plantaris muscle. Frequently a bursa is present below the medial tendon of origin of the gastrocnemius, and the lateral head of gastrocnemius contains a fabella (sesamoid bone) in approximately 30% of the population [42].

To our knowledge, no accurate studies have yet been done on the stabilizing effect of the gastrocnemius muscle on the knee joint. However, the muscle can actively stabilize the posterior and especially the posterolateral portions of the joint through its close attachments to components of the arcuate complex [317, 621].

1.7.2
Lateral Collateral Ligament

The lateral (fibular) collateral ligament is a rounded cord 5–7 cm long running from the lateral femoral condyle obliquely downward and posteriorly to the head of the fibula [1, 65, 67, 167] (Figs. 1-17, 1-35, 1-37, 1-38).

There is an approximately 1-cm-wide interval between the lateral capsule and lateral collateral ligament that is traversed by the tendon of the popliteus muscle. Posterior fibers from the lateral collateral ligament blend with the deep capsular layer to form the aforementioned arcuate popliteal ligament, which for that reason is alternately known as the "short fibular collateral ligament" (Figs. 1-29 and 1-31).

The lateral collateral ligament has much the same orientation as the PCL, while the course of the medial collateral ligament corresponds to that of the ACL [448, 450] (Fig. 1-39).

There is diversity of opinion in the literature as to the functional significance of the lateral collateral ligament. While some authors regard it as a major lateral stabilizer of the knee [343, 479], others claim that it performs no essential stabilizing function [167, 279, 321].

The distal portion of the lateral collateral ligament is enveloped by the biceps femoris muscle, the most important active stabilizer of the lateral part of the joint (Figs. 1-32 and 1-38).

1.7.3
Iliotibial Tract

The annular fibers of the fascia lata enclose and encircle the femoral muscles like a sleeve. On the lateral side the fascia lata is thickened as a longitudinal fiber band called the iliotibial tract, which arises with the tensor fasciae latae from the anterior superior iliac spine (Figs. 1-6 and 1-37).

Distally the fibers divide into an anterior, intermediate, and posterior portion [255, 651]. The anterior fibers blend with the lateral retinaculum, the posterior fibers accompany expansions from the biceps femoris into the crural fascia, and the midportion of this "trifurcation" of the iliotibial tract passes distally over the joint space of the knee to insert anterolaterally on the tubercle of Gerdy (Fig. 1-37).

Proximal to the knee joint there are strong connecting fibers that bind the iliotibial tract to the femoral shaft. These are named "Kaplan fibers" after the author who first described them [342] (see Fig. 1-6).

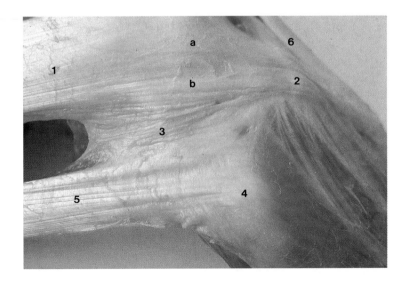

Fig. 1-37. Lateral view in approximately 30° flexion, with the fascia of the thigh removed. Attachment of the iliotibial tract *(1)* on the tubercle of Gerdy *(2)* with the anterior *(a)* and middle *(b)* groups of fibers, bulge of lateral collateral ligament *(3)*, fibular head *(4)*, biceps femoris muscle *(5)*, patellar ligament *(6)*

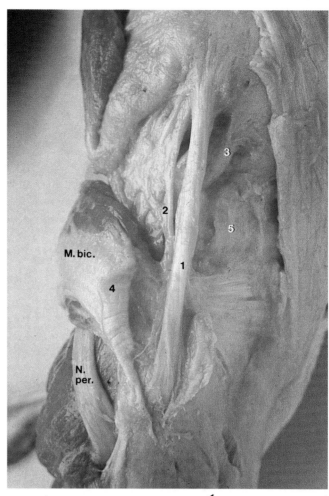

Fig. 1-38. Lateral view in extension. Lateral collateral ligament *(1)*, arcuate popliteal ligament *(2)*, and popliteus tendon *(3)*, which runs below the superior part of the lateral collateral ligament. The superficial layer *(4)* of the biceps femoris muscle *(M. bic.)* has been divided. Anterior part of lateral capsule *(5)*. The close proximity of the peroneal nerve *(N. per.)* to the biceps femoris *(M. bic.)* must be considered in all surgical procedures in this region

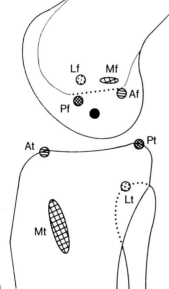

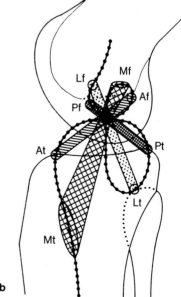

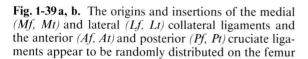

Fig. 1-39 a, b. The origins and insertions of the medial *(Mf, Mt)* and lateral *(Lf, Lt)* collateral ligaments and the anterior *(Af, At)* and posterior *(Pf, Pt)* cruciate ligaments appear to be randomly distributed on the femur *(f)* and tibia *(t)* around their common point of intersection *(●)* (a), In fact, they all lie on the Burmester curve as shown in (b)

Studies on the distal femoral fixation of the iliotibial tract indicate the presence of a three-part fiber system. A supracondylar portion runs obliquely distally and inserts on the femur above the lateral condyle. Another fiber bundle runs transversely and connects the superficial tract with the posterolateral femur. A third, curved fiber system extends between the tubercle of Gerdy and the posterolateral femur [398]. Distance measurements between the tubercle of Gerdy and the three different femoral insertions of the iliotibial tract have shown that only the posterior, curved fiber group remains isometric over the full range of knee-joint motion [398]. This discrepancy in the behavior of the three fiber systems presumably accounts for the frequent loosening of the surgically fixed iliotibial tract (tractopexy).

The iliotibial tract glides anteriorly in extension and posteriorly in flexion, its mobility being restricted by the Kaplan fibers. Due to the fixation of the tract by the Kaplan fibers and its attachment distal to the joint space, a portion of the iliotibial tract is removed from the range of action of the tensor fasciae latae and is regarded as a separate ligamentous structure. Recent authors have applied the terms "tractotibial ligament," "iliotibial ligament" or "lateral anterior femorotibial ligament" to this structure [255, 470, 651].

The iliotibial tract, whose development paralleled the assumption of an upright gait, serves as a lateral iliofemoral tension band [342]. Its function as a static lateral stabilizer of the knee is even more important than the active, dynamic function that is imparted to the tract by its connection with the tensor fasciae latae [255, 321, 342, 651]. The iliotibial tract prevents lateral opening of the joint space, checks internal rotation, and prevents anterior displacement in 90° flexion with the tibia internally rotated. The anterior fibers that are distributed to the patella, known also as the iliopatellar ligament, prevent medial subluxation of the patella [651].

The iliotibial tract has a special significance in tests for the pivot-shift sign, as described in Sect. 3.4.

1.7.4
Biceps Femoris Muscle

The long head of the biceps femoris muscle arises from the ischial tuberosity and the short head from the midportion of the linea aspera of the femur. The tendon of insertion runs distally and anteriorly and splits around the inferior third of the lateral collateral ligament. The tendon consists of three layers: a lateral layer that is superficial to the lateral collateral ligament, an intermediate layer which splits around the collateral ligament, and a deep layer that is medial to the ligament [427] (Fig. 1-38).

The superficial insertion fans out in three directions, sending an anterior expansion to the crural fascia and the tubercle of Gerdy [427, 680], a direct intermediate expansion that blends with the fasciae of the peroneal muscles, and a posterior expansion that blends with the fasciae of the calf muscles (Fig. 1-37). The intermediate layer envelops the lateral collateral ligament from the medial and lateral sides and inserts with the ligament upon the fibular head. The deep layer divides into an anterior part that inserts on the tubercle of Gerdy and a posterior part that inserts on the fibular head medial to the collateral ligament [427] (Fig. 1-38).

Analogous to the semimembranosus muscle on the posteromedial side, the biceps femoris muscle stabilizes the posterolateral part of the joint, checks internal rotation, and acts as an external rotator of the tibia.

1.8
Proprioception

Besides mechanical stabilization, the capsuloligamentous structures of the joints perform a neuromuscular function owing to the presence of small nerve terminals (receptors) first described by Krause [374] in 1874 [62, 89, 94, 171, 222, 230, 498, 604]. These receptors, called proprioceptors, constitute a peripheral, internal sensory organ of the joint in question.

1.8.1
Classification

The proprioceptors are classified histologically as free (unmyelinated) receptors or corpuscular receptors (e. g., Ruffini corpuscles, Vater-Pacini corpuscles, Meissner corpuscles, Krause's bulbs, Merkel's disks).

Receptors can be classified as follows on the basis of their physiologic function:

1. Mechanoreceptors (touch, pressure, stretch)
2. Chemoreceptors (pH, hormone levels)
3. Pain receptors
4. Thermoreceptors
5. Osmoreceptors

This detailed classification should not create the impression that the specificities of the receptors are fully known. Neither has it been established whether each type of receptor can respond to just one or more than one type of stimulus energy. But since many different receptors occur in a very small area, it may be assumed that a high degree of specialization exists [653].

Based on extensive studies in the knee joints of cats, Freeman and Wyke [183] classified the joint receptors into four types. The basic features of this classification are believed to be valid for the human knee joint as well:

Type I: *Ruffini corpuscles.* These receptors are arranged in clusters in the superficial layer of the fibrous capsule. They are supplied by terminal branches from a myelinated afferent axon. The type I receptors are low-threshold static and dynamic mechanoreceptors that respond to stretch [183]. They are sensitive to static joint position, intra-articular and atmospheric pressure changes, and to the direction, amplitude, and speed of active or passive joint movements. The axons that supply the Ruffini corpuscles do not give off branches to other receptors, so these endings are considered to

be highly specific. Type I receptors also occur in tendons and aponeuroses that merge with the joint capsule, on the surface of the ligaments, and at the insertion sites of the menisci.

Type II: *Vater-Pacini corpuscles.* These receptors occur in the fibrous capsule of all joints and are most abundant around blood vessels. They respond to the acceleration or deceleration of joint motion.

Type III: *Golgi corpuscles.* The Golgi corpuscles are among the largest receptors present in ligaments. They are slowly adapting, plate-like mechanoreceptors that occur on the ligament surface and whose long axis is oriented parallel to the long axis of the ligament. They are supplied by myelinated afferent fibers which lose their myelin sheath upon entry into the end organ [183, 653].

Type IV: *Unmyelinated nerve endings.* This receptor type usually consists of a lattice-like arrangement of unmyelinated nerve filaments and free nerve endings with no corpuscular attachments. They occur in the fibrous capsule, in perivascular tissue, and in the fat pads. Free nerve endings also occur in the ligaments.

The plexus-like nerve filaments are believed to mediate pain sensation [653]. They occur in the synovial membrane, in the meniscus, and in the ligaments.

1.8.2
Distribution of Proprioceptors in the Knee Joint

The first studies on the location of proprioceptors in the knee joint were performed in cats. The major initial work was done by Andrew [11], Boyd [61, 64], Freeman and Wyke [183], and Gardner [200].

1.8.2.1
Anterior Cruciate Ligament

While mechanoreceptors were first detected morphologically in the ACL of the cat [183, 199, 200], Schultz et al. [583] were the first researchers to detect them in the ACL of the human knee. They identified fusiform nerve endings with a single axon in addition to Golgi tendon organs (type III receptors). The receptors were located on the ligament surface, where they can register the greatest potential changes associated with flexion and rotational movements of the joint. The peripheral ligamentous fibers show the greatest degree of tightening and loosening in response to knee motion.

Zimny et al. [723] found an extensive intraligamentous neural network in the human ACL. In addition to free-ending nerve fibers, they identified Ruffini endings and Pacini corpuscles (type II receptors). The greatest receptor density was noted at the proximal and distal ends of the ligament [585, 723]. Cerulli et al. [88, 89] found mostly free nerve endings and a few corpuscular receptors in the middle third of the ligament and at its femoral attachment.

Though it had been assumed that these receptors influence the activity of the synergists of the ACL, Grüber et al. [229] were the first, in 1986, to demonstrate electrophysiologically the existence of a reflex arc between the ACL and the ischiocrural muscles. The irreversible disruption of this reflex arc, known as the ACL reflex, by rupture of the ACL is probably one reason for the frequently unsatisfactory results of ACL reconstructions.

All proprioceptive studies of the ACL indicate that this ligament has more than a purely mechanical stabilizing function, and that it additionally performs an important function in proprioceptive control [88, 89]. Thus, rupture of the ACL leads not only to a loss of stability with disintegration of the rolling-gliding mechanism but also to the loss of its proprioceptive protective function.

This has important clinical implications, for a reconstruction of the ACL can do no more than replace the purely mechanical function of the ligament. Its proprioceptive function is permanently lost and cannot be restored by any therapeutic procedures. It may be possible, however, to preserve any residual receptors that are still present. Since the receptor density is high at the femoral and tibial insertions, a rationale exists for preserving the ligament stumps. Unfortunately, many surgeons routinely resect all of the tibial stump when performing an ACL replacement in order to improve exposure and facilitate drilling of the tibia. We always make an effort to preserve as much of the ligament stump as possible so that the remnant can be sutured to the graft. Our goal is to re-expose the proprioceptors in the area of the tibial insertion to motion-related stresses so that they can provide a residual proprioceptive protective function.

Thus, Feagin [159] recommends the operation of Wittek for ruptures of the ACL for patients who have deferred ACL reconstruction, for young patients with open epiphyseal growth plates and for older patients. In this technique the ruptured ACL is sutured to the PCL as a means of restabilizing and restoring nutrition to the damaged ligament. This procedure can be performed through a small arthrotomy (< 5 cm), and with special instruments and devices it may even be accomplished arthroscopically. However, the main value of this procedure, which is not meant to be definitive [159], probably relates less to its stabilizing effect than to the restoration of tension to the proprioceptors, which, though not reattached at their anatomic site, can continue to mediate important protective reflexes for the knee joint. In arthroscopic examinations it is not unusual to find the ACL apposed and fused to the PCL as an incidental finding following conservative treatment for an unrecognized rupture of the ACL. It is likely that knee-joint function in these patients is not so severely impaired as in cases where the ACL fails to find a new insertion after its rupture. Further studies are still needed in this area.

1.8.2.2
Medial Collateral Ligament

With isolated lesions of the medial collateral ligament, it is common for a painful limitation of extension to develop one day after the injury. Palmer [514] found that stimulation of the femoral attachment of the medial collateral ligament induced a strong contraction of the semimembranosus, sartorius, and vastus medialis muscles. This multisynaptic reflex arc confirms the presence of proprioceptors at the femoral origin of the ligament. When these receptors are stretched, the synergistic muscles (see above) contract to prevent overstretching of the ligament. A first- or second-degree ligament injury near the insertion leads to a sustained excitation of the receptors and thus to an increased contraction of the corresponding muscles, whose overt manifestation is a painful limitation of extension.

1.8.2.3
Meniscus

Cerulli et al. [87, 88] were the first researchers to demonstrate Golgi-type proprioceptors in the human menisci as well as free nerve endings and corpuscular endings. The free-ending nerve fibers were most numerous in the basal third of the menisci, while the corpuscular receptors (Golgi corpuscles, Ruffini corpuscles, Pacini corpuscles) were most abundant in the anterior and posterior horns. Accordingly, the menisci are counted among the knee structures that perform a proprioceptive protective function in addition to their passive role. This fact should emphasize the essential functional importance of the menisci for the knee joint and provide a rationale for reattaching or partially resecting damaged menisci instead of "simply removing" them. Above all we feel that the base of the meniscus, which contains numerous proprioceptors, should be preserved.

1.8.3
Therapeutic Implications

Since proprioceptors occur in all important capsuloligamentous structures of the knee joint, therapeutic considerations should not be limited to the mechanical function of the ligaments. Ultimately, the capsule and ligaments are able to tolerate excessive or violent stresses only by virtue of proprioceptive control mechanisms, which enable synergistic muscles to prevent overstretching and tearing of the ligaments.

This proprioceptive protective function must be taken into account when treatment is planned and carried out. All too often the operatively treated knee joint is opened through a very extensive arthrotomy, especially in ligament reconstructions. To get optimum exposure, many surgeons completely dislocate the patella laterally and release all of the vastus medialis obliquus muscle from its patellar insertion. While care is always taken to avoid injury to stabilizing structures, little if any thought is given to the proprioception of the joint capsule. This purely mechanistic attitude has led to "drastic" operations in which entire knee joints are skeletonized to effect isolated ligament repairs. In chronic instabilities, it has been common practice to release, transpose, and/or redirect many ligamentous components. Thus it is not unusual for reconstructions of the ACL to result in alarmingly extensive arthrotomies, frequently involving both the medial and lateral sides of the joint (Fig. 1-40).

In reality, only a small arthrotomy is needed to provide surgical access to the ACL. Moreover, there is no need for the surgeon to dislocate the patella laterally or release the vastus medialis obliquus. A limited arthrotomy 4–6 cm long will yield adequate exposure (Fig. 1-41 a, b). Advances in arthroscopic techniques have even made it possible to repair or replace the cruciate ligaments arthroscopically. With proper technique, only two small puncture wounds are required. Somewhat larger incisions are required at the femoral and tibial attachments of the ligament (Fig. 1-41 c).

The unacceptably high incidence of prolonged postoperative pain and swelling in the femoropatellar joint after extensive arthrotomies, the frequency of unsatisfactory outcomes, and new discoveries about ligamentous healing have led increasingly to a functional and "biological" way of thinking in the surgical treatment of ligament injuries. Extensive, mutilating arthrotomies that destroy the proprioceptors are avoided.

The larger the arthrotomy, the more proprioceptors are destroyed.

The most important factor for favorable ligament healing is early functional therapy (mobilization). The operative treatment of individual structures, such as the medial collateral ligament, is by no means superior to conservative treatment. Decades ago, Palmer [514] stated that the nonoperative treatment of collateral ligament injuries was just as effective as surgery. In 1972 Pässler [516] described a motion splint for functional therapy of the knee joint following ligament repairs and reconstructions.

Dahners [107] states that ligaments heal much more favorably when the knee is mobilized than when it is immobilized. The ligaments become larger, stronger, stiffer, contain more collagen, are more cellular, and display a better collagen architecture. In biochemical studies of immobilized ligaments, Gamble et al. [197] showed that the collagen-producing fibroblasts revert from an anabolic to a catabolic state under conditions of immobilization.

All of these findings provide a rationale for the early mobilization and functional therapy of capsuloligamentous injuries. If the injury has made the knee joint "unstable" (usually due to rupture of the ACL: positive Lachman test with a soft end point), the central complex (cruciate ligaments) should be operatively stabilized so that early mobilization will be possible. The ruptured peripheral capsuloligamentous tissues should heal completely under this regimen. At operation the joint is entered through a small arthrotomy to minimize trauma and to avoid needless "iatrogenic" destruction of proprioceptive elements.

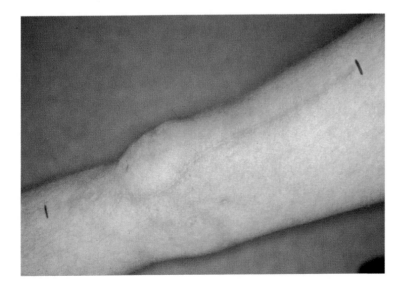

Fig. 1-40. Scar over 50 cm long following open ACL reconstruction

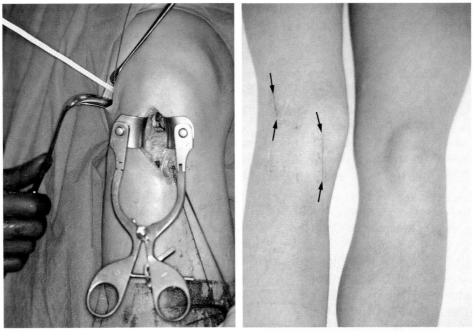

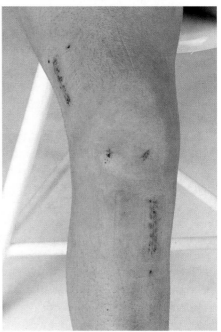

Fig. 1-41 a–c. Autogenous reconstruction of the ACL (middle part of the patellar tendon, bone-ligament-bone graft) is possible via a small arthrotomy (5-6 cm). Arthrotomy is performed after partial resection of the infrapatellar fat pad in the area where the graft is removed. The introduction of the augmentation device (e.g. Kennedy LAD, see **a**) and the bone-ligament-bone graft into the joint, as well as the femoral fixation of the bone block are carried out through a small lateral incision (2-3 cm) just proximal of the lateral femoral condyle (**a**). Medial and lateral retinacula are not dissected with this technique. Scars left by this open ACL reconstruction *(arrows)* (postoperative day 21) (**b**). Scars left by an arthroscopic synthetic ACL reconstruction (postoperative day 10) (**c**)

1.9
Biomechanics and Biometry

The foremost goal of all organic and metabolic functions is to sustain the capability for movement. The central nervous system, muscles, circulation, and respiration all work together solely to achieve this goal. Without movement, the organic functions would have no purpose.

The human knee joint is the product of an evolutionary process spanning 400 million years [141]. Yet, despite a vast body of clinical and experimental investigation, we still know appallingly little about the conditions that exist within moving biologic systems (joints). Accordingly, an attempt must be made to elucidate the internal principles of these structures. Our relative ignorance of the true nature of articular movements is demonstrated by the widely known maxim from anatomy and biomechanics that "Since function affects anatomy, we can deduce the function of a part from its anatomy." This "medieval" concept has been internalized by many biologists and medical professionals as well as by physicists and mathematicians [455].

To date there have been numerous attempts to analyze the patterns of articular motion using classical geometry. Most of these attempts have met with little or no success. This led Knese, in 1950, to conclude with resignation that "The articular members, specifically those of the knee joint, cannot be made to conform to any geometric principle" [from 454]. In a 1985 article on "Walking Machines," the biomechanics expert Wolfgang Baumann summarized the dilemma of present-day biomechanics by noting that "We know a great deal about movement, about walking and running, especially in sports. But in the final analysis, we know nothing at all. The internal principles of movement continue to be a riddle" (after Menschik [455]).

Clearly, one basic problem is that the scientists were either too much the physician and not enough the mathematician and philosopher, or conversely were oriented too much toward mathematics and physics and too little toward medicine.

The Viennese scientist Alfred Menschik may be credited with making the most fundamental contributions to our present-day understanding of biologic motion systems, especially the knee joint. Menschik, in whom the talents and interests of the orthopedist are combined with those of the mathematician, physicist, and philosopher, has enabled us to advance our understanding of biomechanics past the stage of the crossed four-bar linkage (see Fig. 1-7) – a simplified, two-dimensional model of cruciate-ligament function which disregards the role of the collateral ligaments.

1.9.1
Basic Considerations

In laying the conceptual foundation that will free us from antiquated ideas, it is helpful to review the following statements of Menschik [455]:

1. No serious discipline in theoretical physics or the natural sciences can doubt that living creatures, including human beings, are a product of our physical world. Consequently, there cannot be a separate physics for living organisms with its own laws. If this were the case, we would have to have a "superphysics" that could relate both systems (physical world and living organisms) to each other. Thus the term "biomechanics" is misleading, for there is no separate mechanics for biologic systems. It is more correct to speak of mechanical principles as they are manifested in biologic systems.
2. Recurring movements, regardless of whether they occur in technology or in biologic systems, must obey certain laws. Without those geometric and kinematic laws, there could not be recurring, reproducible movements either in technology or in living organisms.
3. Joints, including the knee joint, are optimized motion systems. We cannot analyze such systems until we have discovered the basic, elemental principle of the joint.

Geometry has disclosed but few of the principles that govern movements in space. This is due in part to a "human problem," i. e., the fact that mathematicians recognize the interesting problem of biologic motion systems but do not consider it a true geometric problem. One reason for this, in turn, is the attitude of physicians who regard the joints as "a product of nature's wisdom" or "a creation of God." This kind of thinking makes it difficult to perceive the essential problem. It must be realized that the observable phenomenon – the "how" – has its causes in a "what." This may seem abstract at first, but it can be understood by citing some examples. One historical example is the astronomer Kepler (1571–1630). From our current perspective, Kepler was only partly successful. By describing planetary motion with mathematical formulas, he was able to perceive the "how," but he attributed the cause of the motion, the "what," to divine intuition. A century later Newton (1686) described the cause of planetary motion, the "what," in terms of mathematical physics by formulating his law of gravitation, thereby ending the "dualistic thought" that dominated medieval physics. Similarly, the goal of the analysis of biologic motion systems must be to elucidate the "what," the cause of the articular motion [454].

Menschik [454] states that only an analysis of the "what" can lead to the true understanding of an unknown motion system. If we ask "Why does the knee move?" we may get the reply "because the muscles contract." A similar question could be posed with regard to a different, known motion system such as the automobile. If we ask "Why does the car move?" we might be told "because the driver is pressing the gas pedal." This reply is correct as far as it goes, but it does not satisfactorily answer the question. The cause, the "what" of the motion systems, is not apparent from any of the answers given.

Guided by these basic considerations, Menschik [448–454] developed his system of biometry as a successor to traditional biomechanics, which, as we have seen, has not led to appreciable success.

Menschik published Part One of his results on the "Mechanics of the Knee Joint" in 1974, followed shortly thereafter by Parts Two and Three. In Part Three [450] Menschik describes how, following a suggestion of Dr. Jank, his colleague at the Second Geometric Institute of Vienna Technical College, he was able to analyze his previous kinematic data on the relationship between the cruciate and collateral ligaments and deduce the kinematic law underlying his empirically acquired data. More than 100 years earlier, the mathematician L. Burmester had worked on a similar problem. Menschik [450] writes: "Burmester examined those points on the gait plane which lie momentarily at the vertex of their path for a given imposed, uniplanar range of motion, i. e., points that lie on circular paths at the given point in time. Burmester called the resulting curve the 'circle-point curve,' which present-day geometry describes as the 'vertex cubic.'"

Subsequently Menschik, in collaboration with Jank, plotted the vertex cubic for the knee joint.

In 1982 Werner Müller [470] of Switzerland made Menschik's calculations and conclusions accessible to an expanded circle of interested colleages. Using copious illustrations, Müller was able to portray the interrelationship between clinical and kinematic phenomena and derive important therapeutic implications.

In 1987 Menschik published his book *Biometry* [454] in which he presents his knowledge, calculations, and proofs regarding the design principles of the knee joint, the hip joint, leg length, and body size. The term "biometry," coined by Menschik, is not synonymous with kinematics or biomechanics. Biometry is concerned with techniques for identifying and analyzing the design features of moving biologic systems. Thus it goes well beyond traditional "motion geometry," or kinematics. Biomechanics is concerned with investigating, observing, and recording motion and analyzing the results mathematically; it is not concerned with the actual cause of the movement. Thus, Menschik's biometry represents the farthest advance to date in the analysis of the knee joint as a biologic motion system.

1.9.2
Analysis of an Unknown Biologic Motion System

The recurring, reproducible movement of the knee joint is made possible by the existence of specific physical laws which govern the movements. For example, if all the soft tissues are removed from a knee specimen except for the cruciate and collateral ligaments, and the joint is then moved through its habitual range of motion, it will be found that the obligatory movement of the system is preserved. Division of both collateral ligaments causes valgus and varus laxity, but the intact cruciate ligaments preserve the obligatory joint movement. However, severing the cruciate ligaments severely disrupts the motion sequence, and the familiar drawer sign is elicited.

It may be concluded, then, that the cruciate ligaments are a basic physical prerequisite for the obligatory movement of the knee joint. Accordingly, we can regard the crossed four-bar linkage as the first geometric construction to appreciate the functional significance of the cruciate ligaments.

If the femur is held stationary while the tibia is moved as it is constrained to do so by the intact cruciate ligaments, the tibia will follow a curved path of motion around the femoral condyles (Fig. 1-42). In this case the tibia represents the "moving system" and the femur the stationary or "resting system." By connecting the successive centers of rotation (points of crossing of the cruciate ligaments), we can draw a curve called the "resting pole curve." Conversely, if the tibia is fixed while the femur is moved, a different curve called the "motion pole curve" is traced out by the successive crossing points of the cruciate ligaments (Fig. 1-42).

Under these conditions the two articular surfaces remain in contact despite the difference in their circumferences, the point of contact moving backward from an anterior position in extension to a more posterior position with increasing flexion. This type of movement is made possible by a simultaneous rolling and gliding of the femoral condyles upon the tibial plateau.

Thus it is clear that, besides the cruciate ligaments, the shape of the articular surfaces has an important bearing on the obligatory movement of the knee joint. Often it is claimed that the two articular surfaces of the knee joint are "completely incongruent" and that movement is possible only by virtue of the "wisdom of nature". According to Menschik [454], however, the articular surfaces are not a biologic problem but are a logical consequence of mathematic and geometric laws.

If we examine the movements of the knee joint (Figs. 1-42 and 1-43), we notice that the articular surfaces envelop each other. For our purpose, then, we may replace the term "articular surface" with the term "enveloping surface." Thus the two most important parameters that constrain and direct articular motion are the paired cruciate ligaments and the enveloping surfaces.

If we project the origins and insertions of the cruciate ligaments onto a flat surface (e. g., a sheet of paper) so that they follow circular paths, we find that all the points on the moving system (tibia) describe sixth-order curves (Table 1-8). Holding the tibia stationary in a position of, say, 45° flexion, we find that all the vertex points of the arcs lie on the vertex cubic (Burmester curve of the moving system). The locus of the centers of curvature of all the points on the vertex cubic is called the pivot cubic (Burmester curve of the resting system). The straight lines connecting points on the vertex cubic with points on the pivot cubic pass through the instant center of the motion system. A major advantage of this model is that it takes into account the collateral ligaments of the knee, the "connecting lines" between the vertex cubic and pivot cubic being represented anatomically by the fibers of the medial and lateral collateral ligaments.

Thus, while the areas of attachment of the ACL, PCL, and collateral ligaments may appear to be more or less randomly located (Fig. 1-39a), they in fact conform to the geometric and kinematic principles of the Burmester curve (Figs. 1-39b and 1-43). The instant center of rotation P during flexion and extension is always located at the point of

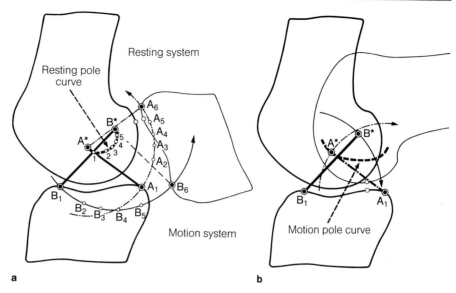

Fig. 1-42a, b. Resting pole curve (**a**) and motion pole curve (**b**); see text for further details (from [454])

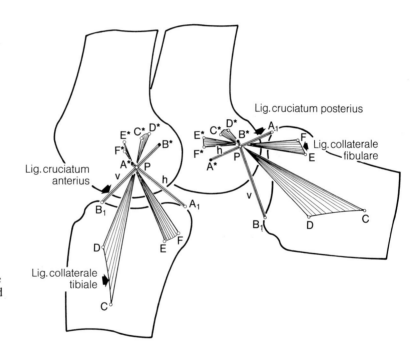

Fig. 1-43. Movement of the knee joint in flexion and extension. The crossing point of the collateral and cruciate ligaments coincides with the instant center of rotation P (from [454])

Table 1-8. Parameters of joint morphology

1. Distance between the centers of rotation of the cruciate ligaments on the frontal plane
2. Relative positions of the attachments of the cruciate ligaments
3. Length of the cruciate ligaments
4. Difference in the lengths of the cruciate ligaments
5. Length of the tibial plateau
6. Shape of the tibial plateau
7. Accessory movements of the cruciate ligaments, e.g., during automatic rotation

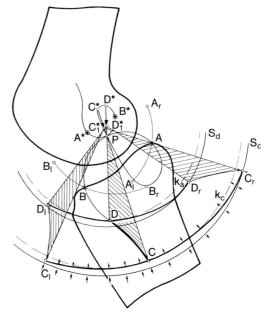

Fig. 1-44. Laxness of the medial collateral ligament in moderate flexion. The ligament becomes tight in extension *(dl, cl)* and at a high flexion angle *(dr, cr)* (from [454])

crossing of the cruciate ligaments and the collateral ligaments (Fig. 1-43).

During flexion and extension of the knee, many points of ligament insertion describe arcs that do not exactly match the idealized paths in the model. This accounts for the relative laxness of the ligaments when the knee is in moderate flexion (Fig. 1-44).

This kinematic principle and its implications apply to all joints that possess cruciate ligaments [448, 450]. However, the obligatory movement of the knee joint is additionally a product of the collateral ligaments, whose origins and insertions also lie on the Burmester curve (Fig. 1-44).

The biomechanical principles described above can account for other interesting phenomena as well. Since the flexion axis of the knee changes its position during flexion and extension, there is an associated change in the length of the force and lever arms. In engineering terms, we could describe the articular mechanism as a "variable-ratio gear." It enables a person to rise smoothly from a squatting to a standing posture while expending an almost constant muscular effort, i.e., without having to exert inordinate force to overcome resistance at any one point. An ideal braking and spring mechanism is provided that would not be possible with a "simple hinge joint" [450].

Menschik [450] believes that the mechanics of the four-bar linkage also serves to stabilize the intra-articular volume. The necessary volume shift from the anterior to the posterior side that occurs during flexion thus represents a "synovial pump system" that maintains lu-

brication of the joint and assists cartilage nutrition. The cartilage is further protected by the constant shifting of the femorotibial contact point as the flexion angle changes.

We can regard the cruciate and collateral ligaments of the knee joint as a four-rod mechanism that allows movement in flexion, extension, and rotation. If a fifth rod is added to the mechanism, it will fixate the system at the position in which the extra rod is added. Nature has provided the quadriceps muscle with the patella and patellar ligament as a "fifth rod" that can be added to or removed from the system by muscular effort. When the quadriceps muscle is tense, its kinematic effect is to fix the joint in the corresponding position of flexion. In other words, the knee joint cannot flex further when the quadriceps muscle is tense [450].

1.10
Radiographic Anatomy

The physician examining the knee must be well acquainted with radiographic anatomy so that he can identify the source of bone fragments, establish the anatomic location of other bony lesions, and perform accurate measurements, e.g., on stress radiographs.

1.10.1
Anteroposterior Projection

The two femoral condyles differ in size, the medial condyle being larger than the lateral and presenting a more regular shape. The lateral condyle bears a small impression on its lateral aspect to provide a gliding surface for the popliteal tendon. Superior to the medial epicondyle is the adductor tubercle, which appears as a bony prominence.

The intercondylar eminence, whose medial tubercle is higher than the lateral in almost 80% of cases [327], and the elevated position of the lateral tibial articular surface relative to the medial surface are useful landmarks for differentiation.

The radiolucent space between the femur and tibia is formed by the cartilage covering the femorotibial articular surfaces. It is customary for radiologists to call this feature the "joint space," though this is actually a misnomer [367].

Because of the posterolateral position of the proximal fibulotibial articulation, approximately one-third of the head of the fibula is overlapped by the lateral tibial condyle. In 10%–33% of cases [42, 67, 470] the lateral head of the gastrocnemius muscle contains a fabella that is projected onto the lateral femoral condyle.

Generally the examiner will have no problems identifying the anatomic structures of the knee and differentiating them from one another in the AP radiograph.

1.10.2
Lateral Projection

The features on lateral radiographs can be somewhat more difficult to interpret than on AP views [307] (Fig. 1-45). The boundary unsharpness of the condyle more distant from the casette (usually the medial femoral condyle), though sometimes difficult to appreciate, provides a simple means for medial/lateral differentiation [647]. Another useful landmark is the limiting grooves (condylopatellar grooves) that occur at the junction of the tibial and patellar surfaces of the femur (Figs. 1-2, 1-3, 1-45) and are thought to represent impressions from the anterior horns of the menisci [167, 307, 470, 536]. The medial limiting groove lies on the superior third of the femoral condyle, where it appears as an irregular concavity and may present only as a slight radiolucency. The lateral limiting groove is on the middle third of the condyle, due to the smaller size of the lateral meniscus, and appears as a relatively constant indentation [307, 536]. The limiting groove is poorly marked in about 10% of the adult population and is not yet present in children and adolescents [647]. It is especially prominent in patients with ACL or PCL insufficiency, which permits an abrupt angulation of the knee into hyperextension with a disruption of the normal rolling-gliding sequence [690] (see Fig. 1-46). The difference in the prominence of the medial and lateral grooves is based on biomechanical factors. The more anterior or inferior position of one condyle is not useful for differentiation because the position of the condyles varies greatly with the position of the knee and the radiographic projection [536, 647].

The roof of the intercondylar notch appears as a dense line (Blumensaat's line) that forms a 40° angle with the axis of the femoral shaft [54]. A fabella, if present, lies apposed to the posterior aspect of the lateral femoral condyle.

In contrast to the femoral condyles, the tibial condyles show rotational variations in the lateral projection which can complicate lateral/medial differentiation on stress as well as nonstress radiographs. The most useful fea-

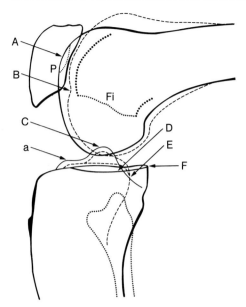

Fig. 1-45. Anatomic structures visible on the lateral radiograph (medial-to-lateral projection) in 90° flexion with neutral tibial rotation. Lateral structures are indicated by broken lines, the fibula by a dotted line. The solid lines represent medial structures, the patella *(P)*, and important landmarks *(A–F)*,
A = Limiting groove of medial femoral condyle, projected above the lateral groove in 90° flexion. *B* = Limiting groove of lateral femoral condyle, projected below the medial groove in 90° flexion, appears as a constant indentation. *C* = Medial intercondylar tubercle (higher), *D* = concavity of medial tibial plateau, *E* = junction of lateral intercondylar tubercle with posterior tibial surface (smooth curve), *F* = junction of medial tibial plateau with posterior tibial surface (angular), *Fi* = roof of intercondylar notch (Blumensaat's line), *a* = third intercondylar tubercle (variable)

tures in this regard are the posterosuperior contours of the tibial plateau.

The medial tibial plateau is concave and in lateral projection appears longer than the convex lateral tibial plateau [167, 168, 307, 341, 536]. The posterior borders of the upper tibia show characteristic differences: The medial plateau has a sharp, angular junction with the posterior tibial surface, whereas the lateral plateau blends with the posterior tibia in a smooth, convex arc and merges posterolaterally with the roof of the proximal fibulotibial joint [307, 447]. The lateral intercondylar tubercle also provides a useful differentiating landmark owing to its posterior location and its in-

volvement in the smooth, convex junction with the posterior tibial surface (Fig. 1-45).

The posteromedial border of the tibial plateau appears relatively uniform as the rotational position of the tibia is changed. However, identification can be difficult in strong external rotation due to overlapping of the more inferior medial plateau by the lateral plateau (Fig. 1-47, 30° external rotation). By contrast, the appearance of the posterolateral border of the tibial plateau varies greatly as a function of tibial rotation. In external rotation the laterally situated roof of the proximal fibulotibial joint appears as a feature of variable prominence that bounds the lateral tibial plateau posteriorly. In internal rotation this feature is replaced by the smooth, convex junction of the lateral intercondylar tubercle with the posterior tibia [307] (Fig. 1-47, 30° internal rotation).

Jonasch [326] reports that a "third intercondylar tubercle" of variable prominence occurs in 6% of knee joints in the area of the anterior intercondylar fossa.

The medial tibial plateau can be identified by the sharp anterior convergence of its boundary lines. This kind of differentiation cannot be made on the lateral side.

The femoral surface of the patella usually appears slightly concave on lateral radiographs and presents a double contour due to the superimposed borders of its medial and lateral facets. The contour of the patellar crest projects posteriorly beyond both. The posterior surface of the patella often bears an indentation (Haglund's depression) that has been variously interpreted with regard to its pathologic significance [26].

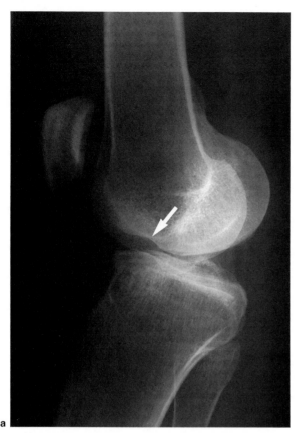
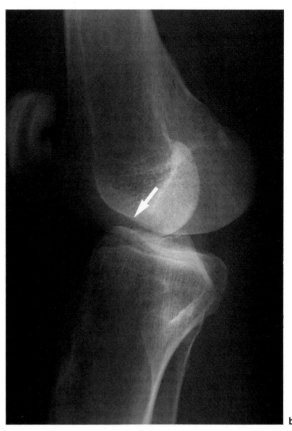

Fig. 1-46a, b. Deep limiting groove on the lateral femoral condyle with marked hyperextension due to chronic posterior instability and constitutional hyperlaxity (**a**). The contralateral knee is also hyperextensible, but the lateral limiting groove *(arrow)* is considerably smaller (**b**)

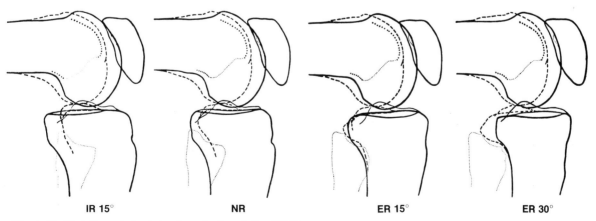

IR 15°   NR   ER 15°   ER 30°

Fig. 1-47. Rotation study, lateral projection (after [624])

1.10.3
Tangential Projection (Sunrise View)

This view demonstrates the "radiographic joint space" of the femoropatellar articulation. Medial/lateral differentiation is readily established by the longer lateral patellar facet. The medial patellar facet varies considerably in its prominence (see Chaps. 5 and 6).

1.11
Congenital Anomalies and Malformations of Ligamentous Structures

There may be rare cases in which one or more ligamentous structures of the knee joint are not present due to a congenital anomaly. This possibility should definitely be considered in cases where minor trauma in a child has led to an unstable knee joint with positive laxity tests.

Congenital aplasias have been described for:

1. The anterior cruciate ligament [122, 575, 652] (Fig. 1-48)
2. The anterior and posterior cruciate ligaments [336].

Congenital dislocation of the knee is a very rare condition in which a familial, constitutional component has been described (Fig. 1-49) [177]. In all congenital anomalies a search should be made for associated lesions due to the frequent coexistence of tibial and fibular dysplasias, patellar dislocations, femoral dysplasias, foot deformities, scoliosis, and congenital dislocation of the hip [177, 652]. Hypoplasia or even aplasia of the intercondylar eminence noted on a survey film may suggest the presence of a congenital intra-articular malformation [122]. Knee disorders may also exist in the setting of congenital diseases and chromosome abnormalities (Table 1-9).

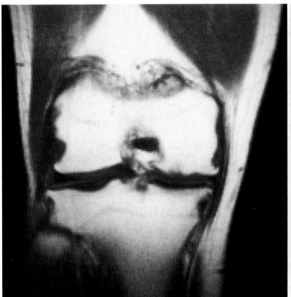
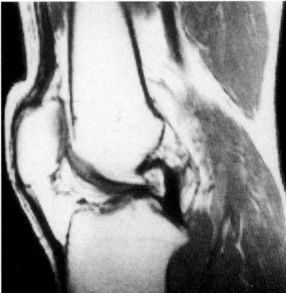

a　　　　　　　　　　　　　　　　　　　　　　　　　　　　　　　　b

Fig. 1-48a, b. Congenital aplasia of the ACL. The patient, a 29-year-old male, consistently avoided athletic activities because of his knee, which felt unstable during exertion. MR imaging shows pronounced degenerative changes with marginal excrescences in both articular compartments (**a**). The sagittal scan reveals a giant osteophyte (**b**) constricting the intercondylar notch

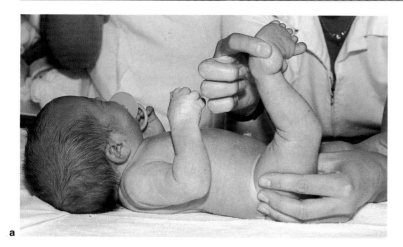
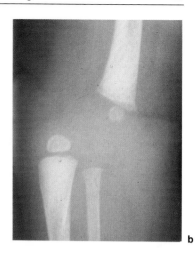

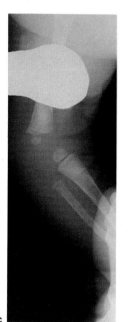
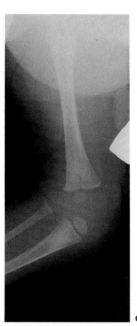

Fig. 1-49a-d. Bilateral congenital dislocation of the knee. Examination discloses a markedly hyperextensible knee joint with clubfoot (**a**). Radiographic appearance (**b**). The varus and valgus stress radiographs (**c** and **d**) show maximum lateral and medial opening of the joint space

Table 1-9. Knee disorders associated with congenital diseases and syndromes

Spina bifida
- Genu recurvatum, extension contracture

Osteogenesis imperfecta
Ullrich-Turner syndrome
Blount's syndrome
- Genu varum

Bonnevie-Ullrich syndrome
Larsen's syndrome
- Hyperextensibility of the joints

Fèvre-Languepin syndrome
- Pterygium genu

Dreyfus' syndrome
- Hyperextensibility of the joints
- Bi- and multipartite patella
- Genu valgum

Klippel-Trenaunay syndrome
- Flexion contractures

Hoffa-Kastert syndrome (Hoffa's disease)
- Lipomatous degeneration of the infrapatellar fat pad with cordlike intraarticular adhesions

Madelung's deformity
Hypercystinuria syndrome
Morquio's syndrome
Pseudo-Fröhlich's syndrome
- Genu valgum

Waardenburg's syndrome (cephalosyndactyly)
- Joint contractures

Rubinstein-Taybi syndrome
- Knee deformities

1.12
Conclusion

Anatomic studies reveal that almost all the ligamentous structures of the knee joint have connections with musculotendinous units. Thus we cannot draw a strict dividing line between active (dynamic) and passive (static) stabilizers. Müller [470] refers to this as the "principle of dynamization" of articular ligaments, while Bonnel et al. [59] speak of a "three-dimensional active rotatory stabilization." All structures but the ACL have musculotendinous attachments – the lateral meniscus and arcuate popliteal ligament to the popliteus muscle; the oblique popliteal ligament, medial collateral ligament, medial meniscus, and posteromedial capsule to the semimembranosus muscle, etc. These attachments enhance the functional importance of the muscles that insert about the knee joint, giving them both a direct and indirect stabilizing function which imparts a primary tension to the ligaments and helps protect them from peak loads. Thus, the muscular status is an important consideration in every repair or reconstruction of capsuloligamentous structures. Intense, preliminary physiotherapy may be indicated to develop the muscles that will stabilize the repair.

Anatomic and kinematic principles are a central concern in ligament reconstructions of the knee, which should be performed in a manner that preserves proprioception. New or altered parameters should not be introduced into the kinematic system. The fixation or transposition of ligaments to "extra-anatomic sites" is an outmoded practice that often results in limitation of motion or residual instability.

General Clinical Diagnosis

2
General Clinical Diagnosis

The clinical evaluation of the knee joint consists of:

I. History

II. General clinical diagnosis
    - Inspection
    - Function testing
    - Palpation

III. Special clinical diagnosis
    - Evaluation of the ligaments (laxity testing)
    - Evaluation of the menisci
    - Evaluation of the femoropatellar joint

With a detailed history and careful clinical examination, nearly all extra- and intraarticular lesions of the knee joint can be identified. The diagnostic goal at this stage is to establish the nature and extent of the injury or disease [34, 235]. Arthrography or arthroscopy should be considered as diagnostic adjuncts only after noninvasive options have been exhausted.

Diagnostic arthrotomy is obsolete.

Even an extensive medial or lateral arthrotomy cannot expose all portions of the joint space, which are easily evaluated through an arthroscope. It should be added, however, that the number of diagnostic arthroscopies can be reduced by paying greater attention to taking down a careful patient history and to physical examination.

The use of a standard report form is recommended for all general and special clinical examinations, both for documentation purposes and to ensure a thorough, systematic evaluation.

2.1
History

A good patient history can disclose the presence of most knee dysfunctions and provide a basis for instituting further, appropriate diagnostic and therapeutic measures. Besides eliciting basic information (Table 2-1), the examiner should question the patient concerning associated disorders or other coexisting ailments that may precipitate knee problems or influence management.

The basic questions to be asked of patients include:

1. How did the injury occur? The leading cause of knee diseases is athletic activity (Fig. 2-1) [285, 378, 466, 626]. The sports listed in Table 2-2 are commonly practiced by inadequately conditioned "weekend athletes." Deficient preparation, poor motor coordination, and inadequate muscular development place these individuals at particularly high risk for injuries. The relative slowness of musculoliga-

Table 2-1. Essential trauma data in knee-injured patients

1. Time of injury
2. Mechanism of injury
3. Behavior after the injury (able to ambulate? able to engage in sports? swelling?)
4. Pain? (location? time of onset?)
5. Current complaints (pain? giving way? locking? snapping? crepitus?)
6. Previous treatment after the injury? (immobilization? operation? intraarticular injections?)
7. Previous knee injuries (operation? previous complaints?)

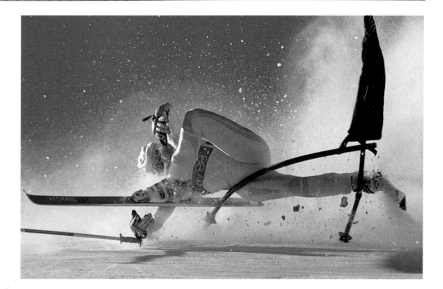

Fig. 2-1. A skier falls in the giant slalom during the 1988 Winter Olympics in Calgary, Canada, seriously injuring the left knee joint (complex capsuloligamentous injury) (photo: H. Rauchensteiner)

Table 2-2. Sports that frequently lead to knee injuries

1. Soccer
2. Skiing
3. Track and fields athletics
4. Tennis
5. American football
6. Rugby
7. Riding
8. Gymnastics
9. Martial arts (judo, karate)
10. Basketball
11. Volleyball
12. Squash

mentous and tendon reflexes has also been cited as a factor predisposing to sports-related injuries in these individuals [531].

In some sports the development of a new, special technique is associated with a rise in the incidence of knee injuries. A recent example is the cross-country skiing technique (the "Siitonen step" or skating), which causes increased stretching and irritation of the medial capsule and ligaments. There are even some sports in which "knee-damaging moves" seem part and parcel of the game. An example is the block thrown against the extended leg, which is used in rugby and American football as a means of bringing down an opponent.

Automobile and motorcycle accidents usually lead to severe, complex injuries that are not confined to the knee [475, 679].

True injuries require differentiation from apparent "injuries" that occur without a corresponding mechanism. Patellar dislocation can occur in healthy knees, while lesions of the menisci, capsule, and ligaments can occur in knees with preexisting degenerative change [202, 234, 257, 610]. The accurate differentiation of "true" and "false" injuries based on the patient's history can be of key importance in cases involving insurance claims.

2. Cause of the injury. Particular attention should be given to the question of whether the mechanism described by the patient could account for the presenting joint injury. Especially in cases of meniscus injury, there is likely to be significant preexisting degenerative damage so that even a mild or incidental trauma can produce a meniscal tear. Where insurance claims are involved, it is frequently the task of the evaluating physician to establish the definitive cause of the complaint.

3. Previous knee disorders? Previous operations? Previous therapy? An awareness of preexisting knee problems and of any prior operative or nonoperative treatment is crucial to the planning of further diagnostic and therapeutic measures. Many patients give a prior history of complete meniscectomy, an operation which, unfortunately, was practiced far too often in the past and was viewed as the "usual" treatment for a torn meniscus. If the meniscectomy was done some years previously, there may be significant degeneration of cartilage and bone in the corresponding joint compartment.

The patient should also be questioned about previous injuries, diseases, and swellings. Not infrequently, asking specifically about a previous aspiration will show that the patient has had an effusion, that blood-tinged fluid was aspirated from the knee, and that the leg was subsequently immobilized in plaster for four to six weeks. This should raise suspicion of a previous partial or complete tear of the ACL, in which case the most recent trauma cannot be considered the sole cause of the presenting injury.

4. Knee function before the injury. Preexisting knee problems are identified, and the patient's expectations are assessed before further diagnostic or therapeutic measures are instituted (Table 2-3). While a professional athlete will wish the knee restored to full function, an older patient with preexisting degenerative disease will probably desire the restoration of painless or less painful ambulation.

Sometimes patients report that "my knee has always snapped," or "I haven't been able to walk well for the last few years anyway" (degenerative changes), or "sometimes I had the feeling of something moving or catching in my knee" (meniscal lesion, ligamentous lesion, loose body), thus establishing the presence of a preexisting abnormality.

2.1.1
Time of Injury

In acute injuries the interval between the trauma and examination should be kept as short as possible. It is best to perform the examination within the first 6 h after the injury. If more

Table 2-3. Questions on the preinjury functional status of the knee

1. Able to engage in sports? (what kind? how often?)
2. Able to run? (how far?)
3. Able to walk? (how far?)
4. Feeling of giving way (when, how often?)
5. Intraarticular sounds (what kind? how often? when?)
6. Locking or catching? (how often? when?)
7. Pain? (when? how often? where? how long?)
8. Previous knee effusion (when? after an injury? after exercise?)

than 8–12 h have elapsed, the pain is often so severe that the physical examination is made much more difficult by reflex muscle spasm and by guarding of the joint. The slightest manipulation or change of joint position in these cases can be excruciating. Even the aspiration of effusion in these patients may do little to alleviate pain.

If a diagnosis cannot be made on the day of the injury or the day after, it need not be forced during the initial examination (e.g., by the night-duty emergency room staff). However, every effort should be made to establish a definitive diagnosis within one week of the injury, as the surgical repair of injured ligaments is technically easier during this period and is generally more successful.

A preliminary diagnosis should be formed during the initial examination, even if the patient complains of severe pain. Several days later, when acute pain and muscular guarding have subsided, the patient can be reexamined under more favorable conditions. Under no circumstances should the patient be allowed to "drop from sight." If within a week there is no significant pain reduction, radiographs are negative, and there is suspicion of a severe intraarticular injury, examination under anaesthesia and diagnostic arthroscopy should be performed in a setting where definitive operative treatment, if indicated, can also be carried out.

Plaster immobilization for more than six days is contraindicated when a definitive diagnosis has not been made.

In open injuries with osseous involvement, a prolonged time interval between trauma and treatment greatly increases the risk of infection. Cuts and lacerations of the skin most commonly occur anterior to the patella. If more than 8h old when seen, they should not be sutured but simply covered with a moist dressing due to the risk of infection. If there is bursal involvement, the affected bursa should be excised, the wound adequately drained, and the entire limb immobilized on a splint.

If the injury has been present for some time, such as a capsuloligamentous disruption sustained several weeks or months previously, secondary damage to initially uninvolved structures (cartilage, meniscus, medial and lateral ligaments) should be anticipated [267, 352, 357, 650].

2.1.2
Mechanism of the Injury

A major goal of history taking is to reconstruct the mechanism of the injury, because typical trauma-producing mechanisms are associated with characteristic patterns of injury [234, 287, 466, 470].

An accurate analysis of the trauma mechanism should address the following questions:

1. Direct or indirect trauma? Local skin changes such as impact marks, hematomas, and abrasions are characteristic of direct injuries and usually are not seen with indirect trauma (caused, for example, by twisting of the tibia) (Fig. 2-2).

2. The direction of the traumatizing force. Violence to the lateral aspect of the knee is manifested by direct skin damage on the lateral side and often by indirect injury to medial ligamentous structures. An anterior trauma causes direct damage to prepatellar and pretibial soft tissues (impact marks, hematomas, abrasions) and indirect damage to posterior and central articular structures (see Fig. 2-10 and 2-26b).

3. The magnitude of the force. The greater the force of the trauma, the greater the potential for ligamentous disruption. However, ligaments can withstand even very large forces without injury if the force acts from one direction for a very brief time [470].

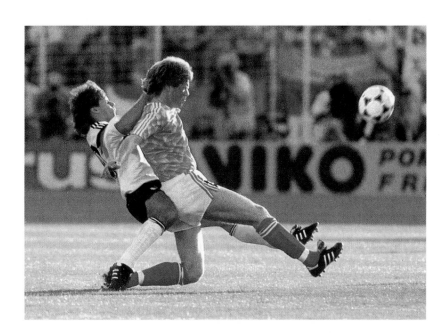

Fig. 2-2. The knee joint of the athlete is frequently exposed to the traumatizing effects of direct and indirect forces (photo: S. Simon)

4. Velocity of the trauma. As early as 1893, Hönigschmied [289] showed experimentally that slowly applied forces tend to cause bony ligament avulsions while more rapid forces tend to tear the ligaments within their substance. This is easily understood when we consider that rapidly applied forces are not effectively distributed and will abruptly stretch the ligament past its point of rupture. A slowly applied force, on the other hand, can be transmitted to the insertion sites on the bone, where it may exceed the fracture strength of the bone and tear out the bony ligament attachment. Indirect trauma in children and adolescents most commonly produce bony ligament avulsions.

5. Position of the knee joint during the injury. The state of tension of the capsule and ligaments depends chiefly on the joint position. When a trauma occurs, primary injury occurs to the structures responsible for stabilizing the knee joint in that position. If the trauma mechanism causes a forced external rotation of the tibia, for example, the structures that stabilize the knee against external rotation will be injured first. Thus, the pattern of the injury can be easily deduced by looking at the functional anatomy of the injured area and the force components acting upon that area. Because the elastic reserve of a ligament is proportional to its total length, short ligaments rupture first.

Abrupt direction changes during running (cutting moves) are necessary in all sports played with a ball (basketball, soccer, tennis, squash). The "side-step cut" can injure the medial joint structures, while the "cross-over cut" threatens the structures on the lateral side [12].

Dashboard injuries are a frequent consequence of automobile accidents. The extent of the injury depends on the level of the dashboard, the velocity of the impact, and the tibial rotation that is induced by the impact [475]. For the motorcycle driver faced with an impending collision, it is essential to decelerate and reduce the kinetic energy of the vehicle and driver as quickly as possible. The portion of the energy not eliminated by braking becomes active on impact as a deforming and disrupting force [679]. The forces are mostly absorbed by the vehicle chassis and by the body parts closest to the front of the vehicle, especially the flexed knee joints, which form natural "bumpers" in the seated driver or passenger (see Fig. 2-9).

Motorcycle accidents often lead to complex ligamentous injuries, sometimes with associated fractures of the limb, pelvis, acetabulum, or skull. The possibility of knee involvement should always be considered even in cases of multiple trauma where there is obvious clinical evidence of a fracture of the femoral shaft or tibia [683].

Hyperextension injuries of the knee are frequently associated with tearing of the ACL and/or portions of the posterior capsule. Bony and subchondral depressed fractures may also occur. With a depression in the area of the limiting groove, laxity tests are indicated to evaluate for rupture of the ACL (Fig. 2-3).

The principal mechanisms of injury to the knee joint are listed in Table 2-4 along with the structures that are liable to be injured [56, 128, 149, 234, 285, 327, 402, 428, 486, 664, 666, 667, 686, 708].

2.1.3
Locking

Locking is a frequent symptom of knee injuries and may even form the principal complaint. The condition may be sustained or intermittent. Locking immediately after the injury may be difficult or impossible to distinguish from resistance to full extension caused by muscle spasm.

Intermittent locking can have various causes (Table 2-5, Fig. 2-4). Arthroscopy is often necessary to establish a diagnosis in patients with negative radiographic findings and normal meniscus tests.

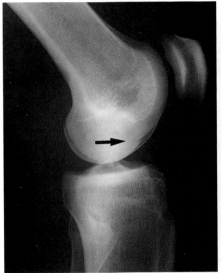
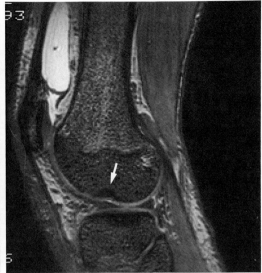

Fig. 2-3a, b. The cortex is depressed in the area of the lateral limiting groove (lateral notch fracture) (**a**). MR scan shows a small chondral depression with a sub-chondral contusion (hemorrhage) (**b**). A positive Lachman test confirmed the radiologic impression of an ACL rupture

Table 2-4. Typical mechanisms of knee injury and their effects

1. Hyperextension
   - Posterior instability
   - Isolated ACL rupture
   - Rupture of ACL and posterior capsule
2. Hyperflexion
   - Meniscus injury (posterior horn)
   - ACL rupture
3. Forced internal rotation
   - Meniscus injury (lateral meniscus)
4. Forced external rotation
   - Meniscus injury (medial meniscus)
   - Medial collateral ligament, possibly with ACL rupture
   - Patellar dislocation
5. Varus trauma
   - Lateral instability
6. Valgus trauma
   - Medial instability (frequent)
7. Flexion-varus-internal rotation
   - Anterolateral instability
8. Flexion-valgus-external rotation (most frequent trauma)
   - Anteromedial instability
9. Dashboard injury
   - Isolated PCL rupture
   - Rupture of PCL and posterior capsule
   - Posterolateral instability
   - Posteromedial instability
   - Patellar fracture
   - Proximal tibial fracture
   - Tibial plateau fracture
   - Acetabular and pelvic fractures

Table 2-5. Potential causes of intermittent locking

1. Meniscal lesion (bucket handle tear, tab tear)
2. Loose body (cartilage, osteochondral fragment)
3. Enlarged villus of infrapatellar fat pad
4. Exophyte in osteoarthritis (rare)
5. Ruptured ACL fibers (behaves like meniscal tab)
6. Patellar subluxation
7. Plica syndrome (hypertrophied mediopatellar plica)
8. Chondromatosis
9. Pigmented villonodular synovitis
10. Anomaly of lateral meniscus (discoid meniscus)

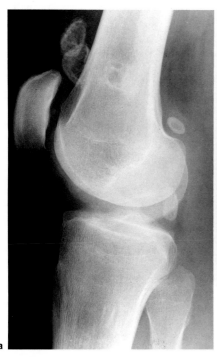
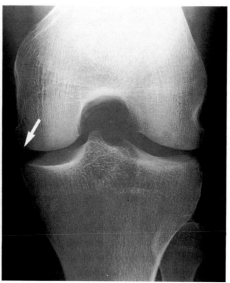

Fig. 2-4a, b. Multiple large loose bodies in chondromatosis (**a**). A small, easily overlooked loose body is visible in the medial joint space (**b**)

2.1.4
Snapping

Snapping of the knee (Table 2-6) should not be confused with loss of extension or intermittent locking (see Table 2-5). Snapping is said to be present when the knee catches suddenly and briefly during flexion or extension. Usually the transient resistance is overcome with an audible click or snap. This contrasts with true locking of the knee, which prevents full extension until relieved by shaking or by a particular movement.

The "snapping knee" phenomenon can occur at various ages. Snaps are frequently noted in children two to three years of age and generally have no pathologic significance. Snapping usually does not cause complaints until adolescence or the end of the growth period.

Numerous intraarticular lesions may be responsible for a snapping knee (Table 2-6). Extraarticular causes may involve the abrupt slipping of a tendon over exostoses on the medial tibial plateau (semitendinosus muscle, sarto-

Table 2-6. Differential diagnosis of snapping knee (intraarticular causes)

1. Discoid meniscus
2. Meniscal lesion
3. Patellar subluxation
4. Fixed loose body
5. Old partial tear of ACL
6. Meniscal cyst
7. Enlarged synovial villus
8. Cyst on ACL or PCL (rare)

rius muscle) or over the fibular head (biceps femoris). Snapping of the semitendinosus tendon occurs over the medial femoral condyle and can be elicited by 20°–30° active or passive flexion of the knee [412].

Structural changes in the tendons or their gliding surfaces can also lead to abrupt slipping or jerking movements. The heads of the gastrocnemius muscle, the insertion of the semimembranosus muscle, and the tendons that converge in the pes anserinus may acquire fibrinous deposits and steplike thickenings as a result of inflammatory processes in the surrounding bursae, causing a snap to occur during motion [613]. An enlarged anserine bursa can act like a mechanical stop to hinder normal gliding of the semitendinosus and sartorius tendons. Postoperatively, the gliding of tendons, capsule, and ligaments can be hampered by the presence of internal fixation material (e. g., on the upper tibia or distal femur) or by pseudobursae that form in response to the material. However, a torn or discoid meniscus continues to be the most frequent cause of a snapping knee.

2.1.5
Pain

Pain is the most frequent symptom of knee disorders. It is not true that severe pain signifies a major injury while mild pain implies a minor injury. Ligamentous injuries that involve little or no ligament disruption frequently cause protracted pain that seems paradoxical. However, when we consider that partial tears and overstretching of ligaments lead to hemorrhage into the ligament substance which exerts pressure and tension on tiny nerve fibers within the ligament, we can understand why so-called "minor injuries" may be followed by significant pain. By contrast, a complete ligament rupture severs the fine sensory nerve fibers and allows blood to flow from the torn vessels into the joint (hemarthrosis) and/or into the subcutaneous fat. An intraligamentous hematoma does not form, there is no nerve compression, and the severed nerves are unable to transmit pain. As a result, instability tends to be the major presenting feature of complex ligament disruptions, whereas pain is more characteristic of bruises, contusions, and partial ruptures.

Other useful diagnostic clues are provided by the time of onset of pain (immediately after the injury or several hours or days later), the quality of the pain (stabbing, cutting, twinging, burning, throbbing), and its pattern of occurrence (at night, after exercise, intermittent, random).

Points and areas of tenderness noted on palpation yield the most important diagnostic information during initial evaluation (see Sect. 2.4.4).

2.1.5.1
Reflex Sympathetic Dystrophy

Reflex sympathetic dystrophy (RSD) should be suspected in patients who report excruciating, burning pain following an injury or operation [48, 55, 97, 134, 236, 350, 506, 584]. A history of a precipitating event can always be elicited, although the severity of the trauma is extremely variable. Even very minor knee injuries can incite the development of RSD.

A great many synonyms are recognized for this disorder, including causalgic syndrome, Sudeck's posttraumatic osteoporosis, posttraumatic dystrophy, reflex dystrophy, algodystrophy, posttraumatic acute bone atrophy, hyperesthetic neurovascular syndrome, and traumatic vasospastic disease. Here we shall use the term reflex sympathetic dystrophy (RSD).

The diagnostic criteria for RSD are as follows:

1. History of trauma (e. g., patellar fracture, arthroscopy, minor injury).
2. Change in the character and location of the primary posttraumatic pain.
3. Triad of autonomic, motor, and sensory disturbances with the cardinal symptoms of soft-tissue swelling (especially on the extensor side), weakness, and spontaneous pain.
4. Disturbance of arterial perfusion (temperature disparity on comparison with the unaffected side).

Unfortunately, RSD is not usually considered in the differential diagnosis of a painful knee. Once radiographic changes such as patchy decalcification have appeared, permanent losses of function may be inevitable despite intensive therapeutic efforts.

The knee is the fourth most commonly affected joint, accounting for 10% of all RSD cases [214]. All the bony joint members need not be affected by the dystrophy, which is more likely to involve isolated structures such as the patella or the medial or lateral femoral condyle (Fig. 2-5). Quadriceps atrophy is usually present [48].

Primary treatment consists of active and passive physiotherapeutic exercises below the pain threshold. Standing stress therapy may be used in patients with severe pain that precludes other types of exercise. Physiotherapy may be supported by pharmacologic agents such as calcitonin (e. g., Karil) or alpha-receptor blocking drugs (intravenous sympathetic blockade with guanethidine).

Psychotherapeutic referral is indicated in selected cases. As always, the prevention of RSD centers on a nonpainful diagnostic workup and treatment with special emphasis on atraumatic postoperative care.

2.1.5.2
Pain Originating Outside the Knee

With knee pain of undetermined origin, diseases external to the knee joint should be excluded. In older patients, osteoarthritis of the hip or lumbar spine is frequently responsible for knee complaints. But a number of other diseases can lead to pain in the knee region (Tables 2-7 and 2-8).

Besides causes of pain resulting from damage to the knee joint, referred pain due to postural defects, spinal deformities, pelvic tilt, leg shortening, and foot deformities should be excluded.

It is not unusual for patients to have difficulty localizing their pain to the knee joint

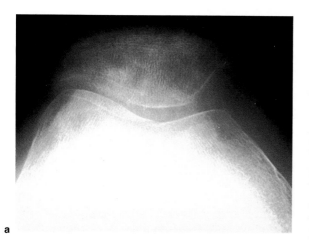
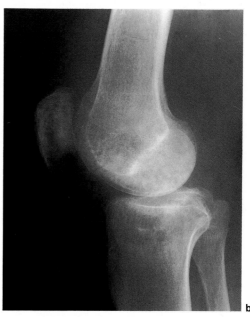

Fig. 2-5a, b. Reflex sympathetic dystrophy. Localized involvement of the patella and femoral condyles following diagnostic arthroscopy (**a**), and involvement of the entire joint following blunt trauma (**b**)

Table 2-7. Potential causes of pain about the knee [262]

1. Tumors
   - Benign (lipomas, hemangiomas, chondromas, xanthomas, etc.)
   - Malignant (synovialoma, osteosarcoma, chondrosarcoma, etc.)
2. Neurologic disorders (tabes)
3. Ulcerative colitis
4. Whipple's disease
5. Hemochromatosis
6. Hemophilia
7. Endocrine disorders (hyperparathyroidism, acromegaly, thyroid disease)
8. Cushing's syndrome (or prolonged cortisone therapy)
9. Paraneoplastic process (bronchial carcinoma)
10. Panchondritis (rare)

Table 2-8. Potential causes of pain in the knee joint [141]

1. Infectious diseases with no demonstrable pathogenic organisms in the joint
   - Infectious hepatitis
   - Measles
   - Scarlet fever
   - Gonorrhea
   - Brucellosis
   - Salmonellosis
   - Tuberculosis
   - Rheumatoid arthritis
   - Reiter's syndrome
   - Löfgren's syndrome (acute Boeck's disease)
   - Herpes virus
2. Inflammatory rheumatic diseases
   - Secondary chronic arthritis
   - Rheumatoid arthritis
   - Collagen diseases
   - Bekhterev's disease
3. Metabolic diseases
   - Gouty arthritis
   - Hyperlipidemia
   - Alkaptonuria

even when the pain is caused by a knee disorder. Therefore diseases of the S1 and S2 spinal roots and of the sacroiliac joints should additionally be considered. In some cases knee pain is the first and only symptom of root compression at S1 or S2. With a primary posterolateral disc herniation, the knee pain typically increases during walking and sitting. Coughing and sneezing also precipitate or exacerbate the pain. These symptoms are also seen in ankylosing spondylitis (Bekhterev's disease), but the pain in the latter condition is worse in recumbency and in the early morning hours and does not increase with exercise.

Retroperitoneal masses (hemorrhage, tumor, abscess) also can incite a persistent knee pain that is refractory to treatment [631]. In this case there is often a demonstrable reduction or loss of sensation on the thigh.

There is a danger of misdiagnosing the condition as "osteoarthritis of the knee" or "knee attrition," especially if corresponding radiographic findings are obtained.

2.1.5.3 Knee Pain in Children

Special consideration should be given to pediatric knee pain (Table 2-9), which is too easily dismissed as being exertion- or growth-related when it persists for longer than expected following an apparently minor injury. In children the pain may even radiate to the opposite side [77].

Because serious diseases may underlie knee pain in children, knee pain occurring spontaneously or persisting long after a minor trauma requires careful diagnostic evaluation. Blood tests are always indicated, since unexplained joint pain can be an early sign of a malignant systemic disease (e. g., leukosis).

Table 2-9. Differential diagnosis of knee pain in children. (After Deigentesch, in [77])

1. Appendicitis
2. Brodie's abscess
3. Osteomyelitis
4. Tumors (osteochondroma, chondromyxofibroma, osteoid osteoma, osteoclastoma, fibrous dysplasia, Ewing's sarcoma, fibro-osteosarcoma, solitary bone cyst)
5. Villonodular synovitis
6. Leg length discrepancy (long-leg arthropathy)
7. Aseptic necroses of bone
   - Blount's disease (proximal tibial epiphysis)
   - Sinding-Larson-Johannson syndrome (patellar apex)
   - Base of patella
   - Osgood-Schlatter disease (tibial tuberosity)
   - Perthes' disease (hip)
8. Slipped capital femoral epiphysis
9. Osteochondritis dissecans of the hip
10. Hip dysplasia
11. Systemic rheumatic diseases
12. Systemic malignant diseases (e.g., leukosis)

2.1.5.4
Chronic Knee Pain

Patients with prolonged, unexplained pain in the region of the knee joint should be examined with utmost care. Treatment should never be abandoned due to lack of response to local conservative therapy (e. g., physiotherapy, radiation) or surgery. This is especially true in cases where a definitive diagnosis has not been established. We must avoid placing patients in situations where they go from doctor to doctor, their complaints becoming less plausible with each visit and ultimately prompting referral to a psychologist or psychiatrist. This "therapy" can have tragic consequences for these patients (Fig. 2-6).

Certainly it cannot be denied that psychosomatic disturbances can have causal importance in knee complaints. However, a psychosomatic etiology should never be assumed until an organic cause of the pain has been reliably excluded. All available diagnostic modalities should be utilized in this process. Whole-body radionuclide bone scanning, for example, is a proven method of screening for local foci outside the knee joint.

Thus, refractory complaints are an indication for interdisciplinary consultation involving an abdominal surgeon, neurologist, urologist, radiologist, gynecologist, and nuclear medicine specialist for the purpose of excluding disorders that are not initially considered by the orthopedist or traumatologist (see Tables 2-7 and 2-8).

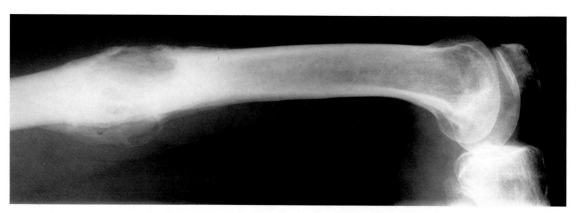

Fig. 2-6. Woman 27 years of age with a malignant bone tumor in the middle third of the femur. The patient had a three-year history of knee pain that had been unsuccessfully treated by two general practitioners, five orthopedists, two neurologists, one surgeon, and two internists. Her knee had been radiographed several times. Finally she was referred to a psychiatrist. Only after the appearance of a marked swelling in the thigh did the patient, labeled a "malingerer," again seek medical attention

2.1.6
Giving Way

Many patients complain of a spontaneous buckling or "giving way" of the knee joint, often accompanied by severe pain. The knee may give way for no apparent reason, and the patient may even fall down. Most patients are unsure whether the buckling preceded the pain or whether the pain came first.

The primary diagnosis suggested by giving way is ligamentous disruption, but other potential causes should be included in the differential diagnosis (Table 2-10).

If giving way occurs while walking uphill or downhill, a retropatellar lesion should be suspected. But if it results from changing direction, and the knee joint simultaneously catches momentarily and is then able to move again, the most probable diagnosis is a ligament disruption (ACL insufficiency), meniscus lesion, or patellar subluxation [12, 405].

2.2
Inspection

Inspection of the patient begins as soon as he arrives at the office or clinic.

In accident victims, the vital functions are evaluated first. In patients with multiple injuries, first priority is given to the detection and treatment of life-threatening conditions (intracerebral, intrathoracic, or intra-abdominal hemorrhage; thoracic and pelvic fractures; fractures of the femur, tibia, or humerus).

Further management depends on the findings. The measures for an open knee injury differ considerably from those for a closed knee injury (see below).

If the patient presents on foot, the gait should be evaluated (limp? walking aid? full heel-to-toe evolution of the step?). If possible, this should be done without the patient's knowledge. In patients who are evaluated in connection with insurance claims or trade association membership, it is not unusual to see

Table 2-10. Potential causes of giving way

1. Ligamentous lesion
2. Meniscal lesions
3. Mediopatellar plica
4. Patellar dislocation
5. Chondromalacia
6. Retropatellar osteoarthritis
7. Femorotibial osteoarthritis
8. Loose bodies
9. Discoid meniscus
10. Enlarged villus of retropatellar fat pad
11. Quadriceps atrophy (e.g., after prolonged cast immobilization)
12. Psychogenic (rare)

the gait pattern change after the patient leaves the examination room.

The inspection and the rest of the clinical examination are performed in an examining room with the lower extremities undressed.

2.2.1
Open Injuries

With an open injury of the knee joint or open fracture of the femur, patella, and/or tibial plateau, inspection of the wound should be delayed until the patient has been taken to the operating room. In the outpatient facility the wound should be sterily draped, if this has not already been done, and the patient prepared for operation as rapidly as possible (Fig. 2-7, Table 2-11).

Laxity testing and extensive palpation are performed only under sterile operating-room conditions following the induction of general anesthesia.

Depending on the severity of the injury, the goals of treatment are to preserve the limb, prevent infection, and establish coverage of the skin defect (Table 2-11). With an open injury that is grossly contaminated or is old and inadequately treated, suction irrigation should be instituted as part of the initial management. As with intra- and periarticular infections following an injection, arthroscopy, or aspiration, the systemic intravenous administration of a potent antibiotic (e. g., Cefotaxim, Cefuroxim) is indicated.

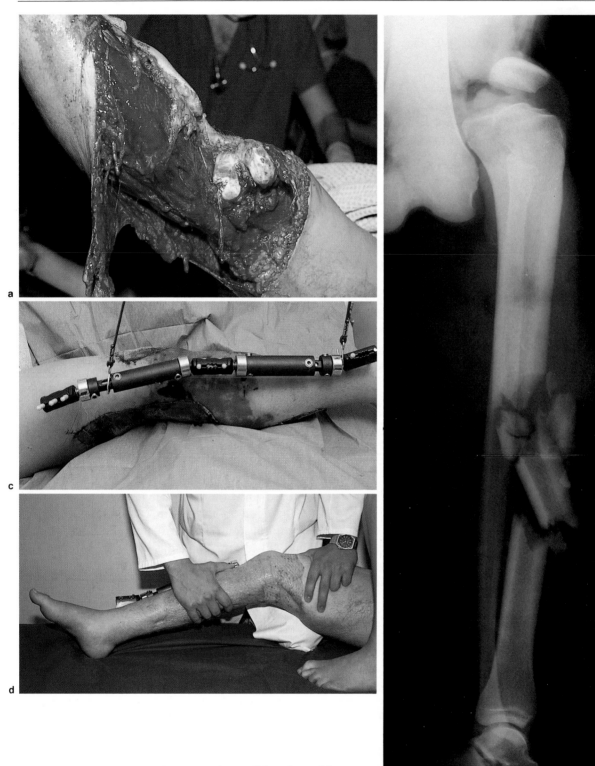

Fig. 2-7 a–d. Complete grade-3 open knee dislocation with a comminuted fracture of the tibia and soft-tissue degloving in a 19-year-old female. Posttraumatic appearance with exposed femoral condyles (**a**), radiographic appearance (**b**), status at 10 days after operation (**c**). At six months (**d**) the patient has active flexion to 75° with adequate stability (mildly positive Lachman test)

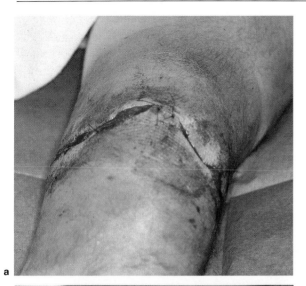

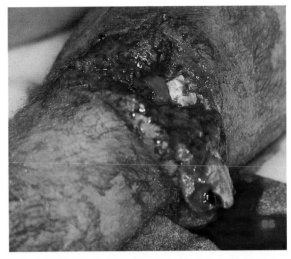

Fig. 2-9. Grade-3 open knee injury (comminuted patellar fracture, shear fractures of both femoral condyles) in a 21-year-old motorcyclist. Blades of grass, glass fragments, and a live caterpillar were removed from the wound at operation

Table 2-11. Management of a severe open knee injury

1. Circulatory stabilization
2. Exclusion of associated injuries
   Radiographic examination: pelvis, lumbar spine, chest, skull
3. Immediate preparation for operative treatment
4. Operative treatment
   Priority 1: Preserve the limb
   Priority 2: Prevent infection
   Priority 3: Repair the skin defect

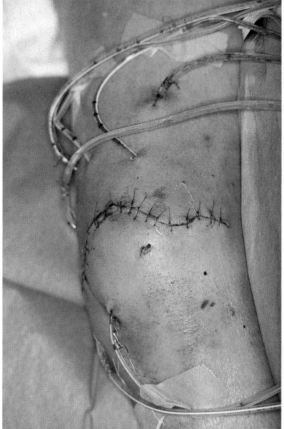

Fig. 2-8a, b. Grade-3 open knee injury sustained in a motorcycle accident (22-year-old male). When hospitalized three days after inadequate primary treatment with approximating sutures, the patient had septic fever, leukocytosis, and local signs of infection (**a**). The wound was debrided, partial synovectomy was performed, and suction irrigation was established (**b**). At 30 days postinjury there was a healthy scar with some motion loss at terminal flexion and extension

An open comminuted fracture and disruption of the joint-stabilizing bony and ligamentous structures should be stabilized by external fixation using a half-frame type of device. With extensive open fractures of the femur and/or tibia that involve the knee, the fixation device should be mounted across the joint to facilitate nursing care and immobilization of the knee (Fig. 2-7c). Multiple operative measures are often required.

Generally it will take several weeks to achieve closure of the skin defect. Once this has been accomplished, the mobility of the knee joint should be restored; this may necessitate surgical arthrolysis. A ligament recon-

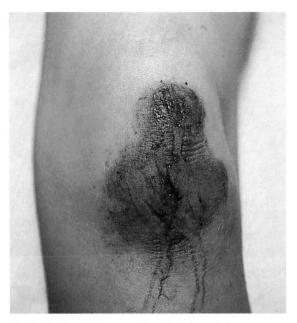

Fig. 2-10. Severe prepatellar abrasion, the most common (!) knee injury. Such wounds should always be examined for disruption of the prepatellar bursa

Prepatellar wounds should be examined to exclude bursal involvement. If the prepatellar bursa has been breached by the trauma (Fig. 2-10), it should be completely removed during primary treatment.

2.2.2
Effusion and Other Swelling

Generalized swelling of the knee usually represents an acute effusion that develops immediately after the trauma and is obvious on inspection (Figs. 2-11 and 7-15a). Additionally there may be localized swellings at various sites that require palpation or special diagnostic studies for their evaluation (Fig. 2-12). The potential causes of localized swelling about the knee joint are listed in Tables 2-12 to 2-15.

struction, if required, may be undertaken only after satisfactory full-thickness skin coverage has been established.

Complete dislocations of the knee (Fig. 2-7) do not always result in severe instability as one might assume, because a large portion of the capsuloligamentous complex, having been torn from the femur or upper tibia like a cap or hood, remains intact and can heal as a unit [470].

2.2.3
Muscular Atrophy

With long-standing ligamentous injuries, meniscal lesions, or prolonged immobilization, careful inspection will reveal atrophy of the quadriceps muscle group and especially of the vastus medialis. Zippel [724] considers quadriceps atrophy to be the most important and also the most common feature of an old meniscal lesion.

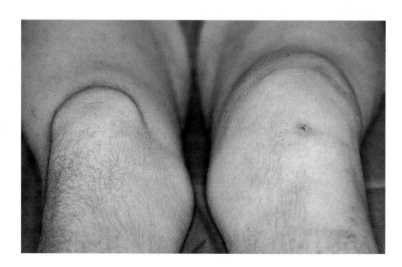

Fig. 2-11. Effaced contours of the left knee joint in a three-day-old injury. There is a small, unresolved prepatellar abrasion that must be allowed to heal before definitive operative treatment is performed

Table 2-12. Causes of local swelling on the anterior side

1. Prepatellar bursitis
2. Infrapatellar bursitis
3. Osgood-Schlatter disease
4. Enlarged infrapatellar fat pad
5. Meniscal cyst
6. Tumors
7. Lipomas
8. Synovialoma
9. Tendon sheath fibroma (rare)

Table 2-13. Causes of local swelling on the lateral side

1. Cyst of the lateral meniscus
2. Enlarged infrapatellar fat pad
3. Baker's cyst behind the biceps femoris insertion
4. Tumors
5. Degenerative osseous changes

Table 2-14. Causes of local swelling on the medial side

1. Degenerative joint diseases (osteophytes on medial tibial plateau, medial femoral condyle)
2. Flap tear of meniscus
3. Ossification at origin of medial collateral ligament (Stieda-Pelligrini shadow)
4. Meniscal cyst (rare)
5. Bursitis at insertion of pes anserinus (fluctuant swelling distal to joint space with no limitation of motion, pain on flexion)
6. Tumors
7. Gouty arthritis

Table 2-15. Causes of local swelling on the posterior side

1. Baker's cyst
2. Lipoma
3. Aneurysm (rare)
4. Muscular hernia (semimembranosus, biceps femoris)
5. Tumors (liposarcoma)
6. Tumoral calcinosis

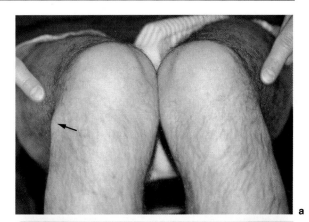
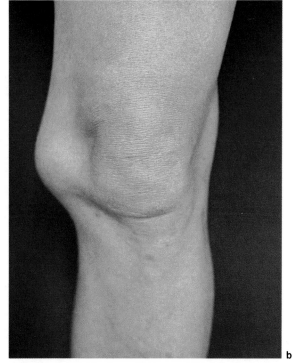

Fig. 2-12a, b. Cyst of the right lateral meniscus (**a**). Tumor (gouty note) at the medial joint line (**b**)

Smillie [610] states that quadriceps atrophy is a consistent feature of all internal knee injuries and even describes the vastus medialis muscle as the "key to the knee joint." That is the area in which initial signs of muscular atrophy should be sought. Localized atrophy is appreciated more easily by inspection (Fig. 2-13) than by measurements of muscle girth. The potential causes of quadriceps muscle atrophy are listed in Table 2-16.

Atrophy of the vastus medialis muscle is especially marked after lesions of the ACL [33,

513]. The fact that the atrophy is difficult to relieve by conditioning even after an alloplastic or autologous reconstruction suggests that a proprioceptive feedback mechanism may be involved.

Any atrophy of the vastus medialis weakens the medial patellar checkrein, resulting in a relative functional predominance of the vastus lateralis with increased lateralization of the patella [276, 524].

The potential consequences of quadriceps atrophy, together with the favorable effect of guided mobilization on ligament healing (see Sect. 1.8.3), provide a rationale for instituting

Table 2-16. Potential causes of quadriceps atrophy

1. Meniscal lesions
2. Painful extension loss
3. ACL insufficiency
4. Chondromalacia
5. Mediopatellar plica
6. Patellar dislocation
7. Femoropatellar pain syndrome
8. Prolonged immobilization
9. Chronic pain
10. Sympathetic reflex dystrophy
11. Neurogenic
12. Reflex atrophy due to long-standing knee effusion

functional therapy of the knee joint following operative or nonoperative treatment measures.

Functional therapy of the knee means mobilization!

Any prolonged immobilization of the knee leads to shrinkage of the joint capsule. The consequent loss of motion interferes with cartilage nutrition and predisposes to chondromalacia (Fig. 2-14).

Regarding the type of physical therapy that is indicated for the rehabilitation of quadriceps atrophy, we do not feel it is appropriate to strengthen the quadriceps by active extension against a high resistance from a large flexion angle. It is still common practice among physiotherapists to attach a sandbag or other weight to the foot with the knee flexed 90° and then instruct the patient to straighten the knee. Due to the long lever arm of the tibia, this action can generate extremely large compressive forces in the femoropatellar joint that may exceed 1000 kg/cm². Thus, quadriceps strength-

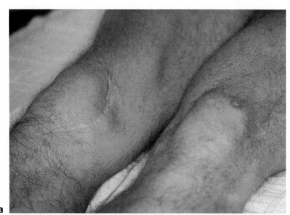
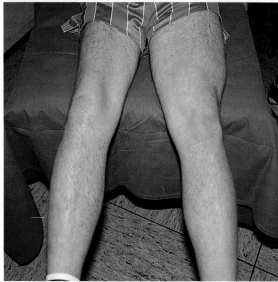

Fig. 2-13a, b. Localized atrophy of the right vastus medialis muscle following knee trauma with rupture of the ACL (**a**). General quadriceps atrophy in a patient who favored the right knee for 12 weeks due to pain (**b**)

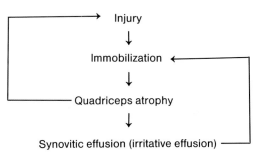

Fig. 2-14. Vicious cycle associated with "nonfunctional therapy" (modified from [610])

ening exercises should always be initiated from a small angle of flexion. In patients with ACL insufficiency, exercises should stress conditioning of the hamstrings, which are linked to the ACL by the "ACL reflex" described by Grüber et al. [229]. In all flexion angles, tightening of the hamstrings reduces the tension on the ACL [546]. Quadriceps contraction, on the other hand, increases tension on the ACL, especially in the range from $0°–45°$ flexion, as Arms [15] and Renström [546] have shown. For this reason intensive quadriceps exercises are contraindicated in early rehabilitation following surgical ACL repairs [275, 335, 470, 546], since the quadriceps muscle acts as an antagonist to the ACL when the joint is near extension. Active near-extension anterior drawer test (active Lachman test, see Fig. 3-46) and the active pivot shift are elicited by contraction of the quadriceps. These signs are useful in diagnosing a deficient ACL (see Sects. 3.9.2 and 3.9.6 and Figs. 3-47, 3-48 and 3-54).

Elongation of the ACL is produced not only by isometric quadriceps exercises performed near extension but also by downhill walking, which can create very high tension in the anteromedial part of the ligament [275].

Isolated tears of the ACL have even been noted after maximal contraction of the quadriceps muscle. This has been seen, for example, in downhill ski racers who straighten up suddenly after crossing the finish line in a crouched position [470].

2.2.4
Skin Changes

The location of cutaneous wounds, impact marks, and hematomas provides useful clues to the nature and direction of the trauma-producing force (Fig. 2-15). Cutaneous changes can range from superficial abrasions to deep cuts, lacerations, and extensive soft-tissue defects. Management depends on the status, age, and extent of the skin injuries. With an unresolved wound not yet covered with scab, the risk of infection contraindicates surgical intervention, including arthroscopy, until the wound has completely healed. A draining wound should be given primary, definitive surgical treatment, any joint fistula excised, and suction irrigation continued for three to five days (Fig. 2-16).

Trophic disturbances like those associated with impaired arterial blood flow, post-thrombotic syndrome, or varicosis are identified and taken into account during further treatment (Fig. 2-17). These changes may contraindicate prolonged immobilization of the limb. In the presence of systemic disease with cutaneous changes such as psoriasis (Fig. 2-18), hypercholesterolemia (Fig. 2-19), or folliculitis affecting the thigh region, it is determined whether these changes have therapeutic implications (e. g., require postponement of operation, contraindicate operative treatment) or whether the disease itself (e. g., psoriasis arthropathica) underlies the joint problems.

On the enening prior to or the morning of the operation, the condition of the skin should always (!) be reviewed to confirm that it is acceptable. If it is found that vesiculation, pressure sores, or other skin changes have developed due to an overly tight or poorly fitting compression dressing, plaster cast, or tape bandages, surgery should be postponed due to the risk of infection (Fig. 2-20).

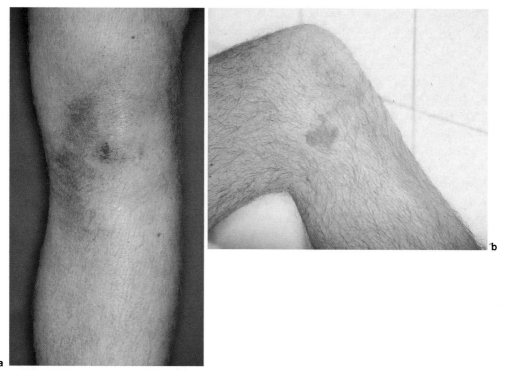

a

Fig. 2-15a, b. Medial hematoma, small prepatellar abrasion, and diffuse prepatellar redness signifying incipient prepatellar bursitis. The latter was also evidenced by coexisting lymph node enlargement (**a**). The small, circumscribed hematoma on the medial side following a direct lateral (!) trauma signified a medial capsuloligamentous rupture. Clinical examination disclosed moderate valgus laxity in 20° flexion (**b**)

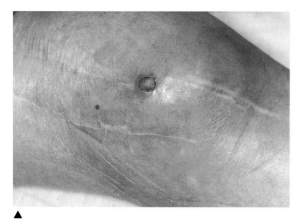

▲
Fig. 2-16. Draining fistula associated with chronic joint infection following a total knee replacement

▶
Fig. 2-17. Conspicuous varicose trunks in the left leg and incipient trophic skin changes on the right lower leg

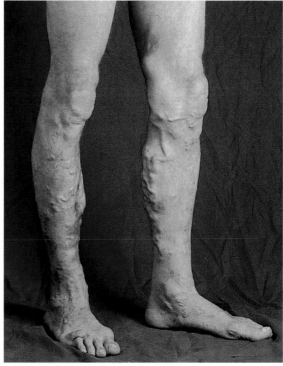

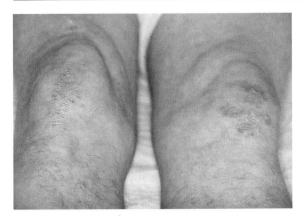

Fig. 2-18. Prepatellar skin changes in psoriasis

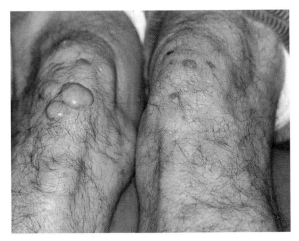

Fig. 2-19. Multiple prepatellar xanthomas in a patient with familial hypercholesterolemia

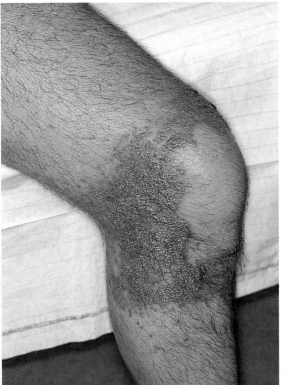

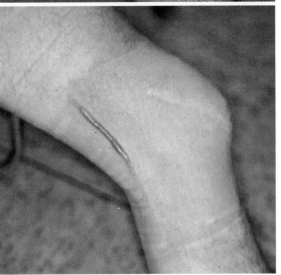

Fig. 2-20 a, b. Extensive pyodermia following self-treatment with ointment and bandage (**a**). Tension bulla caused by an overtight compression dressing applied after percutaneous aspiration of the knee (**b**)

2.2.5
Loss of Extension

Restricted knee extension may be noted immediately after an injury or may be slowly progressive. Intermittent extension loss is described as a "catching" or "snapping" of the knee [610, 613] (see Table 2-6 and Sect. 2.1.4).

An acute extension loss can have various causes (Table 2-17) but is most commonly due to a meniscal lesion. Even injury to structures not primarily responsible for extension of the knee joint can decrease the range of extension.

The painful extension loss frequently seen after sprains or partial ruptures of the medial collateral ligament is usually a "morning-after"

condition that develops 10–18 h after the injury. Typically it is relieved by a brief period of immobilization or by analgesia [513, 514]. Most patients report that they were able to continue their normal activities after the trau-

Table 2-17. Differential diagnosis of acute extension loss

1. Meniscal injury
2. Rupture of patellar ligament
3. Rupture of quadriceps tendon
4. Complete or partial rupture of ACL
5. Intraarticular effusion of rapid onset
6. Pain (guarding)
7. Loose body (osteochondral fracture, chondromatosis)
8. Patellar dislocation
9. Patellar fracture
10. Muscular fiber tear

Table 2-18. Differential diagnosis of extension loss of gradual onset

1. Medial collateral ligament injury ("pseudolocking")
2. Femorotibial osteoarthritis (osteophytes)
3. Retropatellar osteoarthritis
4. Hypertrophy of infrapatellar fat pad
5. Abnormal laxity of reserve extensor apparatus (retinacula)
6. Intraarticular tumors
7. Prolonged immobilization
8. Capsular fibrosis
9. Iatrogenic
   - Improperly attached ACL
   - Soft-tissue irritation by internal fixation material
10. Hypertrophy of reconstructed, repaired, or augmented ACL
11. Infrapatellar contracture syndrome
12. Cyst on ACL (rare)
13. Villonodular synovitis
14. Fixed loose body
15. Scar contractures
16. Bony deformities (femur, tibia, foot)
17. Neuromuscular disorders
18. Psychogenic

ma but that, on the following morning, they were unable to straighten the knee. This "pseudolocking" is frequently misdiagnosed as a meniscus injury.

Acute limitations of extension are distinguished from the congenital, slowly progressive, iatrogenic, and postoperative forms (Table 2-18, Figs. 2-21 and 2-22).

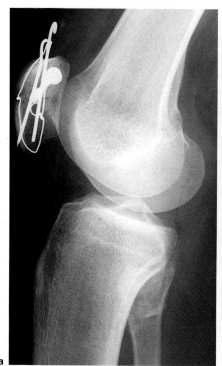 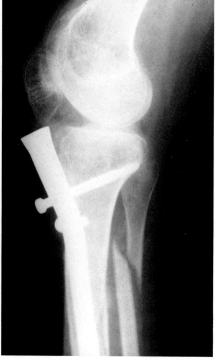

a   b

Fig. 2-21a, b. Restricted knee extension secondary to soft-tissue irritation caused by internal fixation material in the fractured patella (**a**) and by locking nail fixation of the tibia with coexisting patella baja (**b**)

The extension loss caused by soft-tissue irritation (Fig. 2-21) is usually reversible after removal of the internal fixation material or elimination of the scar contracture. By contrast, extension losses following ACL reconstructions in which the tibial insertion has been placed too far anteriorly will persist for as long as the substitute ligament remains intact, i. e., until it becomes elongated or torn.

Though rare, a congenital anomaly such as a pterygium in the popliteal fossa will cause significant extension loss and flexion deformity (Fig. 2-23). Pterygium genu is usually a bilaterally symmetrical anomaly that is more pronounced on the tibial side of the joint and most commonly extends from the ischial tuberosity to the calcaneus (28%) or to the Achilles tendon (25%). The muscles in the pterygium usually arise from the semitendinosus and less frequently from the semimembranosus [695]. Depending on the severity of the malformation, there will be some functional impairment of the knee joint. Patients with a

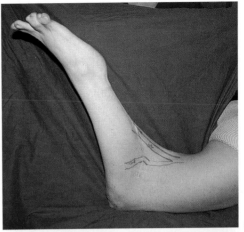

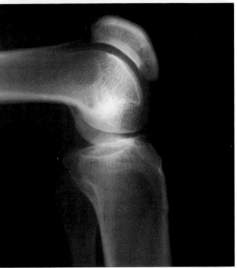

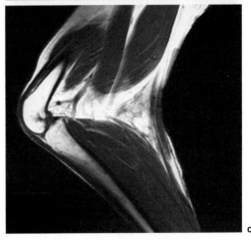

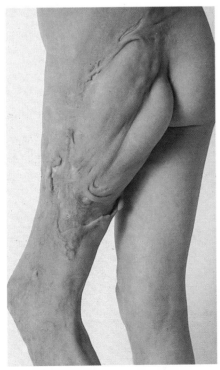

Fig. 2-22. Flexion deformity of the knee caused by scar contractures in the thigh

Fig. 2-23a–c. Bilateral pterygium genu in Fèvre-Languepin syndrome. In the prone position, the full extent of the flexion contracture can be appreciated. The nerve course in the pterygium is indicated (**a**). The patella shows marked elongation and anterior convexity (**b**). The extent of the pathologic changes is demonstrated by the MR scan (**c**). The pterygium is traversed by muscles and blood vessels

very pronounced pterygium genu walk with a "duck waddle" gait.

Radiographs demonstrate typical osseous changes resulting from the prolonged deformity. Round femoral condyles, a convex tibial epiphysis or tibial plateau, and an elongated patella are characteristic findings (Fig. 2-23 b) [695].

Pterygium genu is most commonly seen in the setting of Fèvre-Languepin syndrome and occasionally in Rossi or caudal regression syndrome.

A true pterygium is traversed by tendons, muscles, and nerve cords, which serve to distinguish it from a simple skin duplication (web) or scar contracture [695].

A knee operation or direct trauma may incite a fibrous hyperplasia with the development of adhesions in the anterior part of the joint. An extension deficit is caused by the inability of the quadriceps muscle to act as a knee extensor at very small flexion angles due to the adhesions between the patellar ligament and surrounding soft tissues, including the infrapatellar fat pad (Fig. 2-24). Paulos et al. [521] report that a low-riding patella (patella baja) is present in 17% of these cases. The treatment of this condition, known as infrapatellar contracture syndrome, consists of intraarticular and possibly extraarticular debridement with lysis of adhesions followed by intensive physicotherapy.

An extension loss may develop after the replacement, augmentation, or reattachment of the ACL even though optimum femoral and tibial insertion sites have been chosen for the

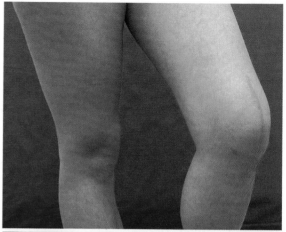

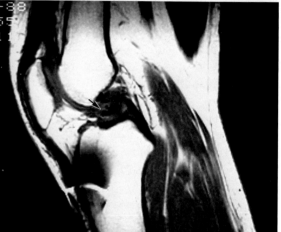

Fig. 2-25 a, b. Extension deficit 11 months after a tear of the ACL treated by primary surgical repair and augmentation with the semitendinosus tendon. There is diffuse swelling of the entire joint (**a**). The MR scan shows small globular structures representing fibrosed tissue in front of the cruciate ligament (**b**). Following arthroscopic resection of the hypertrophied portions and thinning of the ligament with enlargement of the intercondylar notch, eight weeks intensive physical therapy was sufficient to restore full extension

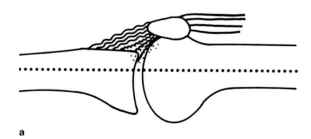

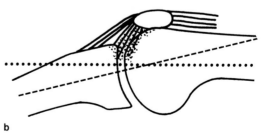

Fig. 2-24 a, b. Infrapatellar contracture syndrome and secondary patella baja. The patellar ligament is lax in extension (**a**) and tightens with slight flexion due to the presence of intraarticular adhesions (**b**). Little active flexion is possible, although the range of passive extension often is not decreased

ligament [190]. Hypertrophy of the graft or sutured ligament probably results from small, fibrosed hematomas in the anterior portion of the joint and ligament. The hematomas may be caused by repeated microtraumata like those associated with forced extension exercises. The fibrosis leads to thickening of the graft, which then abuts against the intercondylar notch, blocking the knee short of full extension. The diagnosis can be confirmed by arthroscopy or preferably by MR imaging (Fig. 2-25). The treatment of choice is arthroscopic removal of the hypertrophied tissue, thinning of the graft if it appears to be too thick, and enlargement of the intercondylar notch (notchplasty).

2.2.6
Spontaneous Posterior Drawer

Simple inspection of the tibial tuberosities with the knees flexed 90° and the feet on the examination table in the supine patient can disclose a severe ligamentous injury. Unless proven otherwise, a posterior sagging of the tibial tuberosity (Posterior sag sign) on one side is considered presumptive evidence of a ruptured or deficient PCL (Fig. 2-26).

2.2.7
Limb Axis

The limb axis can yield important information on the underlying disorder. In an athletic patient with genu varum who complains of pain on the medial side of the knee, a lesion of the medial meniscus should be suspected (Fig. 2-27). On the other hand, lesions of the lateral meniscus and patellar dislocations are more common in patients with genu valgum. Genu valgum is most commonly seen in children and in the elderly, especially females (Fig. 2-28). Genu recurvatum and/or genu valgum are regarded as predisposing factors for patellar dislocation. Smillie [610] notes that the combination of a high-riding patella (patella alta) and genu recurvatum predisposes not only to patellar dislocation but to other injuries as well.

When an axial deformity of the limb is noted, its cause should be ascertained so that symptomatic therapy (e. g., partial medial meniscectomy) can be combined with causal therapy (correction of the deformity) if the patient so desires.

The limb axis is also an important consideration in ligamentous reconstructions, since lateral stabilization is essential in patients with genu varum but is of minor importance in patients with genu valgum [49, 485].

It should also be considered whether the axial deformity is unilateral or bilateral. Ligament insufficiencies can exacerbate or mimic a unilateral angular deformity of the leg (Fig. 2-29).

2.3
Function Testing

Tests of joint function yield valuable diagnostic information in recent as well as older injuries and are performed before selective palpation is carried out.

2.3.1
Mobility

The normal range of motion of the knee joint as measured by the neutral-0 method (extension/flexion) is $5°-10°/0°/120-150°$. The active and passive ranges of motion are tested and documented. Any pain that is noted at this stage may already signify a meniscal lesion (Fig. 2-30).

When the range of motion is restricted, it is helpful to evaluate the end point of motion. If it feels soft and elastic, i. e., if different or increasing ranges of motion are noted on repeated testing, the motion loss is usually a result of pain or muscle spasm. If the end point feels springy or firmly elastic (with a constant range of motion on repeated testing), an entrapped

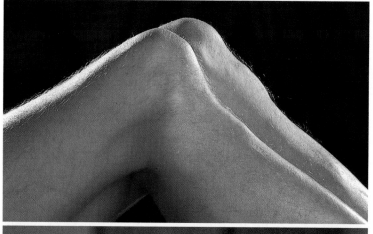

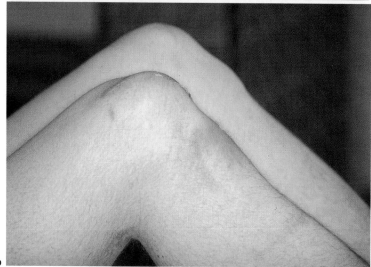

Fig. 2-26a, b. Sighting across the tibial tuberosities reveals a posterior sagging of the right proximal tibia (spontaneous posterior drawer) (**a**). The pretibial abrasion in this fresh injury signifies a direct trauma (dashboard injury) (**b**)

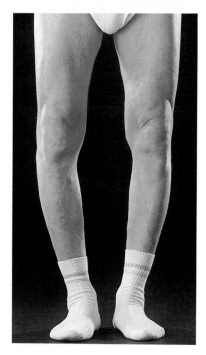

Fig. 2-27. Genu varum

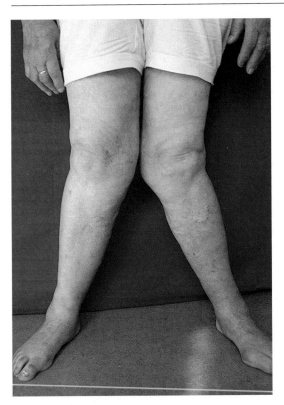

Fig. 2-28. Genu valgum

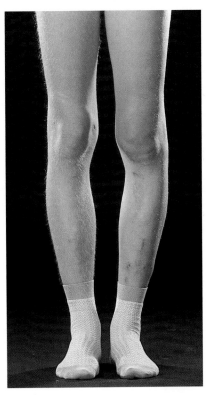

Fig. 2-29. Varus component and excess recurvatum with a external rotation tendency of the left tibial plateau. Simple inspection raises suspicion of a posterolateral instability (see Fig. 3-43)

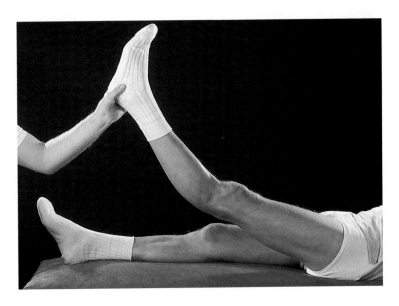

Fig. 2-30. Test of maximum extension. Hyperextensibility may signify a lesion of the posterior capsule or cruciate ligaments

meniscus or loose body should be suspected. A firm, hard end point is consistent with intra-articular adhesions, osseous deformity, or other articular deformity. The range of motion does not increase on repeated testing [234].

The active and passive ranges of internal and external rotation are determined in the sitting position with the knee flexed to 30°, 60°, and 90° (Fig. 2-31).

Increased external rotation of the tibia with the patient supine and the knee flexed 60° (exorotation) points to a lesion of the popliteus muscle [235].

2.3.2
Rigidity Tests

Shortening and contractures of the flexor and extensor muscles may be responsible for a variety of knee complaints.

It is known that the distensibility of a muscle, such as the quadriceps, decreases as the muscle increases in size. One effect of this "quadriceps contracture" is to reduce the mobility of the patella. Many of these patients complain of anterior knee pain after exertion or even after prolonged sitting with the knee flexed [316, 518]. Thus it is important to test the distensibility of the quadriceps muscle and especially of the biarticular rectus femoris (see Figs. 5-3a and b). For this examination, called the rigidity test, the patient lies prone on the examining table. While the patient keeps the pelvis flat, the examiner slowly flexes the knee until the heel approaches the buttock (Fig. 2-32). The distance between the heel and buttock is measured. With a normally distensible quadriceps, the heel will almost touch the buttock. The heel-buttock distance should not exceed 10 cm in men or 5 cm in women [518]. In many patients with anterior knee pain, the

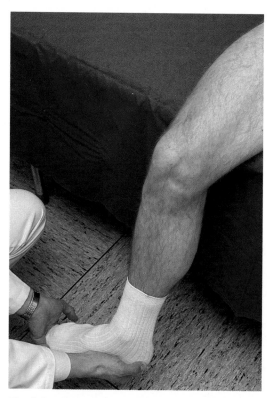

Fig. 2-31. Test of maximum range of external rotation in 90° flexion

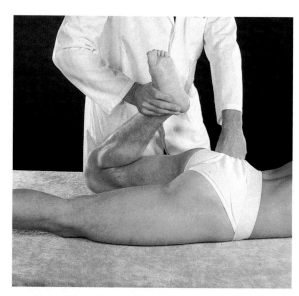

Fig. 2-32. Test of quadriceps rigidity. Though the thigh muscles are well developed, the quadriceps is shortened. The heel-buttock distance is 20 cm

heel-buttock distance is increased. The patellar hypomobility that is associated with a "rigid" quadriceps leads to a rise of the retropatellar pressure, and this pressure rise can account for the symptoms described. Thus, in cases of femoropatellar pain syndrome (anterior knee pain) or presumed retropatellar chondromalacia, shortening of the quadriceps muscle should always be excluded. Often symptoms can be markedly improved and the need for invasive treatment avoided simply by performing regular quadriceps stretching exercises.

2.3.3
Muscular Function

Chronic knee disorders often lead to pathologic findings in tests of muscular strength and function. In conditions affecting the tendons and especially in insertional tendinopathies, resistance tests will elicit pain in the area of attachment of the affected muscles. The following muscle groups are tested:

1. Extensor muscles (quadriceps)
Test: Extension against a resistance (Fig. 2-33).
  Anterior pain: consistent with suprapatellar or infrapatellar insertional tendinopathy, supra- or infrapatellar bursitis, injuries and lesions of the quadriceps tendon and patellar ligament.
  Medial pain: consistent with medial parapatellar insertional tendinopathy, plica syndrome, medial meniscus injury.
  Lateral pain: consistent with lateral parapatellar insertional tendinopathy, iliotibial tract friction syndrome.

2. Flexors (semimembranosus, pes anserinus, biceps femoris, gastrocnemius)
Test: Flexion against a resistance.
  Pain in popliteal fossa: consistent with Baker's cyst, semimembranosus bursitis, injury of posterior capsule and PCL, bursitis in area of pes anserinus.
Test: Flexion and external rotation against a resistance.
  Lateral pain: consistent with biceps femoris insertional tendinopathy at the fibular head, meniscal injury, injury to iliotibial tract.
Test: Flexion and internal rotation against a resistance.
  Lateral pain: consistent with lateral meniscal injury, lesion of popliteus tendon.
  Medial pain: consistent with pes anserinus insertional tendinopathy, pes anserinus bursitis, injury of semimembranosus muscle, semimembranosus insertional tendinopathy, medial meniscal injury.

3. Rotators
The patient is seated and told to rotate the foot externally from a position of internal rotation (test of external rotators) and to rotate the foot internally from a position of external rotation (test of internal rotators).

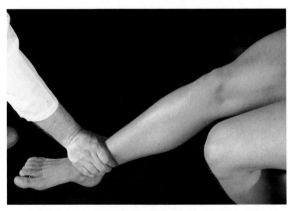

Fig. 2-33. Test of quadriceps muscle strength. The patient is told to straighten the knee against a resistance. The examiner notes the force that is developed and the muscle contours, especially that of the vastus medialis

2.3.4
Sensation

Direct trauma to the lateral side of the knee can contuse or rupture the peroneal nerve, while a varus-producing trauma can stretch it. This provides more than a forensic rationale for testing motor and sensory qualities of the peroneal nerve about the knee.

In previously operated patients who have had an extensive medial arthrotomy, it is common to find pre- and infrapatellar sensory disturbances. Sometimes areas of hypo- or hyperesthesia are present as evidence of damage to the infrapatellar branch of the saphenous nerve. A neuroma is manifested by a painful spot in the scar area that produces an electric-shock-like sensation.

Chronic irritation of the infrapatellar branch of the saphenous nerve caused by a medial meniscus lesion leads to a hyperesthetic area on the medial side, about the size of a quarter, over the course of the infrapatellar branch. Zippel [724] states that this symptom, called Turner's sign, is frequently present with meniscal lesions and disappears following surgical correction of the lesion.

2.3.5
Circulation

Even in closed injuries, direct trauma or over-stretching can cause occlusion or rupture of the popliteal vessels [90, 435]. All vascular injuries should be promptly diagnosed (by palpating the dorsalis pedis, posterior tibial and popliteal arterial pulses) and appropriately treated (Fig. 2-34). When an absent pulse is noted, the vascular lesion should be accurately localized by conventional angiography or digital subtraction angiography (DSA) (Fig. 2-35).

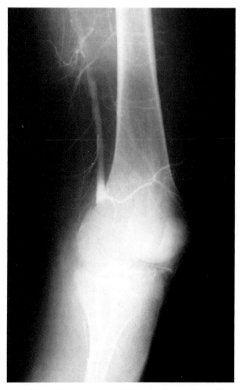

Fig. 2-34. Occlusion of the popliteal artery caused by a direct, blunt knee trauma. The exact location of the vascular lesion is established by angiography

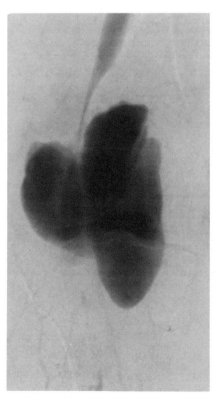

Fig. 2-35. Digital subtraction angiogram showing an arteriovenous aneurysm of the popliteal vessels following arthroscopic resection of the medial meniscus

Like pronounced venous insufficiency, disturbances of arterial blood flow, seen predominantly in older patients, influence the plan of treatment. For example, it may be prudent to shorten the operating time, avoid the use of a tourniquet, and avoid prolonged postoperative immobilization to ensure that the underlying vascular disease is not exacerbated.

A rare condition seen in younger patients is the popliteal artery entrapment syndrome caused by constriction of the popliteal artery in the area of the medial head of the gastrocnemius [82, 411]. The patient complains of intermittent claudication, and clinical examination reveals diminished popliteal and pedal pulses in the affected extremity. The diagnosis is confirmed by arteriography or Doppler sonography.

2.4
Palpation

Palpation provides a means of differentiating among the causes of knee swelling (see Table 2-19) and identifying sites of tenderness. Intraarticular signs such as clicks, snaps, crepitus, scars, and the skin temperature are also evaluated at this time.

2.4.1
Intraarticular Effusion

Intraarticular fluid collections are excluded or confirmed by selective palpation. An effusion is manifested by the "dancing patella" sign. This is elicited by manually compressing the superior, medial, and lateral recesses and pressing the patella against the femur with the index finger. When effusion is present, the patella will spring back to its initial position, and ballooning can be felt on the lateral and medial sides of the joint (Fig. 2-36).

A small effusion is detected by applying the thumb and forefinger lightly to the sides of the patella and stroking downward (distally) on the superior recess with the other hand. The presence of effusion is indicated by a slight separation of the thumb and forefinger.

When an intraarticular effusion is confirmed, radiographs are taken to exclude fractures, osteochondral fractures, bony ligament avulsions, and also degenerative changes in knees with chronic effusion (irritative effusion). Effusions that develop immediately after trauma should raise suspicion of a severe intraarticular injury (ACL rupture) or an injury to bony structures. Every acute posttraumatic joint effusion accompanied by negative radiographic findings and an apparently stable knee should be aspirated to exclude hemarthrosis (see Sect. 2.5 for details).

Table 2-19. Causes of knee swelling

1. Generalized
   - Intraarticular
     • Effusion
     • Transsudate
     • Exudate
   - Capsular
     • Postoperative (e.g., after ligament reconstruction)
     • Synovitis
   - Extraarticular ("soft-tissue rheumatism")
   - Osseous
     • Degenerative changes
     • Tumors
2. Local

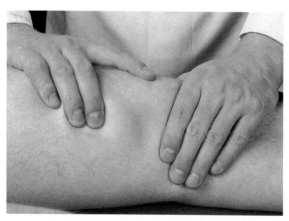

Fig. 2-36. Test for intraarticular effusion ("dancing patella")

The various causes of chronic joint effusion are listed in Table 2-20. In some cases arthroscopy will be necessary to establish a diagnosis (Fig. 2-37).

It should be emphasized that the posttraumatic absence of joint effusion does not exclude a serious knee injury. An extensive capsuloligamentous disruption will allow the fluid to drain into the soft tissues of the lower leg, so that there is no palpable knee effusion ("dry joint") [234, 466, 470]. Only laxity testing in this situation will allow a meaningful assessment of the damage that has occurred.

2.4.2
Extraarticular Swelling

The "dancing patella" sign is not present with extraarticular swelling. Major ligamentous reconstructions are often followed by a generalized extraarticular swelling that may persist for a period of weeks or even months in rare cases (Fig. 2-25a).

Massive swelling of the knee without significant effusion also occurs in pronounced synovitis like that associated with a systemic rheumatic disease.

Generalized extraarticular swellings are less common than localized swellings, which may

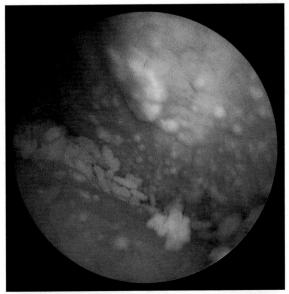

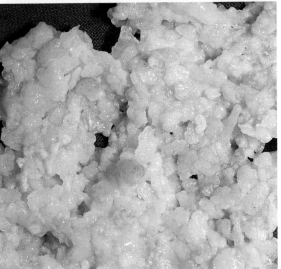

Fig. 2-37a, b. Synovial chondromatosis. Radiographic findings were negative in this patient, who had recurring bouts of knee effusion. Arthroscopy revealed numerous small chondromas in the various joint compartments including the superior recess (a). Treatment consists in removal of the multiple intraarticular bodies followed by arthroscopic synovectomy (b)

Table 2-20. Potential causes of chronic knee effusion [77]

1. Degenerative changes (cartilage, meniscus)
2. Rheumatoid arthritis
3. Ankylosing spondylitis (Bekhterev's disease)
4. Reiter's disease
5. Chondrocalcinosis
6. Chondromatosis
7. Villonodular synovitis
8. Septic arthritis
9. Gout
10. Collagen diseases
11. Ulcerative colitis
12. Gonorrhea
13. Sarcoidosis
14. Hemophilia
15. Neuropathic arthropathies

occur in numerous diseases (see Tables 2-12 to 2-15). These swellings are palpated to evaluate for tenderness, mobility relative to deeper tissues, communication with the joint cavity, temperature, and consistency.

2.4.3
Intraarticular Phenomena

Palpable intraarticular snaps, clicks, or crepitus noted during motion of the knee are suggestive of an old injury or degenerative change. They most commonly originate from the patellofemoral articulation, where a firm scraping, snapping or grating can be detected during palpation, especially when degenerative changes are advanced. The snaps or clicks may be audible to persons standing nearby (see Sect. 10.3).

If snapping or grating is not detected during normal motion of the knee, the patient is told to flex the knee several times, as this often increases the intensity of the sounds (see Fig. 5-6). Often the initial act of flexion will produce a marked snap in the lateral portion of the joint. If this occurs only once and is not painful, it is not considered a pathologic sign. This jumping or snapping phenomenon, which many refer to as "jumping of the iliotibial tract," occurs in a large percentage of healthy individuals.

In the presence of a localized loose body, snapping will be confined to a circumscribed portion of the joint. On the other hand, loose bodies that float freely in the joint space can cause snapping at various sites. When a clip or snap is detected in the joint space, a meniscal lesion should be excluded (see Chap. 4).

2.4.4
Local Pain and Tenderness

A major goal of palpation is to localize sites of maximum tenderness. In many cases this evaluation, together with the special clinical examination, will establish the diagnosis. To be systematic, we shall discuss the significance of pain and tenderness separately for each side of the joint (anterior, medial, posterior, lateral), noting the most important associated symptoms, clinical findings, and special diagnostic techniques.

2.4.4.1
Anterior Pain and Tenderness (Fig. 2-38)

1. Patella

Patellar fracture (longitudinal or transverse): Usually direct trauma. Crepitation? Palpable fracture line? With a transverse fracture, the knee cannot actively extend against a resistance. Radiographic examination, sunrise views.

Hematoma: Negative radiographic findings, direct trauma.

Retropatellar cartilage changes: Retropatellar grinding, history of pain, arthroscopy to confirm damage.

Prepatellar bursitis (traumatic, chronic): Occupational activity (floor tiler, underground miner), athletic activity (wrestling) [474]. Signs of inflammation (redness, heat) and/or fluctuation (see Fig. 2-56).

Chronic ligament instabilities [244]: History, laxity testing.

2. Base of Patella

Bony quadriceps avulsion: Typical radiographic findings, palpable depression.

Quadriceps tendon rupture
History: Spontaneous rupture, usually in older patients without adequate trauma, in patients

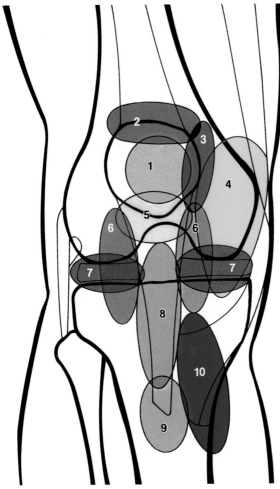

Fig. 2-38. Sites of pain and tenderness on the anterior aspect of the knee. Patella *(1)*, base of patella *(2)*, medial patellar border *(3)*, medial retinaculum *(4)*, patellar apex *(5)*, medial and lateral borders of patellar ligament *(6)*, joint line *(7)*, patellar ligament *(8)*, tibial tuberosity *(9)*, insertion of pes anserinus *(10)*

with systemic diseases, or in athletes. Stabbing pain and weakness of sudden onset, or inability to use the leg.

Findings: Extension against resistance is usually weakened and occasionally is not possible (involvement of medial and lateral retinaculum). Immediately after the injury there is a visible or palpable depression above the patella (Fig. 2-39 a) that later is filled by hematoma, so that an isolated rectus femoris rupture is easily missed (sonography shows hematoma). Bulging on contraction, patella abnormally mobile, femoropatellar gliding surface palpable if entire quadriceps is ruptured, patella baja, absent patellar tendon reflex.

Radiographic signs: Patella baja, anterior tilt of proximal patellar border (Fig. 2-39 c), which often shows osteophytes, calcifications, possible tendon ossification, suprapatellar soft-tissue defect (soft-tissue view).

Bilateral quadriceps tendon rupture may occur in systemic diseases or less commonly after trauma [85, 204, 286] (Fig. 2-39 b).

Suprapatellar insertional tendinopathy: Pain on extension against a resistance, tenderness at the patella-quadriceps tendon junction.

3. Medial Patellar Border (Fig. 2-40)

Bony avulsion (patellar fracture): Usually direct trauma, radiographic examination (differential diagnosis: bipartite patella).

Patellar chondromalacia (common)
History: Trauma? Sunrise views, arthroscopy. Frequently a "catch-all" diagnosis; better known as femoropatellar pain syndrome or anterior knee pain.

Parapatellar insertional tendinopathy (=insertional tendinopathy of vastus medialis): Extension against resistance is painful in the advanced stage; athletes are predominantly affected.

4. Medial Retinaculum

Patellar dislocation: History, genu valgum and/or genu recurvatum, often palpable depression in medial retinaculum? Often hemarthrosis. Positive Fairbank's apprehension test (see Sect. 5.3.1). Sunrise views often show bone flakes chipped from the medial patellar facet or osteochondral fragments from the lateral femoral condyle.

Plica syndrome (medial shelf syndrome, hypertrophied mediopatellar plica): Palpable cord that is mobile relative to the medial femoral condyle. Often "chondropathic" complaints. Diagnosis confirmed by arthroscopy (see Fig. 11-35). Symptoms often resemble those of

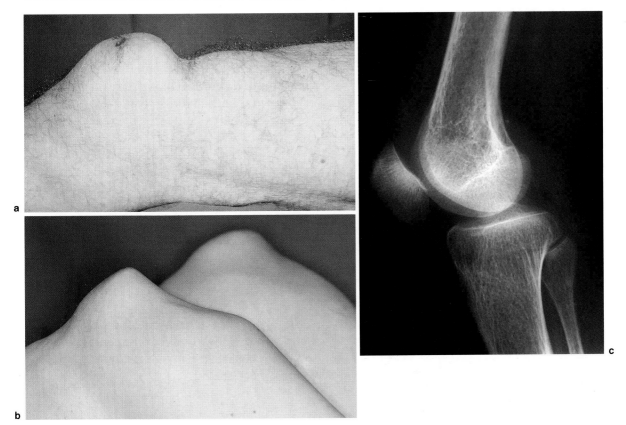

Fig. 2-39 a–c. Quadriceps tendon rupture with associated bulging and depression (**a**). Bilateral quadriceps tendon rupture following minor trauma (**b**). Patient had a several-year history of cortisone medication because of renal insufficiency. Radiographs show marked osteoporosis, patella baja, and anterior tilt of the proximal patellar pole (**c**)

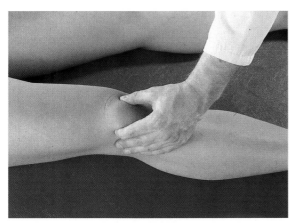

Fig. 2-40. Palpation of the medial and lateral patellar borders

medial meniscal lesion or anterior knee pain. Positive meniscus tests (Apley test, McMurray test), quadriceps atrophy, and pain in the medial and/or lateral joint line are also possible.

5. Patellar Apex

Bony avulsion of the patellar ligament: Extension against resistance is very painful or not possible, characteristic radiographic findings (Fig. 2-41).

Proximal rupture of patellar ligament: Palpable depression. No extension against resistance, patella alta on radiograph.

Jumper's knee (patellar apex syndrome): Palpation reveals marked tenderness over the pa-

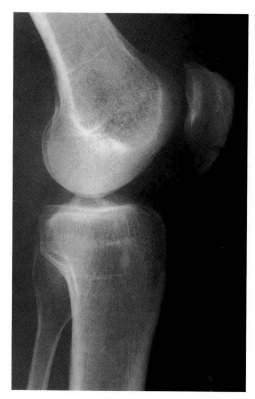

Fig. 2-41. Undisplaced bony avulsion of the patellar ligament

tellar apex. An elongated patellar pole or small ossifications may be palpable at deeper levels. Typically pain increases on extension against a resistance. Five stages of "jumper's knee" are recognized based on subjective criteria (Table 2-21). Sonography can demonstrate the morphologic tendon changes corresponding to the stages of the condition [187, 265] (see Chap. 8).

Radiographs show deformities of the patellar apex ranging from lucency of the insertion zone to thornlike thickenings to grotesque bony excrescences. The condition is attributed to sport-specific factors (vertical forces on the ligament insertion, abrupt stops, floor hardness, quality of athletic shoes) and constitutional factors (femoropatellar joint dysplasia, angular deformities, foot deformities, short ischiocrural and quadriceps muscles, lateralized patella, patella alta, vastus medialis dysplasia) [161, 162, 373, 697].

Tendon ruptures are not uncommon in the late stage (stage V) of the disease [353]. They are usually caused by minor injuries. Jumper's knee may also be the initial manifestation of hyperparathyroidism [415].

Differentiation is required from retropatellar chondromalacia and parapatellar insertional tendinopathies. Jumper's knee frequently coexists with femoropatellar pain syndrome.

Sinding-Larsen-Johannson disease: Lateral radiographs show bony excrescences (traction apophysitis) that may attain grotesque proportions (Fig. 2-42).

6. Medial and Lateral Borders of Patellar Ligament

Irritation of infrapatellar fat pad: Adhesions of the fat pad can lead to twinging anterior knee pain, local tenderness alongside the patellar ligament, or signs mimicking meniscal entrapment. Irritation of the infrapatellar fat pad was described as a separate disease entity by Hoffa in 1904 [348]. Besides congenital and constitutional factors (hypertrophy of the fat pad, lax capsule, vestigial septum in knee joint), causal importance has been ascribed to inflammatory, traumatic, and iatrogenic influences (aspiration, arthroscopy, arthrotomy).

Degenerative diseases: History, typical radiographic findings.

Meniscal lesions: History, positive meniscus tests.

7. Joint Line

Meniscal lesions: History, positive meniscus tests.

Table 2-21. The five grades of "jumper's knee"

Grade I:	Pain after exercise
Grade II:	Pain at start of exercise and afterward
Grade III:	Pain during and after exercise
Grade IV:	Pain precludes exercise (sport), is felt during everyday activities
Grade V:	Rupture of patellar ligament

Meniscal cyst (rare): Local swelling.

Degenerative changes: History, inspection, palpation, radiographic findings.

8. Patellar Ligament

Rupture of the patellar ligament (Fig. 2-43): Patella alta (clinical and radiographic). Palpable gap in the course of the patellar ligament. Knee cannot extend against a resistance. Bilateral rupture is rare but not unknown.

Irritation of the nerve plexus in the patellar ligament [610] ("hyperesthetic gonalgia").

Neuroma of infrapatellar branch of saphenous nerve [610]: Electric-shock-like pain. Usually previous injury or preexisting scars (operation?).

Infrapatellar bursitis (Fig. 2-44): Occupational history (e. g., miner, floor tiler) and athletic history (wrestler). Trauma? Palpable and visible swelling, exclude signs of inflammation. Exact location and extent can be determined by sonography.

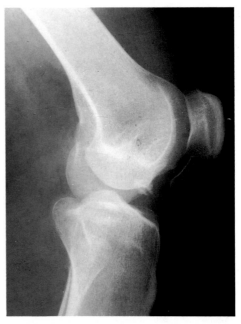

Fig. 2-42. Marked deformity of the patellar apex in Sinding-Larsen disease, coexisting with advanced osteochondritis dissecans

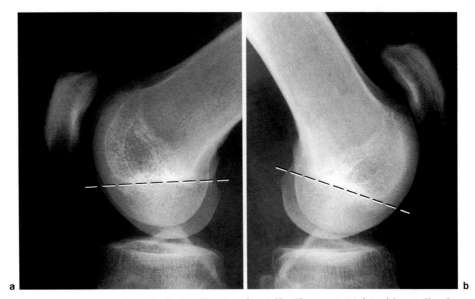

Fig. 2-43a, b. Ruptured patellar ligament *(right)* with patella alta

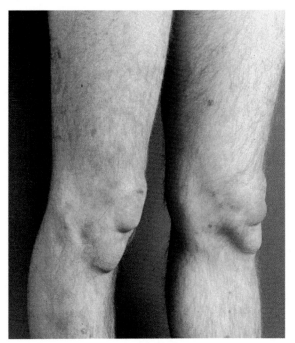

Fig. 2-44. Chronic pre- and infrapatellar bursitis

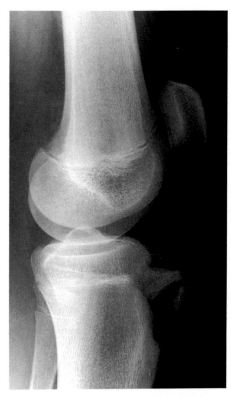

Fig. 2-45. Bony avulsion of the tibial tuberosity with fracture of the avulsed fragment

9. Tibial Tuberosity

Hematoma: Direct trauma. Often dashboard injury (see Fig. 2-26b).

Bony avulsion (Fig. 2-45): Common in adolescents, characteristic X-ray findings.

Aseptic necrosis of bone (Osgood-Schlatter disease): No trauma, characteristic X-ray findings.

Insertional tendinopathy of patellar ligament [162]: Extension against resistance is painful, pain after exercise. Athletes predominantly affected.

10. Insertion of Pes Anserinus

Insertional tendinosis of pes anserinus: Mainly affects athletes (distance runners, swimmers) but may also occur in the setting of degenerative disease. Flexion against a resistance is painful. Pain is intensified by active internal rotation of the foot with the lower leg fixed and the knee flexed.

Degenerative diseases: History, radiographic examination.

Bursitis: Local swelling and Fluctuation. Often combined with insertional tendinosis [640].

2.4.4.2
Lateral Pain and Tenderness (Fig. 2-46)

1. Lateral Femoral Epicondyle

Bony avulsion of the lateral collateral ligament: Pain is increased by varus stress; characteristic X-ray findings.

Sprain of the lateral collateral ligament: Pain is increased by varus stress.

Iliotibial tract syndrome [640] (synonym: iliotibial tract friction syndrome): Mainly affects athletes (cyclists, distance runners, swimmers). Pain usually occurs while running on uneven ground, during mountain training, or when the

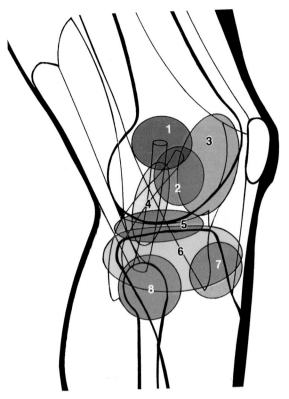

Fig. 2-46. Sites of pain and tenderness on the lateral aspect of the knee. Femoral epicondyle *(1)*, origin of popliteus muscle *(2)*, femoral condyle *(3)*, collateral ligament *(4)*, joint line *(5)*, tibial plateau *(6)*, tubercle of Gerdy *(7)*, fibular head *(8)*

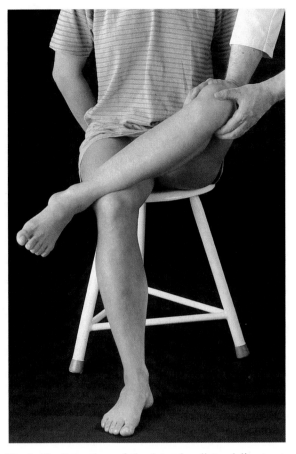

Fig. 2-47. Palpation of the lateral collateral ligament and origin of the popliteus muscle

training regimen is suddenly intensified. Poorly localized pain in the area of the lateral femoral epicondyle provoked by athletic activity is characteristic. Stair climbing can be especially painful.

Local tenderness is elicited by pressure on the lateral femoral epicondyle as the moving knee reaches about 30° of flexion. The pain diminishes with further flexion or extension. It is not uncommon to find a genu varum and/or a valgus position of the calcaneus.

Differentiation is required from iliotibial tract bursitis, a lateral meniscal lesion, and tendinopathy of the biceps femoris or popliteus muscle. It is not unusual for pain to radiate toward the tubercle of Gerdy.

2. Origin and Body of Popliteus Tendon (anterior and posteroinferior to the lateral collateral ligament origin) (Fig. 2-47)

Popliteus tendon injuries: Most common in athletes (martial arts, swimming, running). Popliteus tendon injuries are rarely isolated and usually associated with posterolateral capsuloligamentous disruption. With isolated injury, hemarthrosis is usually the dominant complaint [478].

Popliteal insertional tendinopathy: Site of maximum tenderness is just anterior to the origin of the lateral collateral ligament. Pain is increased by internal rotation and flexion against a resistance.

Popliteal tenosynovitis [434]: Maximum tenderness is just posterior to the lateral collateral ligament between the iliotibial tract and biceps femoris tendon. Pain is increased by flexion and internal rotation against a resistance [706].

3. Lateral Femoral Condyle

Patellar dislocation: Positive Fairbank's apprehension test. There may be cartilage flakes from the medial patellar facet and outer surface of the lateral femoral condyle. Radiographic examination (sunrise views required) (see Figs. 5-13, 5-15 and 5-16).

Degenerative disease: Characteristic radiographic findings (osteophytes).

Lateral Plica Syndrom: (very rare). Lateral counterpart to the medial shelf syndrome (see page 82). Palpable cord (hypertrophied lateral plica) that is mobile relative to the anterolateral aspect of the lateral femoral condyle. Athletes are predominantly affected. Pain and the typical snap phenomen are provoked during sports activity. Differentiation is required but difficult from lateral meniscus lesions and anterior knee pain. Definite diagnosis is confirmed only by arthroscopy.

4. Lateral Collateral Ligament (Fig. 2-47)

Rupture of lateral collateral ligament: Pain is increased by varus stress, alleviated by valgus stress.

5. Lateral Joint Line

Meniscal lesion: Positive meniscus tests, valgus stress (compression of the lateral meniscus) increase pain, varus stress reduces pain (see Chap. 4 for details).

Meniscal cyst: Visible and/or palpable swelling (see Fig. 2-12). Meniscal symptoms may be absent.

Rupture of popliteus tendon (rare) [443].

6. Lateral Tibial Plateau

Segond fragment (lateral bony ligamentous avulsion) (Fig. 2-48): Characteristic radiographic findings accompanied by evidence of severe joint disruption with rupture of the ACL [470, 571, 717]. A more posterior fragment indicates a posterolateral ligamentous avulsion, while an anterior fragment signifies avulsion of the deep insertion of the iliotibial tract.

Degenerative diseases: Radiographic findings.

Injury of popliteus muscle: Site of tenderness is more posterior, with pain radiating to the popliteal fossa (lesion in muscle belly). Pain is increased by internal rotation and flexion against a resistance.

7. Tubercle of Gerdy

Bony avulsion of the iliotibial tract: Radiographic examination.

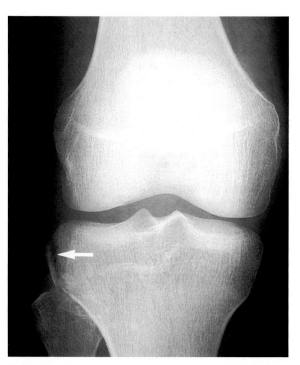

Fig. 2-48. Segond fragment *(arrow).* Evidence of severe intraarticular damage with rupture of the ACL

Insertional tendinosis of the iliotibial tract: Mainly affects athletes (distance runners, cyclists). Often there is genu varum (putting increased tension on the iliotibial tract) or a bony deformity of the foot. If not confined to the Gerdy tubercle, pain may radiate to the entire lateral insertion area of the iliotibial tract (lateral tibial plateau, lateral retinaculum, lateral femoral condyle).

8. Fibular Head

Bony avulsion of lateral collateral ligament: Radiographic findings.

Dislocation of fibular head: Radiographic examination in position of function and in internal and external rotation. May occur without trauma, may cause peroneal nerve irritation [462].

Insertional tendinosis of biceps femoris muscle: Mainly affects athletes. Function testing of biceps femoris: pain caused by flexion and external rotation against a resistance.

Partial or complete rupture of biceps muscle (rare): Local tenderness. External rotation against a resistance is painful.

High fibular fracture: Radiographic findings. Direct or indirect trauma? With indirect trauma (Maisonneuve fracture), a severe medial ankle sprain should be excluded.

2.4.4.3
Medial Pain and Tenderness (Fig. 2-49)

1. Medial Femoral Epicondyle ("Ski Point")

Sprain or partial rupture of medial collateral ligament: The site of maximum tenderness coincides with the rupture site immediately after the injury. Several days later the pain typically radiates to the whole medial side. Valgus stress intensifies pain, varus stress reduces it.

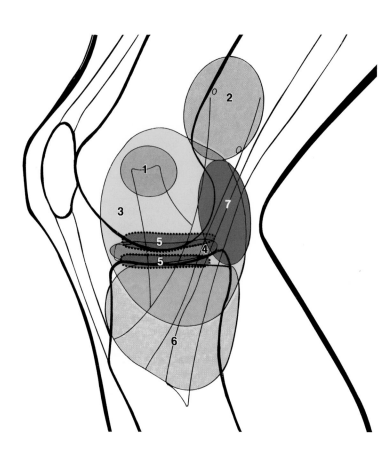

Fig. 2-49. Sites of pain and tenderness on the medial aspect of the knee. Femoral epicondyle ("ski point") *(1)*, proximal to medial femoral epicondyle *(2)*, entire medial side of joint *(3)*, joint line *(4)*, proximal and distal to joint line *(5)*, tibial plateau *(6)*, posteromedial joint region *(7)*

Proximal bony avulsion of medial collateral ligament: Valgus stress causes medial opening in slight flexion. Characteristic radiographic findings (Fig. 2-50). Children and adolescents are predominantly affected.

Stieda-Pelligrini disease (Fig. 2-51): Caused by old medial collateral injury. Small tumorlike hardening is palpable over the medial femoral epicondyle. Radiographs show the Stieda-Pelligrini shadow (type III) caused by calcification in the proximal part of the rupture site and documenting the proximal medial collateral ligament injury (Fig. 2-51b).

2. Proximal to Medial Femoral Condyle (approx. 5 cm)

Saphenous nerve syndrome: Compression of the saphenous nerve (terminal sensory branch of the femoral nerve), which pierces the vastoadductor membrane. Patients report diffuse pain on the medial side of the joint that tends to radiate distally, especially at night. The cause may be direct trauma, an iatrogenic le-

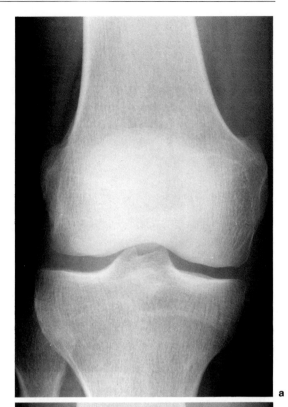

a

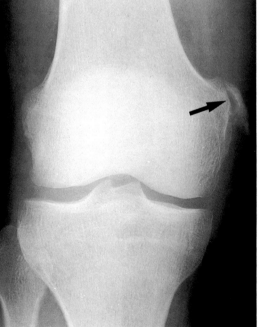

b

Fig. 2-51a, b. Valgus trauma in a 42-year-old male. The posttraumatic radiograph (**a**) showed a normal joint with no osseous changes. One year later the patient complained of pain on the medial side of the knee. Reexamination showed a prominent calcified area at the origin of the medial collateral ligament (Stieda-Pelligrini shadow) (**b**)

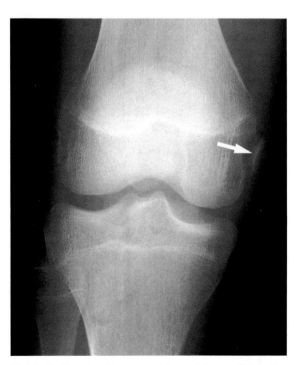

Fig. 2-50. Proximal bony avulsion of the medial collateral ligament

sion (operation), mechanical compression in the area of the vastoadductor membrane (nerve compression syndrome), or phlebitis. Relief of pain by infiltration with local anesthetic confirms the diagnosis [184, 718].

3. Medial Side of Joint

Complete and partial ruptures of the medial collateral ligament: Pain is increased by valgus stress, reduced by varus stress. If the injury is several days old, the pain may radiate to the entire medial side so that a site of maximum tenderness cannot be identified.

Spontaneous osteonecrosis of the medial femoral condyle (Ahlbäck's disease): Characterized by dull or stabbing pain of sudden onset with no apparent cause (no trauma!) that may persist overnight even when the limb is rested. Most patients are over 60 years of age. Radiographs may remain normal for months, but bone scans in early stages will show increased uptake in the medial femoral condyle.

Breaststroker's knee: Mainly affects competitive breaststroke swimmers, characterized by pain over the whole medial side of the joint that increases with age, swimming distance, and shortness of the warmup period. Often the symptoms resemble those of plica syndrome (medial shelf syndrome). In 47% of patients a tense, thickened mediopatellar plica is demonstrable by arthroscopy [562]. Treatment consists in conservative measures (cold applications, etc.) while modifying the kicking technique and instituting a suitably graded training regimen.

4. Medial Joint Line

Fresh or old meniscal lesion (common): History? Positive Meniscus tests.

ACL lesion: Trauma? Usually hemarthrosis. Positive Lachman test.

Degenerative changes (Fig. 2-52): Radiographic findings (osteophytes).

Tibial collateral ligament bursitis [359]: Five bursae are located in close proximity to the medial collateral ligament (between the collateral ligament and capsule, above and below the medial meniscus, between the collateral ligament and tibia) [66]. Inflammation of these bursae leads to tenderness over the medial collateral ligament at the level of the joint line. Mechanical blocking does not occur, however. This condition should be considered in evaluations for meniscal lesions.

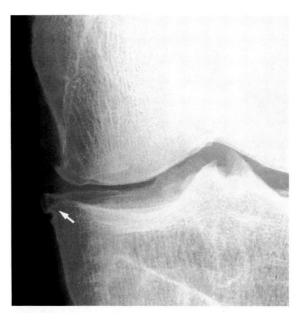

Fig. 2-52. Degenerative excrescences on the medial tibial plateau and femoral condyle. Clinical symptoms resembled those of a meniscal lesion, with medial tenderness over the joint line

5. Proximal and Distal to the Joint Line

Sprain or rupture of the medial capsular ligament: Valgus stress and forced external rotation elicits pain, varus stress reduces it. Difficult to distinguish from meniscal lesions.

6. Medial Tibial Plateau

Distal rupture or partial rupture of the medial collateral ligament: Pain on valgus stress. Valgus trauma?

Tibial plateau fracture: Trauma? Radiographic examination.

Stress fracture (rare): Bone scans are indicated if radiographs are negative and complaints persist.

Bursitis at insertion of pes anserinus: Local fluctuant, tender swelling. Pain on internal rotation of the tibia against a resistance.

7. Posteromedial Joint Region (Fig. 2-53)

Complete or partial rupture of the posterior oblique ligament: Pain on forced external rotation and valgus stress. Trauma?

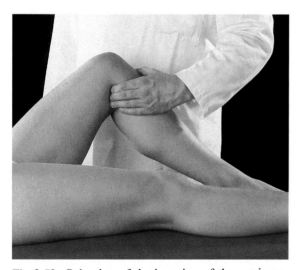

Fig. 2-53. Palpation of the insertion of the semimembranosus muscle and posteromedial capsule

Semimembranosus tendinitis: Localized posteromedial knee pain. Mainly affects athletes during and after exertion (prolonged walking, climbing, running, lifting heavy objects, dancing). Maximum tenderness is in the posteromedial corner just distal to the joint line. Selective palpation of the semimembranosus tendon elicits pain (early stage) or intensifies it (advanced stage). Not infrequently, intraarticular pathology coexists (degenerative meniscal lesions, chondromalacia) [537]. Tenderness at the bone-tendon junction distinguishes insertional tendinopathy of the semimembranosus muscle (see below) from this condition.

Semimembranosus insertional tendinopathy [376]: Pain on internal rotation against a resistance and after athletic activity; fingerpoint tenderness at the bone-tendon junction. Bone scans often show increased uptake on the posteromedial side of the joint.

Semimembranosus tenosynovitis: Older patients, especially females, are predominantly affected. Palpation shows local tenderness in the posteromedial corner just proximal to the joint line. Protective spasm of the medial ischiocrural muscles may occur, producing a kind of pseudolocking. Radiographs show osteophytes of varying size in the area of the semimembranosus groove on the posteromedial aspect of the tibia. This condition may be isolated or may coexist with degenerative joint changes. Differentiation is required from medial meniscal lesions and also from spinal root irritation at L4 (maximum pain is just distal to the joint line) [245]. Bone scans may show increased isotope uptake in that region.

Bursitis at insertion of semimembranosus muscle: Swelling and fluctuation. Sonography shows bursal enlargement.

Pain radiating to the entire medial side of the knee may result from one- to two-day-old injuries of the medial ligamentous apparatus or from osteochondritis dissecans of the medial femoral condyle, which is detected clinically by the *Wilson test:* The knee is slowly extended from a position of 90° flexion and internal rotation. In osteochondritis dissecans, pain is felt between 20° and 30° of flexion due to pressure on the necrotic area and typically is relieved by subsequent external rotation of the tibia (removing pressure from the necrotic zone) [49]. In advanced cases the examination confirms radiologic findings.

2.4.4.4
Posterior Pain and Tenderness

Baker's cyst is a frequent cause of pain or a feeling of pressure on the posterior side of the knee in patients who have not sustained a hyperextension injury and have no significant internal disruption of the knee (Fig. 2-54). The pathogenesis of the cyst is an important consideration in diagnosis and treatment.

Rauschning and Lindgren [535] identified two mechanisms for the production of Baker's cyst, distinguishing a primary (idiopathic) form with a valve mechanism that keeps the inspissated cyst contents from reentering the knee joint [395] from a secondary (symptomatic) form. In the latter type, fluid exchange can occur between the intraarticular space and cyst owing to the similar viscosities of the cystic and synovial fluid. The valve mechanism ("functional stenosis") is based on a difference in the viscosities of the inspissated cyst fluid and the synovial fluid [638].

The two types of cyst call for different treatment strategies. In contrast to the primary form, which generally affects children and adolescents, the secondary form tends to affect older individuals with intraarticular pathology (meniscal lesions, synovial-membrane and cartilage changes). Simple extirpation of the cyst is not curative for the secondary form, and causal therapy requires that arthroscopy be performed to establish the nature of intraarticular disease [401]. In adults with primary cysts, excision is an appropriate treatment after intraarticular pathology has been excluded. An expectant approach is indicated for primary cysts in children and adolescents due to the possibility of spontaneous remission.

If the cyst becomes smaller or disappears when the affected limb is rested (decreasing the production of synovial fluid), it may be as-

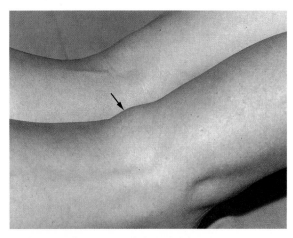

Fig. 2-54. Baker's cyst of the left knee

sumed that the cyst is of the secondary form. Many Baker's cysts are located posterolaterally and require differentiation from biceps femoris bursitis and tumoral calcinosis (Fig. 2-55). Rarely a localized, cystlike swelling in the knee joint may represent a malignant tumor such as liposarcoma [567].

Infrequent causes of posterior knee pain are myogeloses in the gastrocnemius muscle, popliteal artery aneurysms, and gastrocnemius insertional tendinopathies, which by preference affect the medial side of the knee joint. Richter [548] notes the causal significance of "irritation of the gastrocnemius heads" in posterior knee pain. Differential diagnosis should also include arterial and venous disorders, ischialgiform pain due to intervertebral disc disease, and muscular strains and tears.

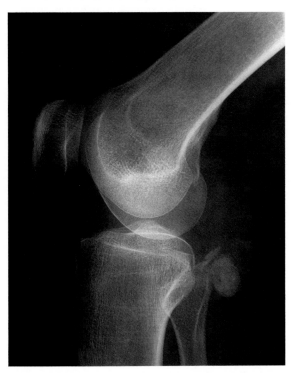

Fig. 2-55. Tumoral calcinosis. Clinical examination showed a popliteal swelling that resembled a Baker's cyst

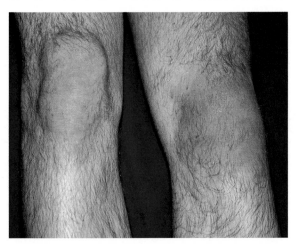

Fig. 2-56. Heat and redness associated with prepatellar bursitis. The patient had been laying garden tiles on the previous day

2.4.5
Temperature

A local temperature elevation in the knee region may result from infection (previous operation? aspiration? open injury?) or an intraarticular effusion.

For local prepatellar heat with swelling of the prepatellar bursa (Fig. 2-56), the bursa is aspirated and irrigated. An antibiotic is administered, the entire limb is immobilized, and a moist dressing (for cooling) is applied. After signs of inflammation have subsided, the bursa should be surgically ("bursoscopically") excised if the swelling persists (chronic bursitis).

2.4.6
Scars

Scars are evaluated for their extent, their mobility relative to deeper tissues, and their condition (irritated or bland). Often the location of a scar will indicate the nature of the previous operation even if the patient cannot recall exactly what was done (Fig. 1-40). In doubtful cases the operation report should be solicited from the colleague who performed the original surgery.

It is not uncommon to find scar tissue that produces an electric-shock-like sensation when percussed. This usually signifies a scar neuroma, and this diagnosis can be confirmed by noting whether the pain is relieved by infiltrating the painful area with a local anesthetic.

2.5
Aspiration of the Knee Joint

In confirmed cases of intraarticular effusion, percutaneous aspiration of the knee joint has value both as a diagnostic and a therapeutic procedure (to alleviate pain).

Since the aspiration involves direct entry into the joint cavity, it should not be done "casually" as an office or bedside procedure but should be performed in an aseptic ambulatory operating room or in an aseptic examination room under sterile conditions. It should be emphasized that, besides intraarticular injections, aspiration of the knee is among the leading causes of intraarticular infection. For this and other reasons we counsel the patient beforehand concerning the potential risks of the procedure (infection) and secure his written consent as we would for a diagnostic arthroscopy.

In cases where osseous injuries are confirmed by standard AP and lateral radiographs, aspiration is beneficial for reducing pain and decompressing the knee joint but has no diagnostic value. Aspiration of the knee is indicated for a fresh bony injury only if surgical intervention is not proposed or will not be possible during the next several days. Immediate preoperative aspiration is not advised, as it poses an unnecessary and avoidable risk of infection.

2.5.1
Aspiration Technique

The patient is placed in the supine position. Usually the knee cannot be fully extended because of the effusion. Caps and masks are worn by the patient, physician, and staff.

The skin is degreased with benzine, and the knee region is prepared with denatured, colored 80% alcohol applied around the whole circumference of the limb and covering an area 15 cm proximal and distal to the joint line. It is best to use a colored antiseptic solution so that the areas of application are well defined. Local anesthesia generally is not required, since aspiration with a No. 1 needle is about as painless as drawing venous blood. Any anxiety expressed by the patient (who may expect a large needle) can usually be dispelled by informing him about the procedure.

Under sterile conditions (sterile drapes and gloves), the needle is inserted on the lateral side of the joint at the level of the proximal half of the patella. Tilting the patella laterally upward before inserting the needle (Fig. 2-57a) facilitates the aspiration by placing the needle tip in an intraarticular space bounded by cartilage surfaces and tense capsule. This prevents obstruction of the needle orifice by soft tissues.

With an effusion of rheumatic origin, there will be some degree of synovial hypertrophy making it difficult or impossible to aspirate the joint successfully. There may also be anatomic problems in these cases such as a narrowed retropatellar space or angular limb deformity. When the aspiration has been completed, the puncture site is dressed with sterile adhesive tape.

The aspiration may be followed by palpation and laxity testing, which now will be less painful and easier for the patient to tolerate. Finally a compression dressing with a peripatellar foam rubber pad is applied to prevent recurrence of the effusion. Further measures depend on the results of the synovial fluid examination and laxity tests.

2.5.2
Examination of the Aspirate

Analysis of the aspirated fluid yields information that is valuable in diagnosing the underly-

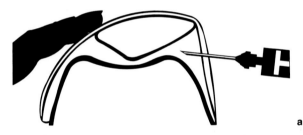

a

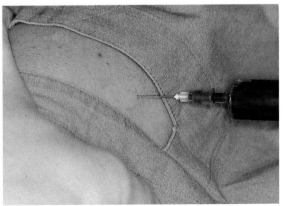

b

Fig. 2-57a, b. The patella is tipped laterally to form a cartilaginous channel for needle insertion that prevents soft-tissue obstruction of the tip (**a**). With the knee draped, the needle is inserted from the lateral side while the index finger of the free hand tilts the patella. The joint is aspirated with a "normal" aspiration needle (**b**)

ing disease. The fluid is evaluated for its volume, color, and consistency and is additionally sent for laboratory analysis (Tables 2-22 and 2-23).

Special biochemical studies of irritative effusions have shown that posttraumatic effusions like those associated with acute meniscal or ligamentous injuries show a substantial rise of alkaline phosphatase activity. By contrast, postoperative effusions contain increased levels of C3c. The lowest parameters are measured in the aspirate from patients with chondromalacia and primary synovial irritation that is not caused by trauma or surgery. The determination of PMN elastase, a sensitive inflammatory parameter, is also valuable for assessing the degree of inflammation that is associated with an existing chondropathy [132]. However, the costly biochemical differentiation of knee effusions continues to be reserved for special scientific inquiries.

It is prudent to inform the patient of the result of the aspiration and synovial fluid examination. Such knowledge can be helpful in view of the fact that even old knee problems with

Table 2-22. Appearance of the aspirate and potential causes of the effusion

Appearance	Potential causes
1. Bloody	ACL rupture Patellar dislocation Meniscal tear (near the base)
2. Bloody with fat globules	Patellar fracture Osteochondral fracture Avulsion of intercondylar eminence Tibial plateau fracture Patellar dislocation Contusion of infrapatellar fat pad
3. Serous	Meniscal lesion Osteoarthritis Chronic ligamentous lesion
4. Turbid and serous	Incipient infection Rheumatic disease
5. Fibrinous	Rheumatic disease
6. Turbid and yellowish	Infection
7. Raspberry colored	Tabetic arthropathy

effusion can have significant implications for diagnosis and treatment.

2.5.3 Hemarthrosis

Hemarthrosis signifies an internal injury of the knee joint (Table 2-24 and Fig. 2-58). Rupture of the ACL is the leading cause of posttraumatic hemarthrosis, accounting for 50% [84, 656] to more than 75% [492, 713] of cases. In 4%–10% of cases there is no identifiable morphologic correlate for the intraarticular hemorrhage [656, 713].

Given the essential function of the ACL, it should be assumed that posttraumatic hemarthrosis with negative radiographic findings signifies an ACL rupture until proven otherwise.

Hemarthrosis in children is frequently associated with bony injuries that are not always appreciated on standard radiographic views. Ligament ruptures and meniscal lesions are not as rare as one might think. Thus, hemarthrosis in children and adolescents should be investigated by arthroscopy to establish the exact cause [148]. If significant pain persists after the joint has been aspirated, it is safe to wait one or two days before repeating the clinical examination and, if necessary, taking additional radiographs [481].

Patellar dislocation is a frequent cause of bloody effusion. Arthroscopy shows bloody imbibition of the synovial capsule, often accompanied by a tear of the medial retinaculum. There may also be osteochondral fractures or cartilage contusions on the medial patellar facet and on the lateral aspect of the lateral femoral condyle [36, 470].

Both the trauma and the resulting intraarticular collection of blood can cause damage to intraarticular structures. The adverse effects of hemarthrosis include:

1. Direct enzymatic damage to the articular cartilage [203]: Destruction of the superficial cartilage layer exposes deeper cartilage layers that release further enzyme systems [98].

Table 2-23. Laboratory findings in the aspirate [77]

Diagnosis	Color	Turbidity	Viscosity	Mucin clot	Leuko-cytes	Lympho-cytes	Erythrocytes (E) Crystals (Cr), Bacteria (Bac)
Normal	Clear		High	Good	− 200	−75	0
Trauma	Bloody Xanthochromic	(+)	High	Good	<10000	−50	E
Irritative effusion	Amber		High	Good	< 2000	−75	0
Rheumatoid arthritis	Yellow-green	(+)	/	/	− 1000	<25	0
Septic arthritis	Creamy gray	+	/	/	>20000	<25	(E), Bac
Gout	Milky or yellow	+	/	/	> 5000	<25	Cr
Chondro-calcinosis	Milky or yellow	(+)	/	/	> 1000	<50	Cr

2. Promotion of degenerative changes [140].
3. Immobilization. Prolonged immobilization intensifies factors 1 and 2 [140]. There is extensive intraarticular scar formation with consequent adhesions and posttraumatic joint stiffness [228].
4. Stretching of the capsule and ligaments by the intraarticular pressure.
5. Damage to the synovial membrane [203].
6. Damage to the collagen matrix: as shown experimentally by Pförringer [525, 526] in the ACL, leading to significant loss of mechanical strength. Prolonged plaster immobilization further reduces the stress tolerance of the ligament.

From the points listed above, we may draw several implications for the management of hemarthrosis:

1. The bloody effusion should be aspirated as completely as possible [228, 525, 526].
2. The aspirated joint should be irrigated, assuming that subsequent arthroscopy or arthrotomy is not proposed.
3. The knee should be mobilized as soon as possible. Prolonged immobilization leads to cartilage damage similar to that caused by hemarthrosis.
4. The patient is cautioned to avoid strenuous exercise for eight weeks. The joint is highly susceptible to injury, even by minor trauma, for up to 16 weeks after the hemarthrosis [525, 526].

Table 2-24. Potential causes of hemarthrosis with normal radiographic findings

1. ACL or PCL rupture
2. Tear in synovium
3. Meniscal tear (near the base)
4. Patellar dislocation
5. Osteochondral fracture
6. Tear of mediopatellar plica
7. Tear or contusion of infrapatellar fat pad
8. Fracture of tibial plateau or femoral condyle
9. Epiphyseal plate injury
10. Anticoagulant medication
11. Knee aspiration
12. Intraarticular injection
13. Hemangioma
14. Hemophilia
15. Pigmented villonodular synovitis
16. Tear of infrapatellar plica
17. No cause

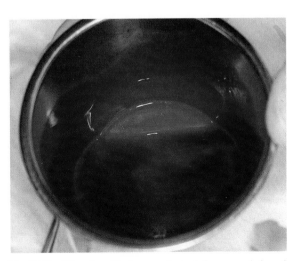

Fig. 2-58. Bloody effusion aspirated from an injured knee. Arthroscopy confirmed a complete rupture of the ACL (see Fig. 11-53)

Special Clinical Diagnosis

3
Evaluation of the Ligaments

A critical question in evaluation of knee injuries concerns the integrity of the capsuloligamentous structures. It is particularly important to exclude an injury of the cruciate ligaments, because an undetected rupture can lead to significant intraarticular damage that is exceedingly difficult to treat [234, 285, 441, 466, 470]. It must be considered that ligament stability is not an end in itself but a prerequisite to achieving integral joint function with adequate closure and stability of the articular surfaces during movement.

In evaluating the ligaments of the knee, it is important to know the functional anatomy of the joint, i. e., the positions in which the joint is stabilized by the structures that are to be tested. The final diagnosis of a capsuloligamentous lesion is based not on a single laxity test but on a combination of varus-valgus testing, active and passive drawer tests, and pivot shift tests. The finding of medial opening with concomitant anterior displacement is neither an acceptable chart entry nor a satisfactory basis for initiating treatment [485].

Thus, labeling a case as a *"sprained knee"* is simply describing a mechanism of injury and is not a meaningful diagnosis.

Prolonged "prophylactic" immobilization of the knee in plaster is not an appropriate strategy [235], and a definitive diagnosis should be established within one week at the latest. Otherwise injuries become obscured and their prompt, adequate treatment is prevented. The motto "when in doubt, cast" should be condemned.

It is sobering to realize that 60% of cruciate ligament ruptures go undetected during the initial clinical examination, despite the fact that 93% of patients seek medical attention within a week after their injury [51]. As the modern diagnostic tests (Lachman test, active quadriceps tests, pivot shift tests) become more widely utilized, it is hoped that serious knee injuries involving the cruciate ligaments will no longer be missed.

3.1
Basic Principles

3.1.1
Theoretical Principles

3.1.1.1
Planes and Axes of Motion, Translation and Rotation

Before we address the various theoretical and practical aspects of clinical laxity testing, it is useful to analyse the kinds of motion that can take place in the knee joint.

All knee movements are defined for the case where the tibia moves relative to the stationary femur. The movements are described in terms of three mutually perpendicular axes, the sagittal, transverse, and vertical, which run parallel to three mutually perpendicular planes, the transverse, frontal, and sagittal (Fig. 3-31). This three-dimensional system of axes and planes is not fixed in space but is constantly moving as a function of knee flexion, tibial rotation, applied forces, individual factors, and the condition of the capsule and ligaments.

Rotation is defined as movement around an axis, *translation* as the sliding of one surface over another on a plane parallel to the axis of orientation [57, 115]. In translation, then, the tibia slides beneath the stationary femur, moving parallel to itself in three-dimensional space. One translational plane is assigned to each of the three spatial dimensions [42, 115] (for details see Sect. 12.4.2).

"Degree of freedom" is the term applied to the ability of a body to rotate around an axis or translate on a plane. Accordingly, there are three degrees of freedom in rotation and three in translation, for a total of six degrees of freedom:

Degrees of freedom in *rotation* (Fig. 3-1 a)

1. *Sagittal* (anteroposterior) axis: abduction/adduction
2. *Transverse* (mediolateral) axis: flexion/extension
3. *Vertical* (proximodistal) axis: internal/external rotation

Degrees of freedom in *translation*

1. *Transverse* plane (motion parallel to the sagittal axis) (Fig. 3-1 b) anterior/posterior translation
2. *Sagittal* plane (motion parallel to the vertical axis) (Fig. 3-1 c) proximal translation (compression)/distal translation (distraction)
3. *Frontal* plane (motion parallel to the transverse axis) (Fig. 3-1 d) medial/lateral translation

3.1.1.2
Motion Spectrum

In examinations of the capsuloligamentous structures of the knee, it must be understood that the mechanisms of knee stabilization act not just in one joint position but in many. This is necessary to ensure that knee function will be adequate in all degrees of freedom and that it can adapt to changing loads. Consequently, evaluations of the anteroposterior and varus-valgus laxity of the knee should be performed in multiple positions of flexion and tibial rotation.

The normal range of knee motion about the transverse axis is from extension to 140° of flexion, and the normal range of tibial rotation is from about 30° of internal rotation to 30° of external rotation, the range of rotation varying with the degree of knee flexion. In theory an infinite number of joint positions may exist over these ranges of motion, each requiring its own pattern of stabilization by ligamentous structures. Thus, different structures are responsible for stabilization at small flexion angles than at large flexion angles. If we additionally consider the possible positions of internal and external rotation that are associated with different degrees of knee flexion, the

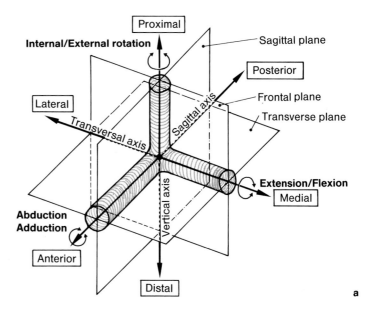

Fig. 3-1 a-d. Three-dimensional model of knee joint motion showing the axes of rotation (sagittal, transverse, vertical) and the planes of translation (transverse, sagittal, frontal) (**a**). Translation of the tibia take place on the transverse plane (**b**), the sagittal plane (**c**), and the frontal plane (**d**)

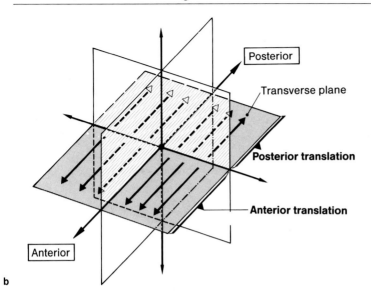

b

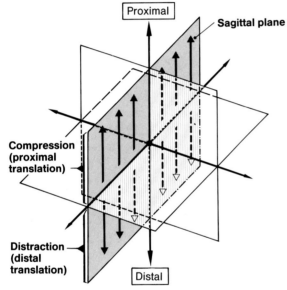

c

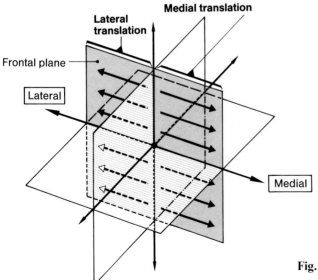

d

Fig. 3-1 b–d. (legend s. p. 101)

stabilization pattern becomes considerably more complex.

For example, if an anterior drawer test is performed only in the "traditional" position of 90° flexion (Fig. 3-2a), the examiner can assess only the laxity of the knee at a single point, i.e., in 90° of flexion. The important range near extension is disregarded. Since the description of rotatory instability by Slocum and Larson [605, 606], it has become customary to perform drawer tests at 90° flexion not just in the neutral position but in positions of internal, neutral, and external rotation (Fig. 3-2b).

But even when the rotation of the tibia is varied, knee laxity is still tested over only a limited range of motion. Considerably more information is furnished by testing laxity in the slightly flexed knee (e.g., by the Lachman test, Fig. 3-2c), although this, too, neglects significant portions of the motion spectrum.

The ideal solution would be to test the laxity of the knee over its entire motion spectrum, following a systematic gridlike pattern (Fig. 3-2d). But while this is qualitatively and quantitatively feasible in research situations, it is too time-consuming to be of practical value in the clinical setting.

Similar considerations apply to tests of varus-valgus laxity, except that in this case testing is customarily performed at small flexion angles. This has led Müller [470] to recommend that valgus-varus testing also be performed in higher degrees of flexion.

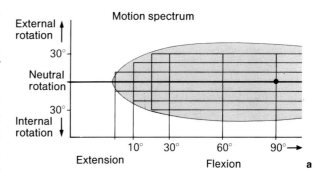

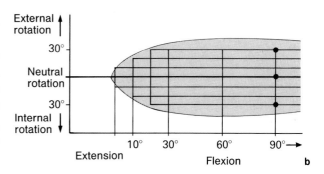

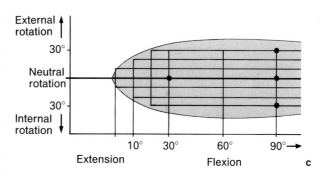

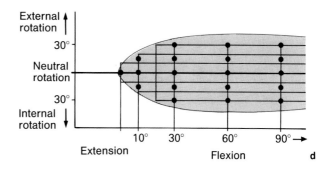

Fig. 3-2a–d. Motion spectrum of the knee joint. Drawer testing in 90° flexion (**a**) evaluates laxity only at one point. Additionally testing in internal and external rotation at the same flexion angle (**b**) provides more differentiated information, at least with regard to rotatory stabilization in 90° flexion. Further testing in 30° flexion (Lachman test) covers an additional point near extension (**c**). Theoretically it would be ideal to test stability over a "grid" covering 19 different joint positions (**d**) (after [633])

3.1.1.3
Laxity and Instability

In examinations of the knee joint it is important to distinguish a physiologic looseness of the ligaments that does not require treatment (physiologic laxity) from an increased (abnormal, pathological) laxity that has been caused by trauma.

Thus, the overall laxity after an injury is the product of the physiologic laxity, which varies from one individual to the next, and the laxity produced by the injury.

Jacobsen [309] determined the physiologic laxity values for the knee joint using a standardized stress radiographic technique (Table 3-1).

"Laxity" is not synonymous with "instability." The latter is said to be present only when the patient experiences a function loss that is subjectively disabling, i. e., experiences a feeling of instability while using the knee and if laxity tests are positive. Minimal trauma may lead to increased joint laxity, as is commonly seen in persons who begin certain kinds of athletic training at a very young age (gymnastics, ballet), or it may lead to a true instability [135]. Differentiation is required from systemic diseases that are associated with increased laxity. Further details on terminology are given in Chap. 12.

3.1.1.4
Increased Laxity

The laxity of the ligaments may be influenced by age, sex, hormonal factors (pregnancy), and by various drugs (penicillamine, prednisone) [629]. Laxity can also be increased by systemic diseases that lead to a disturbance in the collagen metabolism (Table 3-2). In Ehlers-Danlos syndrome, the most common disease of this group, numerous subgroups can be identified according to the degree, biochemical defect, and location of the hyperlaxity (skin, joints, muscles, heart) [136, 629]. Patients typically have hyperextensible joints (knee, wrist, fingers) and hyperelasticity of the skin (Fig. 3-3).

Often it is not possible to assign hyperlaxities to a specific disease group. This kind of hyperlaxity may be regarded as a racial or familial trait.

A general impression of laxity conditions is most easily acquired by asking the patient to extend or flex the wrist and fingers as far as he can (Fig. 3-4) [136].

Table 3-1. Physiologic laxity values measured by Jacobsen [308]. Medial and lateral opening in 20° flexion with an applied force of 9 kg, drawer tests in 90° flexion and neutral rotation with an applied force of 20 kg. m = men, w = women, m/w = both sexes, average displacement = (medial + lateral value)/2

Medial opening	m	5.8–12.1 mm
	w	5.2– 9.8 mm
Lateral opening	m/w	9.2–16.9 mm
Anterior displacement		
Medial condyle	m/w	0.0– 5.5 mm
Lateral condyle	m/w	0.2– 8.8 mm
Average displacement	m/w	0.0– 7.0 mm
Posterior displacement		
Medial condyle	m/w	0.0– 3.4 mm
Lateral condyle	m/w	0.2– 6.0 mm
Average displacement	m/w	0.8– 4.1 mm
Total AP displacement		
Medial condyle	m/w	0.2– 7.5 mm
Lateral condyle	m/w	3.1–12.0 mm
Average displacement	m/w	2.0– 9.5 mm

Table 3-2. Diseases associated with increased ligamentous laxity

1. Ehlers-Danlos syndrome
2. Osteogenesis imperfecta
3. Marfan's syndrome
4. Cutis laxa
5. Larsen's syndrome
6. Homocystinuria
7. Mucopolysaccharidoses (e. g., Morquio type)

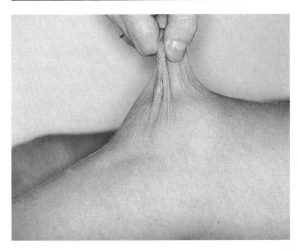

Fig. 3-3. Hyperelastic prepatellar skin in Ehlers-Danlos syndrome

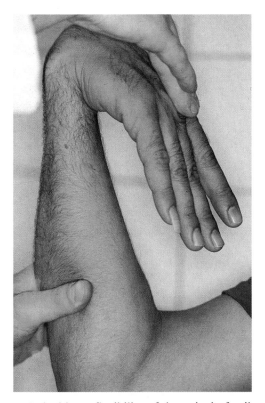

Fig. 3-4. Marked hyperflexibility of the wrist in familial hyperlaxity

3.1.1.5
Laxity Parameters

The laxity of the knee joint depends on a number of parameters besides the condition of the capsule and ligaments (Table 3-3). These parameters should be considered during laxity testing so that the degree and nature of pathologic laxity can be correctly interpreted.

A change in the flexion angle of the knee alters the tension and length of the cruciate and collateral ligaments and of the joint capsule, as stress experiments have confirmed [279, 685]. Markolf et al. [421, 422] found a significant dependence of anterior-posterior displacement, varus-valgus displacement, and range of rotation on the angle of joint flexion, both in cadaver specimens and in living subjects.

It is known from clinical studies that the increased laxity caused by certain injuries is partially or in some cases completely compensated by an adjustment of tibial rotation. By moving the joint to positions in which the injured structures are not primarily responsible for stabilization, it is possible for secondary ligamentous restraints to take over the function of the damaged structures [470, 490].

Fixation of the tibia limits its range of rotation during anteroposterior displacement. Fukubayashi et al. [189] found a 30% reduction of anterior-posterior displacement in the fixated tibia compared with the tibia that is free to rotate. The range of rotation in turn depends on the applied force [596, 708] and the amount of flexion at the hip [598] and knee [28, 421]. When the range of tibial rotation, which varies greatly from one individual to the next, is evaluated on the basis of foot position, it must be remembered that true tibial rotation is only

Table 3-3. Laxity parameters

1. Flexion
2. Tibial rotation
3. Applied force
4. Axial loading
5. Condition of bony structures
6. Voluntary muscle tension
7. Effusion
8. Constitutional factors (age, sex, leg deformity)

about 50% of the observable pedal rotation [596].

The greater the magnitude of the applied force, the greater the laxity that is recorded [189, 490, 639]. Laxity can also be increased by lengthening the lever arm, and thus increasing the torque, for a given applied force. Thus it is important to consider the site of application of the force and the associated center of rotation. Examiner-dependent variables can be minimized by following a consistent, systematic technique.

Axial compression of the tibia and femur, like that produced by the body weight in the standing patient, leads to a marked reduction of abnormal joint mobility under otherwise equal conditions (flexion, rotation, applied force) [292, 335, 423, 685]. A physiologic axial compression is produced by the coiling of the cruciate ligaments that accompanies internal rotation of the knee [470]. On the other hand, even a small amount of axial unloading leads to loosening of the ligamentous structures. This is demonstrated by drawer testing with the tibia hanging over the edge of the examining table (see Fig. 3-12). Often a more distinct positive drawer sign can be elicited under these conditions.

Since the musculotendinous units about the knee not only perform locomotor functions but also contribute greatly to stabilization of the joint, the muscles should be as relaxed as possible when knee stability is tested. Both varus-valgus laxity and drawer displacement are markedly decreased by muscular tension [422]. Especially in recent injuries, there is likely to be significant reflex muscular tension that may create the false impression of a stable knee. According to Müller [470], every laxity test not performed under general anesthesia has only a relative value.

Some authors report differences in laxity values as a function of age and gender (greater laxity in females) [309, 422], while others have been unable to demonstrate a sex-specific correlation [464].

The condition of the bony structures, especially in cases of axial deformity (genu varum, valgum, recurvatum) (see Figs. 2-27 and 2-28) or a tibial plateau fracture (see Fig. 6-37a), can

either increase or decrease the tension on portions of the capsule and ligaments. In laxity testing particular attention should be given to the angular limb deformities that are common in older patients. Besides influencing the evaluation of ligament laxities, these deformities can also have significant therapeutic implications.

Müller [470] calls attention to the relationship that exists between individual joint laxity and the shape of the bony joint members. The greater the radius of the condyles, the more stable is the knee joint in all positions of flexion; the smaller the radius, the more lax the joint.

3.1.2
Principles of the Examination

3.1.2.1
Doctor-Patient Relationship during the Examination

In laxity testing of the knee, it is essential that a trusting relationship be established between the patient and physician. That is because the leg must be manipulated in the very way that elicits the painful sensations which the patient fears or seeks to avoid.

Successful passive laxity testing of the knee (e. g., by the anterior drawer test, Lachman test, pivot shift test, valgus test, etc.) relies on optimum muscular relaxation by the patient. But many patients will relax only when specifically instructed to do so. It is not enough to tell the patient once to "just relax" or "let your leg go loose." Most patients must be told repeatedly to relax their muscles during the course of the examination.

Simple raising of the head by the supine patient will tense the anterior muscle chain, producing a femoral muscle tension that can cause the knee joint to appear stable. This is avoided by telling the patient to relax his neck muscles and keep his head resting on the examining table.

All the tests should be conducted as carefully and accurately as possible. Very often the examiner will be unable to elicit a pivot-shift sign or demonstrate a subluxation at the first attempt. This is perfectly normal and may even be beneficial in reducing the patient's anxiety level. On the other hand, very forcible manipulations will cause the patient to tense his muscles from pain or fear and will hamper the rest of the examination.

Often muscle tension can be reduced by deliberately distracting the patient. This can be done by questioning him about his hobbies, family, job, etc. By taking the patient by surprise and diverting his attention from the knee, it is sometimes possible to demonstrate marked pathologic laxity.

3.1.2.2
Timing the Examination

In acute cases the examination should be performed immediately after the injury or within the first six hours. If 6–12 h have elapsed, the knee can be very difficult to examine as a result of effusion, pain, and muscular guarding. Sometimes it is best to immobilize the knee for several days (after first excluding fresh bone injuries) and then reexamine it when the pain is less severe. In chronic instabilities, the timing of the examination is a matter of less importance.

In acute injuries, standard radiographic projections are obtained before the knee is tested for stability. If the patient complains of severe pain, the knee is examined in less painful joint positions. If there is strong clinical suspicion of a severe capsuloligamentous injury but pain is so pronounced that the examination would have to be deferred for several days, an indication exists for examination under general anesthesia and arthroscopy. Laxity tests may have to be repeated on the following day if the initial examination fails to exclude a ligamentous injury with complete confidence. A particularly serious but common error is to postpone laxity testing for several weeks until the knee joint has reached a "nonirritated state." This policy greatly limits the opportunity for a primary or early secondary operative repair of torn ligaments [235].

3.1.2.3
Active or Passive Tests

It is important to consider the question of whether active or passive laxity tests should be performed first. In all patients, especially those who are anxious, we feel that active tests should take precedence over passive testing (anterior drawer test, Lachman test, pivot shift test). As early as 1919, Hey-Groves [281] called attention to the fact that patients with ACL insufficiency could voluntarily subluxate the upper end of the tibia by tensing the quadriceps muscles with the knee in slight flexion (see Sect. 3.9).

We begin by asking the patient to show us the "instability" that he has been experiencing. Patients with chronic instabilities are only too happy to demonstrate the very phenomenon that the examiner ultimately seeks to provoke with his tests. By tensing certain muscle groups or performing certain movements, patients can recreate the situation that is bothering them or causing them pain (Fig. 3-5). Often this demonstration is striking enough to suggest a very strong presumptive diagnosis. Even with acute injuries, it may be sufficient to observe exactly how the position of the proximal tibia changes when the quadriceps muscle is tensed (see Figs. 3-47 and 3-48).

For these reasons primary attention should be given to the active laxity tests, which can be elicited by the patient himself with a minimum of anxiety or pain.

It is not the mark of a good "knee examiner" to perform his entire repertoire of tests on every knee. A structured, selective approach is indicated.

More diagnostic tests have been devised for the knee joint than for any other joint in the human body. Some of these tests differ only by a subtle change of hand position. As a result, it is often difficult for the inexperienced examiner to position his hands correctly on the patient's knee. In the worst case the examination may proceed in an awkward or clumsy fashion that is noticed by both the examiner and the patient. We therefore urge every examiner to practice his techniques on colleagues, students, or with a friend or spouse and locate the opti-

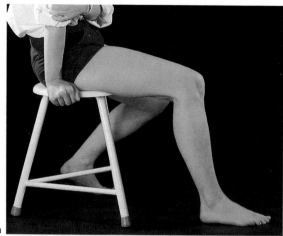

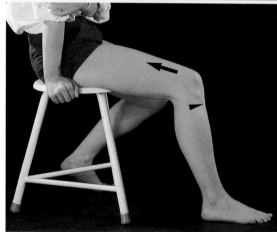

Fig. 3-5a, b. The patient can demonstrate the perceived knee instability in the sitting position with her foot flat on the floor. Initial position (**a**), voluntary anterior displacement (**b**). A true anterior subluxation due to ACL insufficiency can be confirmed only after exclusion of a spontaneous posterior drawer

mum hand placements before proceeding to apply the tests clinically.

3.1.2.4
Evaluation of the End Point

End-point resilience is evaluated in all passive laxity tests (varus-valgus tests, drawer tests). A soft end point implies that the stabilizing ligaments for the given joint position are completely disrupted and that their function has been taken over by secondary ligamentous restraints, whose tension accounts for the soft end point. A hard (firm) end point signifies that the structures being tested are intact or only partially torn and can still exert their stabilizing function through the tension of their intact fibers.

Firm end point = *intact or partial* rupture
Soft end point = *complete* rupture

3.1.2.5
Rules and Goals of the Examination

Certain rules must be followed if the examination is to furnish meaningful information on capsuloligamentous integrity (Table 3-4). Identical examination of the opposite, uninvolved extremity is always indicated to establish a baseline for interpreting the findings. This requires the use of an examining table that is accessible from both sides. If the examining table stands against the wall, it is usually too inconvenient to slide it out into the room, and often the knee closer to the wall is examined inadequately or not at all.

In varus-valgus testing as well as in drawer testing, the following scheme, though commonly utilized, is potentially *misleading:*

Medial opening = medial collateral ligament rupture
Lateral opening = lateral collateral ligament rupture
Anterior displacement = ACL rupture
Posterior displacement = PCL rupture

Use of this scheme as a basis for diagnosis can result in numerous missed cruciate and collateral ligament ruptures, especially when drawer

Table 3-4. Rules and goals of the examination

Rules
1. Note laxity parameters
2. Assess the patient's individual laxity
3. Place the patient in a relaxed position
4. Proceed systematically
5. Evaluate end-point resilience
6. Perform identical examinations in both knees
7. Use an examining table that is accessible from both sides

Goals
1. Abnormal laxity (yes or no?)
2. Injured anatomic structures?
3. Degree of laxity?
4. Type of instability? (e.g., anteromedial, posterolateral)

testing is performed only in 90° of flexion and medial-lateral opening is tested only in extension.

In the sections that follow we shall describe the various tests that are available for evaluating the capsule and ligaments of the knee (Chapter 3), the menisci (Chapter 4), and the femoropatellar joint (Chapter 5). The sequence in which the tests are presented does not reflect their relative diagnostic value. Tests that have been practiced for many years are presented first, while more recent tests generally are described at the end of the section in question.

3.2
Valgus and Varus Test

Valgus-varus testing is indicated not only to exclude a tear of the collateral ligaments but, since it is performed in extension and in slight flexion (10°–20°), also aids in evaluating the posteromedial and posterolateral structures as well as the cruciate ligaments.

With the patient supine and relaxed, the examiner holds the ankle with one hand to support the lower leg and impart a slight external rotation. He places the other hand about the lateral or medial aspect of the knee at the level of the joint line (Fig. 3-6).

Sometimes it is difficult to distinguish between medial and lateral opening, especially in cases where lateral ligament laxity is increased. The inexperienced examiner can easily mistake the greater physiologic varus laxity of the knee (see Table 3-1) for a lateral instability.

Hackenbruch and Henche [234] therefore recommend alternate valgus and varus testing with simultaneous palpation of the joint line. In this technique the examiner secures the ankle between his waist and forearm while palpating the medial and lateral joint lines with the fingertips (Fig. 3-7).

Varus-valgus testing near extension is performed with the tibia externally rotated, because this position uncoils the cruciate ligaments and places increased tension on the collateral ligaments, which then can be examined more selectively [470].

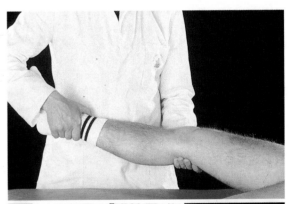

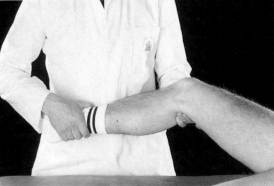

Fig. 3-6a, b. Valgus test in extension (**a**) and slight flexion (**b**) with concomitant external rotation of the tibia

It is not sufficient, however, to test varus-valgus laxity only in slight flexion and extension. In hyperextensible knee joints or in patients with constitutional hyperlaxity, it is also important to perform varus-valgus testing in the hyperextended position (Fig. 3-7c). If marked opening is detected in the presence of an acute or chronic lesion with the knee ex-

tended, a PCL lesion, possibly combined with an ACL lesion, should be strongly suspected [159].

Evaluation of Valgus and Varus Test:

1. Medial Opening in Extension

I *(0):*   Posteromedial capsule (posterior oblique ligament) intact.

II *(slight):*   Lesion of posteromedial capsule and medial collateral ligament.

III *(marked):* Lesion of posteromedial capsule, medial collateral ligament, PCL and possibly ACL. Tear may extend to the posterolateral capsule.

"Extension" refers to the position of straight extension (0°) rather than to the position of maximum extension used in determining range of motion. Maximum extension, even in the hyperextensible knee, places tension on the stretched posterior structures, which can then create a false joint stability during valgus testing. On the other hand, if a valgus stress is applied in hyperextension and the joint opens markedly, it may be assumed that both cruciate ligaments are torn [13].

2. Medial Opening in 20° Flexion

I *(0):*   Medial collateral ligament intact. (Medial stability may be simulated with a sprain or partial rupture of the medial collateral ligament. Generally there is severe pain and reflex muscle tension, especially if the injury is more than 8h old. Valgus testing in these cases is possible only in very cooperative patients or under anesthesia.)

II *(slight):*   Rupture of medial collateral ligament and capsular ligament, possible stretching of the posteromedial capsule.

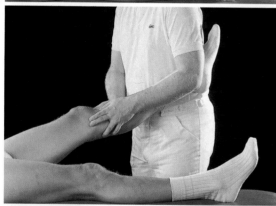

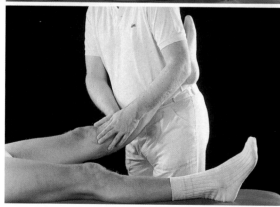

Fig. 3-7a–c. Varus-valgus test with simultaneous palpation of the joint line in flexion (**a**), extension (**b**), and hyperextension (**c**)

III *(marked):* Rupture of medial collateral ligament and capsular ligament, posteromedial capsule, and ACL; possible rupture of PCL.

3. Lateral Opening in Extension

I *(0):*   Posterolateral capsule (arcuate complex) intact.

II *(slight):* Lesion of posterolateral capsule and lateral collateral ligament.

III *(marked):* Lesion of posterolateral capsule, lateral collateral ligament, PCL, iliotibial tract; possible tear of ACL. Tear may extend to the posteromedial capsule.

4. Lateral Opening in 20° Flexion

I *(0):*   Lateral collateral ligament intact.

II *(slight):* Rupture of lateral collateral ligament and capsular ligament, possible stretching of posterolateral capsule.

III *(marked):* Rupture of lateral collateral ligament and capsular ligament, posterolateral capsule and ACL; possible rupture of iliotibial tract and PCL.

3.3
Passive Anterior Drawer Tests

The passive anterior drawer tests (anterior translation tests) are differentiated diagnostic procedures that can be used to evaluate the integrity of the cruciate ligaments and the medial, lateral, and posterior stabilizers. However, a positive anterior drawer sign should not be considered pathognomonic for an ACL rupture, nor does a negative test prove that the ligament is intact. Numerous studies have shown that little or no anterior drawer motion is elicited in 90° flexion when there is an isolated tear of the ACL (see Tables 3-6 and 3-15).

Drawer motion is tested by pulling the proximal end of the tibia anteriorly and pushing it posteriorly. A basic difficulty in these tests is defining the exact starting point (neutral position) from which an anteriorly directed force will elicit a true anterior drawer sign. For example, if there is a PCL tear with posterior sagging of the upper tibia (spontaneous posterior drawer) and the examiner applies an anterior stress, it may appear that a pure anterior drawer sign is elicited when in fact the tibia has merely been pulled forward from a dropped position (caused by the PCL tear) into its neutral position. At that point the ACL becomes taut and limits further anterior displacement (Fig. 3-8).

As in other passive laxity tests, end-point resilience is evaluated (see Sect. 3.1.2.4). The anterior drawer test, performed first, will have a firm end point if the ACL is intact, while the posterior drawer test will have a firm end point if the PCL is intact. The firm anterior end point is particularly marked when the anterior drawer test is elicited from a posterior sagging position of the tibia (spontaneous posterior drawer).

For these reasons, it is prudent to observe the following rule (Müller [470]):

An anterior drawer test may be declared positive only after it has been proven that a posterior drawer is not present.

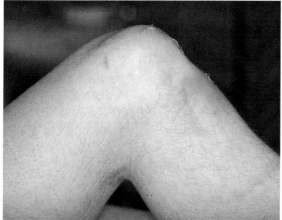

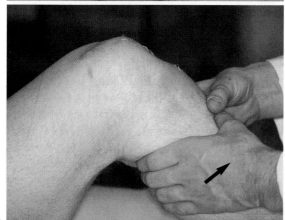

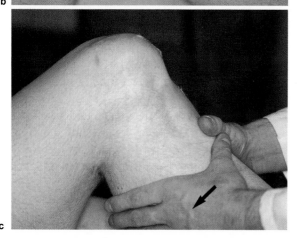

3.3.1
Anterior Drawer Test in 90° Flexion

The anterior drawer test in 90° flexion is frequently negative in acute injuries because many patients cannot achieve 90° of flexion without significant pain [603, 713]. In addition, there is usually a combination of complete and partial ligament ruptures, so that the drawer stress places the partially torn medial and lateral ligaments on stretch. The resulting pain may lead to a negative anterior drawer test and give the erroneous impression of a stable joint. According to Katz [349], the anterior drawer test in 90° flexion is the poorest diagnostic indicator of an ACL tear, especially in acute cases. Testing at a small flexion angle is preferred owing to its simplicity and reliability (see Sect. 3.3.3 for further details).

With chronic ligament injuries, a feeling of instability is the predominant complaint in most cases, and anterior drawer testing in 90° flexion usually can be performed without pain. As it is often difficult to determine the degree of displacement in the passive and active laxity tests, the examiner should position his eyes at the level of the tibial tuberosity and patellar ligament and closely observe the changes in their position (Fig. 3-9) [235].

Fig. 3-8 a-c. Superficial examination of this knee with a pretibial abrasion shows a normal-appearing joint (**a**) with a markedly positive anterior drawer test (**b**) implying an ACL tear. It would be wrong to end the examination here, however, because subsequent posterior drawer testing reveals increased posterior displacement (**c**) signifying a concomitant lesion of the PCL. The findings, then, imply tears of both cruciate ligaments. The careful inspection of both tibial tuberosities (Fig. 2-26 b) would have revealed a spontaneous posterior sag and enabled a correct interpretation of the anterior displacement, which here consists of displacement from the sagging position (PCL rupture) plus the "true" anterior drawer displacement (ACL rupture)

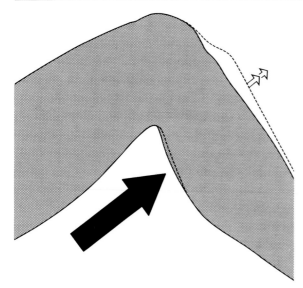

Fig. 3-9. Changes in the position of the tibial tuberosity and patellar ligament during anterior drawer testing

3.3.2
Anterior Drawer Test in 90° Flexion in Various Positions of Tibial Rotation

Since the discovery and description of rotatory instabilities, it has become common practice to test the anterior drawer not just in the neutral position but also with the tibia internally and externally rotated [128, 159, 234, 285, 309, 311, 409, 466, 470, 479, 605, 606]. The tibial rotation tightens or relaxes still-intact ligamentous structures, causing an apparent decrease or increase in the degree of laxity.

In the common anteromedial instability, for example, a marked anterior drawer sign is elicited in 90° flexion with the foot externally rotated, whereas minimal anterior displacement is elicited in internal rotation. Thus, the examiner should always give attention to the rotation of the tibia and secure it in the position desired. Maximum internal or external rotation of the tibia should be avoided, however, because the consequent twisting of the still-intact ligaments can cause the joint to appear more stable than it is.

With the patient supine and relaxed, the hip is flexed to 45° and the knee to 90°. The ex-

aminer sits on the patient's foot to secure it in the desired rotational position (30° internal, neutral, or 30° external). Care is taken that the hamstrings are relaxed during the drawer test (by palpating the tendons) (Fig. 3-10).

Weatherwax [694] described a modified anterior drawer test in which the lower leg is supported in the examiner's axilla (Fig. 3-11). It is relatively difficult to establish a specific position of tibial rotation with this technique, but anterior displacement is easily recognized. The Noyes test can be performed from the same initial position without significantly changing the hand position (see Fig. 3-29). Varus and valgus laxity also can be tested by slightly adjusting the placement of the fingers (Fig. 3-7).

Feagin [159] recommends performing 90° drawer tests with the patient in the sitting position (Fig. 3-12a). Gravity pulls the tibia downward and helps to relax the muscles. The examiner should elicit anterior motion gently and cautiously, placing the tips of the thumbs on the anterior side of the femoral condyles and the balls of the thumbs on the proximal tibia. Feagin claims that anterior displacement of the tibia can be more easily perceived and confirmed using this hand placement (Fig. 3-12b, c, d). The rotational response of the proximal tibia (medial and lateral compartmental translation) also can be evaluated with the hands thus positioned.

Some examiners have abandoned anterior rotatory drawer testing on the grounds that fixing the tibia in a given rotatory position by sitting on the foot (see Fig. 3-10) prevents a full anterior excursion of the tibia when the drawer stress is applied [318]. The fixed rotatory position places tension on the intact capsuloligamentous systems at the sides of the joint. But this also stabilizes the joint during the drawer test. When the tibia is released so that it can rotate freely, a more pronounced drawer sign can be obtained. Free tibial rotation is possible in the sitting patient (Fig. 3-12) and also in the Weatherwax technique (Fig. 3-11).

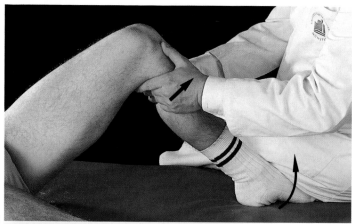

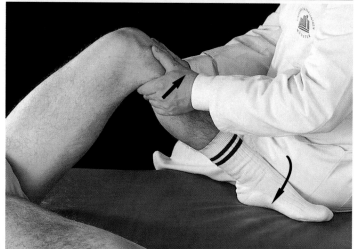

Fig. 3-10a, b. Anterior drawer test in 90° flexion with external (**a**), neutral, and internal rotation (**b**) of the tibia. The examiner sits on the foot to secure it in the desired position of rotation. The forefingers check for relaxation of the ischiocrural tendons on the medial side (pes anserinus, semimembranosus muscle) and lateral side (biceps femoris muscle)

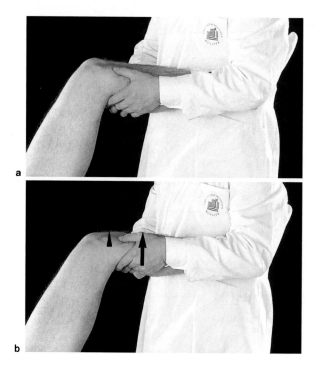

Fig. 3-11a, b. Anterior drawer test in 90° flexion with the hip flexed 90° (**a**). The anterior displacement is plainly recognized in the presence of a chronic ACL insufficiency (**b**)

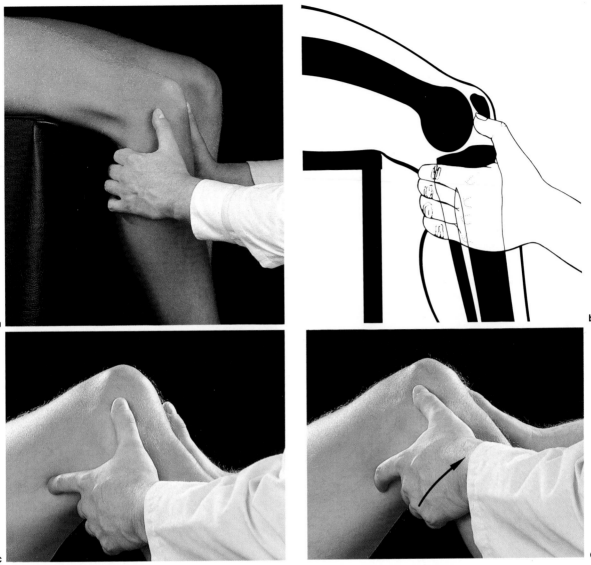

Fig. 3-12 a–d. Anterior drawer test in 90° flexion with the patient seated (**a**). The examiner places the tips of the thumbs on the femoral condyles, the balls of the thumbs on the upper tibia (**b**). The other fingers cup the proximal tibia from the medial and lateral sides and pull it forward (after Feagin [159]). The anterior displacement and rotational response of the tibia are evaluated. Initial position, medial view of the joint (**c**). Anterior stress elicits anterior translation of the tibia with a concomitant external rotation (coupled displacement) (**d**)

Evaluation of Anterior Drawer Test:

1. 90° Flexion with Internal Tibial Rotation

I *(0):* Iliotibial tract and PCL intact. The test is not made positive by rupture of the ACL and posteromedial structures, because the internal rotation "locks" the joint by tightening the posterolateral ligaments, the iliotibial tract, and especially the PCL.

II *(slight):* Rupture of ACL, injury of arcuate complex and iliotibial tract, possible lesion of medial and posteromedial structures.

III *(marked):* Rupture of ACL and PCL (!), lateral and posterolateral structures, lesion of iliotibial tract.

2. 90° Flexion with Neutral Tibial Rotation

I *(0):* Medial and lateral capsuloligamentous structures intact. ACL may be torn.

II *(slight):* Lesion of medial and/or lateral structures. Possible rupture of ACL. With a firm end point, a PCL ligament rupture must be excluded.

III *(marked):* Rupture of ACL and lesion of medial and posteromedial and/or lateral and posterolateral structures. Possible rupture of PCL.

3. 90° Flexion with External Tibial Rotation

I *(0):* Medial and posteromedial structures intact.

II *(slight):* Rupture of medial and posteromedial structures.

III *(marked):* Rupture of ACL, medial and posteromedial structures.

3.3.2.1
Maximum Subluxation Test [319]

This test is performed under general anesthesia. With the patient supine, the knee is flexed to 50°-60°, and the examiner, his hand braced on the contralateral knee, pulls the proximal tibia into maximum anterior subluxation with his forearm. With his free hand the examiner simultaneously palpates the upper end of the tibia to assess the extent of anterior displacement of each tibial plateau (Fig. 3-13). The unfixed tibia is free to rotate so that maximum anterior subluxation can be obtained.

3.3.3
Lachman Test

On May 3, 1875, Georges C. Noulis submitted his doctoral thesis entitled "Entorse du Genou" to the medical faculty in Paris, as was discovered by Pässler and Michel [518 a]. In his thesis, Noulis writes:

"En effet, si l'on met le membre dans la flexion et qu'après avoir fixé la cuisse, on prenne solidement la jambe par la partie supérieure, entre le pouce en avant et les autres doigts en arrière et qu'on cherche à lui imprimer des mouvements d'avant en arrière, on s'aperçoit que les surfaces articulaires sont écartées l'une de l'autre et que le tibia peut se déplacer directement en avant et en arrière. Ces mouvements qu'on observe très-bien quand les deux ligaments croisés sont coupés, s'observent aussi en fléchissant à peine la jambe quand le ligament croisé antérieur est seul coupé. Si au contraire c'est le seul ligament croisé postérieur qui est coupé, il faut pour observer ces mouvements placer la cuisse dans la flexion vers 110°."

Here, Noulis, describes how, with the patient's leg flexed, the thigh can be grasped with one hand and the lower leg with the other hand, keeping the thumbs to the front and fingers to the back. If the lower leg is held in this grip and then moved backwards and forwards, it will be seen that the tibia can be moved directly backwards and forwards. Noulis observed a great deal of tibia displacement when both cruciate ligaments were severed. If only the ACL were severed, tibia displacement could be noted when the leg was only slightly flexed. In contrast, if the PCL were severed, the knee joint had to be flexed to about 110° for extensive tibia displacement to be observed.

With these observations, Noulis not only elucidated the drawer test in large degrees of flexion, and the correct positioning of the hands, but also described *for the first time* examining the drawer using only a slight degree of extension to establish severance of the anterior cruciate ligament. This means that the "Lachman test" could really be called the "Noulis test". Even the opposing reactions of

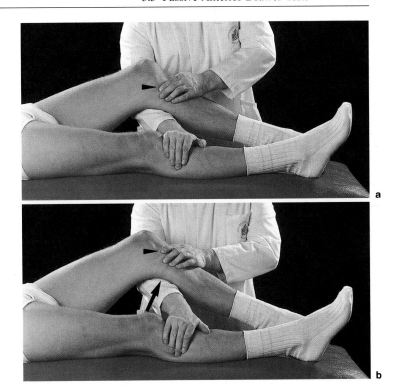

Fig. 3-13a, b. Maximum subluxation test of Jakob [319]. The anterior stress elicits a marked anterior displacement of the tibia with accompanying external rotation (**b**)

the anterior and posterior cruciate ligaments were thus first described by Noulis, since he ascertained that tibia displacement could be observed particularly with only slight flexion when the anterior cruciate ligament was severed, but that this tibia movement could be ovserved especially in a high degree of flexion when the posterior cruciate ligament was severed.

Anterior drawer testing with the knee slightly flexed was also described by Ritchey in 1960 [405]. Since the publication of Torg et al. [661], it has become known as the *Lachman test* or the *Ritchey-Lachman test* [15], and its advantages have become widely recognized [231, 234, 235, 285, 405, 430, 470, 471, 555, 558, 603, 639, 645, 683, 711, 713].

The traditional anterior drawer test with the knee flexed 90° is seldom positive in acute tears of the ACL. The Lachman test, however, is positive in most of these cases, even when applied without anesthesia (Table 3-6). A somewhat higher rate of positives is obtained under general anesthesia. Only the results of Sandberg [564] are inconsistent with this claim. Despite a ruptured ACL, 57% and 41% of the patients in two of his groups did not have a positive Lachman test on clinical examination (Table 3-7).

Dynamic anterior subluxation tests (e. g., the pivot shift test) have about the same low diagnostic sensitivity in acute ACL injuries as does the anterior drawer test in 90° flexion [603, 713] (see Table 3-7).

Table 3-5. Advantages of the Lachman test

1. Highly specific for ACL rupture
2. Not hampered by posterior meniscus horn
3. Not hampered by hemarthrosis
4. Less painful because the muscles are relaxed
5. Not hampered by sprained or partially ruptured medial collateral ligament
6. Elicits greater anterior displacement, not just with isolated ACL rupture
7. Performed in functional position of flexion
8. Can be performed when there is a fracture close to the knee

Table 3-6. Comparison of *positive* Lachman test, anterior drawer test, and pivot-shift test in patients with an ACL rupture (N = number of injured knees, LMT = Lachman test, ADT = anterior drawer test, PST = pivot shift test, NA = no anesthesia, UA = under anesthesia)

Author	Year	Positives (in %)							Type
		N	LMT		ADT		PST		
			NA	UA	NA	UA	NA	UA	
Torg	1976	93	95		40		0		[1]
		43	100		79		28		[2]
DeHaven	1980	35	80	100	9	52	9	63	acute [3]
Jonsson	1982	45	87	98	33	98			acute
		62	97	98	95	98			chronic
Zelko	1982	34	94	100	50	71			
Donaldson	1985	101	99	100	70	90	35	98	acute [4]
		37	98	100	54	81	27	100	acute [5]
Skoff	1985	35	80	100	9	52	9	63	acute [3]
Wirth	1985	246	92		26		11		acute
		216	97	100	27	56	13	68	acute [3]
Katz	1986	9	78		22		89		acute
		13	85		54		85		chronic
Sandberg	1986	92	43	89	40	74	4	86	acute [5]
		32	59	88	34	91	9	81	acute [6]

Notes:
[1] Plus injury of medial meniscus, medial opening; [2] like [1] but without medial opening; [3] complete rupture; [4] partial rupture; [5] isolated rupture; [6] plus injury of medial collateral ligament

Table 3-7. Comparison of *negative* Lachman test, anterior drawer test, and pivot-shift test in patients with an ACL rupture (N = number of injured knees, LMT = Lachman test, ADT = anterior drawer test, PST = pivot shift test, NA = no anesthesia, UA = under anesthesia)

Author	Year	Negatives (in %)						
		N	LMT		ADT		PST	
			NA	UA	NA	UA	NA	UA
Torg	1976	93	5		45			
		43	0		9		70	
DeHaven [1]	1980	35	20	0	73	48	14	37
Jonsson	1982	45	13	2	67	2		
		62	3	2	5	2		
Zelko [2]	1982	34	6	0	50	29		
Donaldson	1985	101	1	0	30	10	65	2
		37	2	0	46	19	73	0
Skoff [3]	1985	35	20	0	73	48	14	37
Wirth	1985	246	2		33		11	
		216	0	0	28	39	7	27
Katz	1986	9	22		78		11	
		13	15		46		15	
Sandberg	1986	92	57	11	60	26	96	14
		32	41	12	66	9	91	19

Notes:
[1] PST with NA not possible in 68%; [2] ADT equivocal in 32% of NA and 50% of UA; [3] PST with NA not possible in 69%

The Lachman test is the most reliable test in the injured knee.

A major advantage of the Lachman test is that it is performed in the functional knee position of 30° flexion. That is the position in which the ACL is an essential stabilizer for activities in which the individual must change direction or come to a stop [12, 404]. It is in these types of movement that ACL insufficiency has its greatest impact by allowing subluxation of the lateral tibial plateau (pivoting). The less functional position of 90° flexion, like that assumed during sitting, requires little sagittal stabilization, so drawer testing in that position is of very limited value from a functional standpoint. Thus, the tests that are performed in a functional (= slightly flexed) knee position (Lachman test, pivot shift test) should be assigned a higher priority in preoperative as well as postoperative evaluations. Knee stability in the slightly flexed position is crucial to a

Table 3-8. Problems in performing the Lachman test

1. Anterior displacement is easier to detect in 90° flexion.
2. Greater chance of confusing anterior and posterior drawer than in 90° flexion.
3. Femur and tibia are difficult to immobilize in obese or muscular patients or by an examiner with small hands.
4. Applied force is difficult to control.

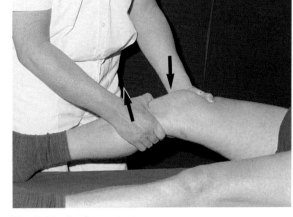

Fig. 3-14. Lachman test

satisfactory outcome of surgery and is manifested by a disappearance of the subluxation sign (pivoting) as the knee nears extension [713].

The clinical conduct of the Lachman test can pose certain problems for the examiner, however, and these are listed in Table 3-8.

With the patient supine on the examining table, the examiner stabilizes the femur with one hand and with the other hand applies pressure to the posterior aspect of the proximal tibia, pulling it forward (Fig. 3-14) [232, 470, 712, 713].

Hackenbruch [234] recommends performing the Lachman test similar to the anterior drawer test (Fig. 3-15). However, his technique allows the flexion angle to change, and it is somewhat more difficult to evaluate end-point resilience.

To record the anterior displacement of the proximal tibia with greater accuracy, Müller

(after [234]) recommends performing the Lachman test in such a way that the examiner can observe the anterior excursion of the tibia. He does this by kneeling beside the patient so that his eyes are level with the tibial tuberosity. One hand is placed on the lateral aspect of the thigh, and the other hand grasps the proximal tibia and pulls it forward (Fig. 3-16). Any anterior displacement of the tibia is easily recognized and recorded. The disadvantage of this technique is that it is difficult to fixate the femur and tibia at the same time, especially when the examiner has small hands.

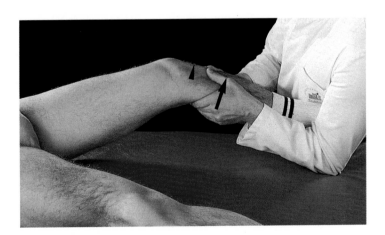

Fig. 3-15. Lachman test as modified by Hackenbruch [234]

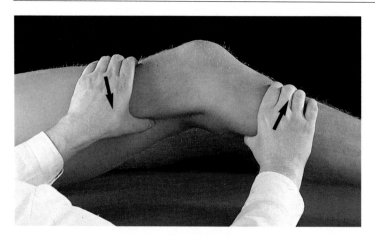

Fig. 3-16. Lachman test as modified by Müller. While applying an anterior stress, the examiner watches for anterior displacement of the proximal end of the tibia

3.3.3.1
Prone Lachman Test

Feagin [159] performs the Lachman test with the patient in the prone position (Fig. 3-17). This technique eliminates the problem of fixating the thigh. Although the patient is relaxed, it can be difficult for the examiner to determine the quality of the end point (Fig. 3-18).

3.3.3.2
Stable Lachman Test

The traditional form of the Lachman test (Fig. 3-14) and the technique described by Müller (Fig. 3-16) can pose problems for the "small-handed" examiner. Simultaneous fixa-

tion of the femur and tibia becomes difficult in very muscular or obese patients [159]. A simple solution is for the examiner to use his own thigh as a "bench" for performing the test. While one hand stabilizes the patient's femur on the examiner's thigh, the other hand applies the anterior drawer stress (Fig. 3-19). Even very obese or muscular patients can be satisfactorily examined by this method. The quality of the end point (soft or firm) is easily assessed.

The following guidelines are helpful for evaluating end-point resilience in the positive Lachman test:

Firm end point with hemarthrosis:
  implies an acute partial rupture.
Firm end point without hemarthrosis:
  implies an old partial rupture or elongation.
Soft end point with hemarthrosis:
  complete rupture.
Soft end point without hemarthrosis:
  old complete rupture, acute complex ligamentous injury (dry joint).

When the end point is firm, a PCL lesion should be excluded by testing for a spontaneous posterior drawer and performing the active quadriceps test in 90° flexion (see Sect. 3.9.3).

A positive Lachman test associated with a soft end point signifies an ACL rupture requiring operative treatment. This may consist of reattachment, repair with augmentation, or pri-

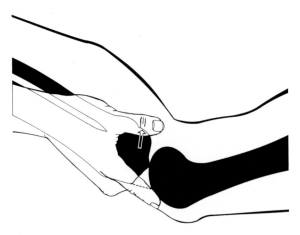

Fig. 3-17. Prone Lachman test of Feagin [159]

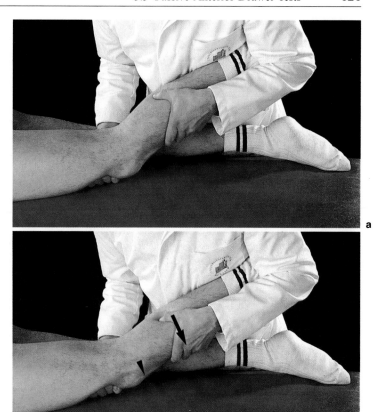

Fig. 3-18a, b. Prone Lachman test. Anterior displacement of the tibia due to rupture of the ACL (**b**)

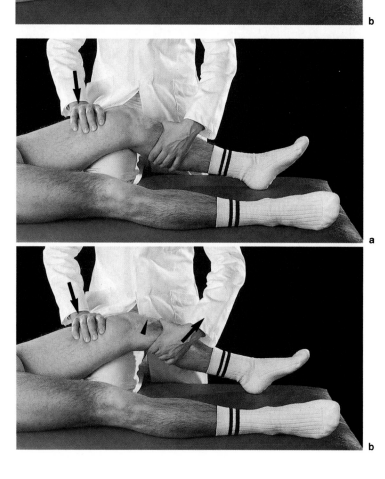

Fig. 3-19a, b. Stable Lachman test. The examiner stabilizes the patient's femur against his own thigh (**a**). This provides a fixation that is constant for each examination and cannot be altered by the patient. With ACL insufficiency anterior displacement of the tibia is plainly visible (**b**)

mary reconstruction, depending on the site of the lesion.

If a careful examination has been conducted that includes the active laxity tests (see Sect. 3.9) and there is doubt as to whether the Lachman test is positive or negative, laxity testing under general anesthesia and arthroscopy are indicated for definitive evaluation.

Some authors recommend Lachman testing in internal, neutral, and external rotation [409], but this is satisfactory only for "small" knees manipulated by an examiner with large hands. For active drawer testing in slight flexion, however, the examiner can hold the tibia in the desired position of rotation (see Fig. 3-46).

3.3.3.3
Graded Lachman Test

Like the anterior drawer test in 90° flexion, the Lachman test can be quantitatively evaluated. Gurtler et al. [232] define four grades in the positive Lachman test:

Grade I: Palpable subluxation. The examiner feels a soft end point on anterior translation of the tibia.
Grade II: Visible subluxation. Characterized by a visible anterior translation of the tibia in addition to the soft end point. The examiner may either place his eyes level with the tibial tuberosity (see Fig. 3-16) or ask a colleague to perform the test.
Grade III: Passive subluxation. Anterior displacement is demonstrated with the patient supine, when the tibia passively subluxates anteriorly. This is accentuated by placing a wooden block or the examiner's forearm behind the knee just distal to the joint line. The junction of the patella and tibial tuberosity will lose its typical contour. The tibia can be passively reduced from its subluxated position by placing a second block or the examiner's other arm beneath the distal femur.
Grade IV: Active subluxation. The patient can actively and voluntarily subluxate the tibia anteriorly by muscular contraction (see Fig. 3-47 and 3-48).

Gurtler et al. [232] measured the following average values for the anterior tibial displacement in the Lachman test:

Grade I: 5 mm   (3–6 mm)
Grade II: 8 mm   (5–9 mm)
Grade III: 13 mm   (9–16 mm)
Grade IV: 18 mm   (13–20 mm)

3.3.4
Finochietto's Sign

The jumping sign ("signo del salto") described by Finochietto [169, 170] has special significance among the laxity tests, for it signifies the coexistence of ACL insufficiency with a lesion of the meniscus.

The disruption of the normal rolling-gliding mechanism of the knee caused by ACL insufficiency results in damage to the posterior horn of the medial meniscus or loosening of its capsular suspension. When the anterior drawer test is performed in 90° flexion, the hypermobile posterior horn of the medial meniscus moves forward, and the femoral condyle rides upon it. This is associated with an audible snap or palpable jerk which indicates a positive test. When the tibia is pushed back posteriorly, the femoral condyle glides back down from the posterior horn. If reposition of the dislocated meniscus is necessary following a positive Finochietto test, a complete posterior detachment of the medial meniscus or a longitudinal or bucket-handle meniscal tear should be suspected (Fig. 3-20).

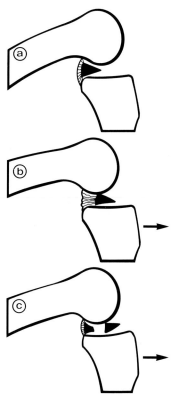

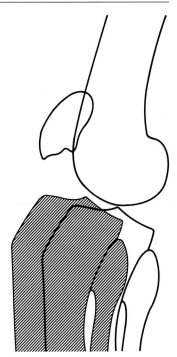

Fig. 3-21. Subluxation of the tibia in the slightly flexed knee due to ACL insufficiency (from Hey Groves [281])

Fig. 3-20 a–c. Finochietto's sign. When the ligamentous suspension of the posterior horn of the medial meniscus is lax and there is a coexisting ACL rupture, the femoral condyle will ride up onto the meniscus from its initial position (**a**) when an anterior stress is applied (**b**). With a posterior meniscal tear, the femoral condyle may lodge between the basal remnant and free portion of the meniscus (**c**) and cause a painful locking of the joint

3.4
Dynamic Anterior Subluxation Tests (Pivot Shift Tests)

As early as 1919, Hey Groves [281] described the characteristic dysfunction of ACL insufficiency as follows (Fig. 3-21): "In active exercise, when the foot is put forward and the weight of the body presses on the leg, then the tibia slips forward. Sometimes this forward slipping of the tibia occurs abruptly with a jerk. Often it is under the patient's control."

Hey Groves also made reference to the typical feeling of instability in the ACL-deficient knee during walking, especially when the patient stops suddenly and unexpectedly, in which case he may even fall to the ground. Since the subluxation signs described in this section were familiar to Hey Groves and were described by him, at least in their essential features, they should not be regarded as "new."

The pivot shift phenomenon is caused by anterior subluxation of the lateral tibial plateau as the knee approaches extension, the cause being a ruptured or deficient ACL. Use of this phenomenon as a diagnostic test procedure was first described not by Galway and MacIntosh [196], as many believe, but by Lemaire in 1967 [386]. Hence it is referred to in this section as the "Lemaire test."

In nearly all dynamic anterior subluxation tests, a valgus stress is applied to the knee with the tibia internally rotated. A positive test is pathognomonic for ACL insufficiency [235, 255, 315, 317, 386, 408, 466]. The test begins with the knee almost extended and the lateral tibial plateau in a position of anterior subluxation (dislocation phase). Flexing the knee to about 30° while applying a valgus stress leads to tilting of the posterior tibial border, a rise of tension in the iliotibial tract, and impingement of the posterior tibial border on the lateral femoral condyle (tension phase). As flexion is increased, this point of impingement is shifted and traction is exerted on the iliotibial tract at a smaller angle, culminating in the sudden relocation of the previously subluxated tibia (reduction phase), usually accompanied by a palpable jerk (Fig. 3-22). Besides the iliotibial tract, factors contributing to the occurrence of this phenomenon are the convex shape of the lateral tibial plateau and the actions of the biceps femoris and popliteus muscles [234, 406, 470, 523].

Contrary to many published reports, a positive pivot shift sign does not necessarily signify an anterolateral instability [195, 404, 442, 607]. This is because a positive test depends on an intact iliotibial tract, but the latter is disrupted in cases of complete anterolateral instability. Thus, the test would be negative in cases of this type, while a positive test is frequently obtained in other types of instability, e.g., anteromedial instability with ruptures of the ACL and medial ligaments [133, 234, 408, 681].

Even when the ACL is deficient, a pivot shift cannot be elicited if there is a complete rupture of the iliotibial tract. There would be appreciable tibial subluxation in the slightly flexed knee, but the typical reduction maneuver could not be demonstrated. Both the subluxation and reduction phases of the pivot shift test may be prevented by a bucket-handle tear of the medial or lateral meniscus or by severe degenerative changes involving the lateral compartment or the intercondylar eminence.

Positive pivot shift tests are known to occur in adolescents with hyperlaxity [138]. Our case records include two young females with positive pivot shift tests in both knees and a positive Lachman test with a firm end point. Both patients have hyperlaxity (mild bilateral recurvatum, hyperextensible fingers and elbows), and both had femoropatellar pain as their presenting complaint.

False-positive pivot shift tests have been described in association with destruction of the lateral meniscus or the presence of a discoid lateral meniscus [138, 480]. When the test is performed preoperatively in the operating room, a false-negative result may be obtained due to fixation of the iliotibial tract by a previ-

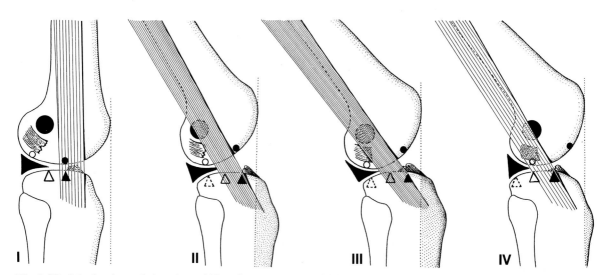

Fig. 3-22. Mechanism of the pivot shift: *Phase I:* Initial position. *Phase II:* Anterior subluxation of the tibia. The iliotibial tract is still anterior to the flexion axis. *Phase III:* Maximum anterior subluxation (shaded area). There is maximal tension on the iliotibial tract, which passes directly over the flexion axis. *Phase IV:* With increasing flexion the iliotibial tract snaps backward over the lateral femoral condyle, where it is posterior to the flexion axis. The tibia is pulled posteriorly (O = flexion axis) (reduced position) (from [470])

ously inflated blood-pressure cuff. A displaced meniscus, a loose intraarticular body, or a disturbance of femoropatellar tracking can mimic dynamic anterior subluxation and hamper differentiation [234].

Eliciting the pivot shift too frequently and too forcibly can lead to cartilage damage or may even convert a partial tear of the ACL into a complete rupture [469].

In examinations of the acutely injured knee, the subluxating forces that are applied in the pivot shift test stretch the frequently injured medial capsule and ligaments. The resulting pain can incite reflex muscle spasms that lead to a false-negative result [406]. On the other hand, a positive test is usually obtained when the knee is examined under general anesthesia [133, 349, 386, 408, 603, 713] (see Tables 3-6 and 3-7).

Even in chronic ligament instabilities, it can be difficult to demonstrate a pivot shift unless the patient is completely relaxed [235, 386]. Thus, as in the drawer tests, it is essential that the patient be positioned in such a way that his muscles are optimally relaxed.

1. False-negative dynamic subluxation tests are common in acute injuries (perform Lachman test).
2. Make certain the patient is completely relaxed during the test.
3. Carefully perform the dynamic subluxation maneuver.

When a positive test is performed, the patient will reexperience the familiar feeling of instability as the lateral tibial plateau slips between subluxation and reduction. Viewing from the lateral aspect, the observer can recognize a positive dynamic anterior subluxation test by the effaced contours at the junction of the patella and patellar ligament with the knee slightly flexed and the tibia subluxated (Fig. 3-23a). The contour of the knee then returns to normal as flexion is increased (Fig. 3-23b). The examiner himself recognizes a positive test by the typical snapping of the lateral side of the joint or of the fibular head that accompanies the change from subluxation to reduction and vice-versa.

It is recommended that the examiner select one or two of the numerous dynamic anterior subluxation tests described below and make them a standard part of every knee examination (Table 3-9). Only after a test has been routinely practiced and mastered is it possible to evaluate the fine distinctions among the different tests and utilize them to best advantage during diagnosis.

Though the examiner may be tempted to perform as many of these tests as he can, this is not justified since a single test that is unequivocally positive provides adequate grounds for diagnosing ACL insufficiency.

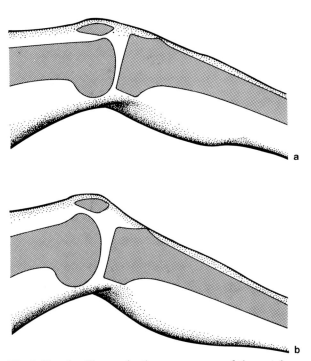

Fig. 3-23a, b. Change in the appearance of the patellar-tibial tuberosity junction with the knee slightly flexed and subluxated (a) and during subsequent reduction (b)

Table 3-9. Dynamic anterior subluxation tests

1. Lemaire test
2. Pivot-shift test of MacIntosh
3. Jerk test of Hughston
4. Slocum test
5. Losee test
6. Noyes test (flexion rotation drawer test)
7. Flexion extension valgus test
8. Nakajima test (N test)
9. Martens test
10. Graded pivot shift test of Jakob
11. Modified pivot shift test
12. "Soft" pivot shift test

3.4.1
Lemaire Test [386]

With the patient supine, the examiner rotates the foot internally while the knee is extended. When the patient has completely relaxed his muscles, the examiner carefully moves the knee through flexion and extension while exerting gentle pressure proximal to the lateral femoral condyle and keeping the tibia internally rotated. Anterior subluxation and reduction of the lateral tibial plateau are plainly recognized in positive cases (Fig. 3-24).

3.4.2
Pivot Shift Test of MacIntosh [195]

The patient is placed in the supine position, and the examiner stands on the lateral side of the involved extremity. With the leg extended, one hand grips the heel and rotates the foot internally while the other hand applies a valgus stress to the proximal tibia. In a positive test the lateral tibial plateau will subluxate anteriorly. As the knee is slowly flexed while the valgus and internally rotating stresses are maintained, the tibia will relocate posteriorly at about 30°–40° of flexion (see Fig. 3-31).

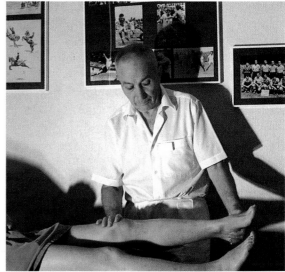

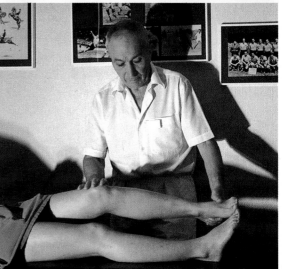

Fig. 3-24a, b. Lemaire test. With ACL insufficiency, the lateral tibial plateau subluxates when the knee is near extension (**a**). When the knee is flexed, reduction occurs (**b**) (Courtesy of M. Lemaire, Paris)

3.4.3
Jerk Test of Hughston

With the knee flexed to about 60°–70°, the examiner grasps the foot with one hand and rotates the tibia internally while applying a valgus stress with the other hand. He then extends the knee gradually. In a positive test, anterior subluxation of the lateral tibial condyle will occur at about 30° of flexion (Fig. 3-25).

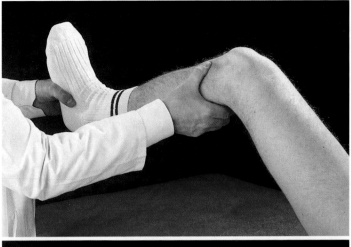

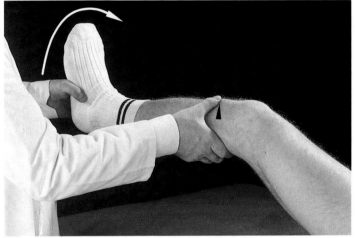

Fig. 3-25a, b. Jerk test of Hughston. Initial position (**a**). As the knee approaches extension, the lateral tibial plateau subluxates anteriorly (**b**)

Dupont [138] prefers to perform the jerk test in external rotation and begins with the knee almost extended (Fig. 3-25b). A positive test in external rotation signifies a global anterior instability, although this is not present in all ACL-deficient knees. In Dupont's series, 97% of patients with a subjectively troublesome anterior knee instability had a positive jerk test in external rotation; 86% had a positive jerk test in internal rotation [138].

3.4.4
Slocum Test

The patient is placed in the lateral decubitus position with the uninvolved side down and the healthy leg flexed at the hip and knee. The involved leg is extended so that the medial side of the foot rests on the examining table; the knee itself is unsupported. The examiner places one hand over the lateral circumference of the proximal tibia from behind, palpating the fibular head with the thumb or index finger. He places the other hand over the distal femur, positioning the thumb on the posterior aspect of the lateral femoral condyle. Both hands then exert gentle pressure to produce valgus angulation of the knee and press it forward into flexion (Fig. 3-26b). With ACL insufficiency, the tibial subluxation will reduce as the knee reaches about 30° of flexion. The examiner detects the reduction with the fingers (e. g., index fingers) placed on the fibular head and lateral femoral condyle (Figs. 3-26 and 3-27).

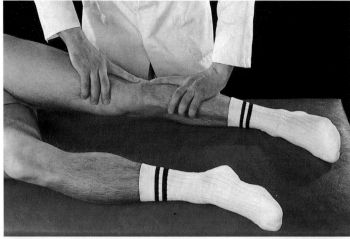

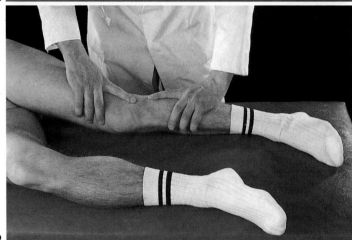

Fig. 3-26a, b. Slocum test. From its anteriorly subluxated position in the slightly flexed knee (**a**) (index fingers point toward each other), the lateral tibial plateau reduces as the knee is flexed (**b**) (index fingers point past each other)

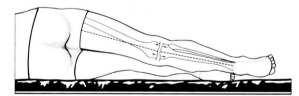

Fig. 3-27. The lateral decubitus position in Slocum's test produces the necessary valgus stress and compression in the lateral joint compartment of the uppermost knee

3.4.5
Losee Test

The Losee test does not involve internal rotation of the tibia. Instead, the examiner holds the medial side of the ankle in a way that produces slight external rotation of the tibia. The other hand is placed on the lateral aspect of the knee with the fingers over the patella and the thumb hooked behind the fibular head. As the knee is slowly extended from a position of 40°–50° flexion, there will be a palpable and visible anterior subluxation of the lateral tibial plateau when ACL insufficiency is present (Fig. 3-28) [403].

The Losee test has assumed special significance among the dynamic anterior subluxation tests owing to the externally rotated position of the tibia. It is important, however, for the examiner to cradle the foot and ankle and not force them into external rotation, since holding them too tightly may prevent anterior subluxation of the tibia. As the knee is extended, the lateral tibial plateau will subluxate anteriorly just short of full extension, producing a corresponding internal rotation of the tibia as a

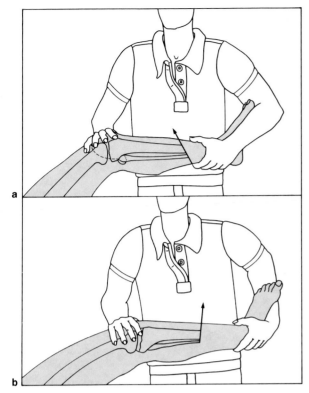

Fig. 3-28 a, b. Losee test. Initial position with the tibia externally rotated (**a**). Subsequent extension elicits anterior subluxation of the lateral tibial plateau (**b**) [403]

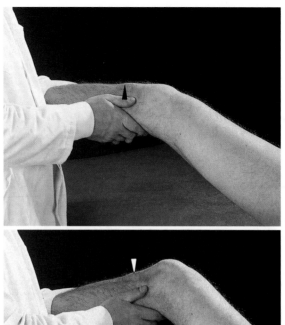

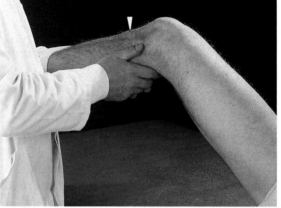

Fig. 3-29 a, b. Noyes test. Subluxated position with effaced knee contours in the presence of ACL insufficiency (**a**). As flexion increases, reduction occurs (**b**) marked by a reappearance of normal patellar ligament contours

whole. This relative internal rotation should not be obstructed by the examiner [403].

3.4.6
Noyes Test (Flexion Rotation Drawer Test)

With the patient supine, the examiner stands on the lateral side of the injured leg and grasps the proximal tibia with both hands. The distal part of the lower leg is held between the examiner's waist and forearm. With the knee flexed about 20°, the examiner elicits a slight anterior drawer while simultaneously confirming relaxation of the hamstrings with the index fingers.

The distal femur is allowed to fall back slightly and externally rotate. As the knee is flexed further, the examiner will detect a palpable internal rotation of the distal femur signifying reduction of the joint (Fig. 3-29). This test differs from those previously described in that the distal femur, rather than the lateral tibial plateau, is tested for subluxation and reduction relative to the fixed tibia.

Thus, the Noyes test combines the features of the Lachman test and the dynamic anterior subluxation test. We have found it useful for the evaluation of acute injuries where there is a marked anterior displacement near extension and there is a desire to avoid excessive valgus pressure.

3.4.7
Flexion Extension Valgus Test

With the patient supine on the examining table, the lower leg is fixed between the examiner's waist and forearm as in the Noyes test. The examiner palpates the joint line and proximal tibia with the thumb and fingers. Valgus stress and axial compression are applied while the knee is flexed and extended. When ACL insufficiency is present, the examiner will feel the anteriorly subluxated tibial plateau reduce with a snap or "clunk" as flexion increases. A relative external rotation of the tibia will also be visible or palpable [248].

In this test the tibia is not forced into a rotated position, so the subluxation sign is easily elicited.

3.4.8
Nakajima Test (N Test)

With the patient supine, the examiner stands on the lateral side of the injured leg and holds the foot with one hand while rotating the tibia internally. He places the other hand over the lateral femoral condyle, positioning the thumb in the popliteal fossa behind the fibular head and pushing the latter anteriorly. From a starting position of 90° flexion, the knee is gradually extended. Anterior subluxation of the lateral tibial plateau at a flexion angle of about 30° is considered positive for ACL insufficiency [476].

3.4.9
Martens Test

The patient is supine, and the examiner stands on the lateral side of the injured leg. One hand grips the leg distal to the knee joint, the index finger against the fibula. As in the Noyes test, the examiner secures the lower leg between the waist and forearm while exerting a valgus pressure. As the examiner pulls the tibia anteriorly, he presses the distal femur posteriorly with the other hand. Starting from an almost

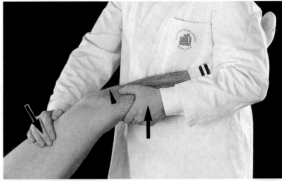

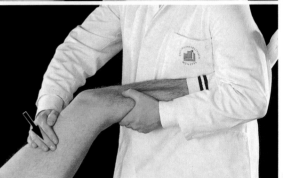

Fig. 3-30a, b. Martens test. Subluxation of the lateral tibial plateau in the slightly flexed knee (raised knee contour) (**a**). Reduction on further flexion (**b**) with reappearance of the normal knee contour

extended position, the knee is gradually flexed until the subluxated lateral tibial plateau reduces posteriorly at about 30° of flexion (Fig. 3-30) [430].

3.4.10
Graded Pivot Shift Test of Jakob

With rupture of the ACL, both the medial and lateral sides of the tibial plateau will translate forward when an anterior drawer stress is applied. MacIntosh was among the first to emphasize the importance of observing motion of the medial tibial plateau during anterior subluxation of the tibia. With an isolated ACL rupture, the anterior translation of the lateral tibial plateau will be greater than that of the medial plateau. However, as the involvement of the medial structures increases, the medial plateau undergoes a greater anterior translation relative to the lateral side [636]. But the greater the anterior translation of the medial plateau, the more plainly the subluxation and subsequent reduction are felt by the examiner. Moreover, the reduction occurs in a somewhat higher degree of flexion [318].

Jakob [319, 320] has devised a graded pivot shift test (see Sect. 3.4.2) which takes into account the translation and rotation of the tibia. In this test the pivot shift is elicited not just with the tibia internally rotated but also in neutral and external rotation (Fig. 3-31).

Classification:

Grade I pivot shift: Test is positive in internal rotation but negative in neutral and external rotation. The subluxation is palpable by the examiner but is not visible.

Grade II pivot shift: Test is positive in internal and neutral rotation but negative in external rotation.

Grade III pivot shift: Test is more severe in the neutral position and markedly positive in external rotation. In internal rotation the subluxation is less obvious (Fig. 3-32). Appearence of positive reversed pivot shift test possible.

A grade III pivot shift is seen in an acutely injured knee only if there is disruption of the posteromedial and posterolateral structures in addition to a complete ACL rupture. It is also found in chronic instabilities where there has been stretching of the secondary ligamentous restraints over time. Patients with a grade II pivot shift and especially those with grade III generally complain of significant instability during uncontrolled loading or uncoordinated movements of the knee.

The test is easy to perform and is like the classic pivot shift test of MacIntosh, except that in the graded pivot shift test the tibia is held in the desired position of rotation.

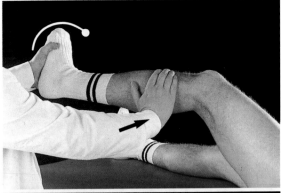

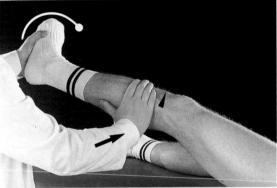

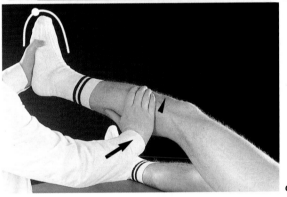

Fig. 3-31 a–c. Graded pivot shift of Jakob. Starting from a position of flexion and internal tibial rotation (**a**), subluxation occurs as the knee approaches extension (**b**), signifying ACL insufficiency. The test is also performed in neutral and external rotation. The subluxation is more pronounced in the neutral position (**c**) than with the tibia internally rotated

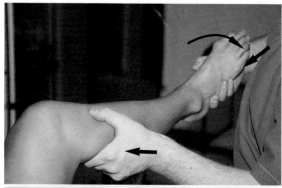

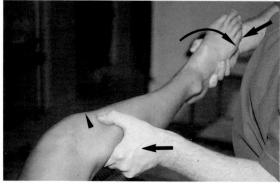

Fig. 3-32 a, b. Grade III pivot shift. The proximal tibia shows marked subluxation as the flexed knee (**a**) approaches extension (**b**) in patient with fresh rupture of the medial collateral, posterior oblique ligament, medial meniscus, and the ACL (preoperative examination under anesthesia)

3.4.11
Modified Pivot Shift Test

Since the iliotibial tract plays a significant role in the occurrence of the pivot shift, it is not surprising that its state of tension before the pivot shift is elicited has an effect on the subluxation that is observed.

This circumstance led Bach, Warren et Wickiewicz [23] to consider the effects of hip position on the pivot shift sign. Since abduction of the hip relaxes the iliotibial tract and adduction tightens it, these authors performed the pivot shift test not just in various degrees of tibial rotation (see Sect. 3.4.10) but also in various hip positions. All knees were tested in hip abduction, neutral, and hip adduction, and with the tibia in internal and external rotation,

so that a total of six positions were evaluated. The authors found that in all the patients with ACL insufficiency, the most pronounced subluxation occurred when the hip was in the abducted position. The subluxation was less pronounced in the neutral position and was least pronounced in adduction (Fig. 3-33 a, b). External tibial rotation increased the pivot shift in abduction and neutral, but not in adduction (Fig. 3-33 c, d). The average pivot shift score ranged from 2.48 (abduction/external rotation) to 0.8 (adduction/internal rotation).

Consequently, the pivot shift is tested first with the hip abducted and with the tibia externally and internally rotated.

The iliotibial tract is involved in both the active and passive stabilization of the lateral side of the joint. The segment of the tract between the Kaplan fibers and tubercle of Gerdy is regarded as a passive component that functions like a ligament. This passive structure, known also as the iliotibial band, can be made tense by the portion of the iliotibial tract that courses on the femur. The tenseness of the passive femorotibial component influences the degree of subluxation that occurs near extension. Internal tibial rotation and hip adduction place tension on the entire iliotibial tract, so that the iliotibial band also becomes tightened. However, this tension restricts the anterior excursion of the proximal tibia during pivot shift testing when the ACL is torn. Conversely, external rotation of the tibia reduces the tension on the iliotibial band and thus allows greater anterior subluxation to occur during the pivot shift test. Even greater subluxation can occur when the hip is abducted, relaxing tension on the iliotibial tract and causing laxity of the iliotibial band. In this situation the tract no longer functions as an active retractor of the proximal tibia and acts only as a tether by virtue of its anatomic orientation and its attachment to the lateral femoral shaft.

3.4.12
"Soft" Pivot Shift Test

Pivot shift testing usually provokes a reflex muscle tension that may prevent a successful conduct of the test. This is due mainly to the various force components that are exerted upon the knee. Besides applying a valgus stress and securing the foot in the desired rotational position, the examiner applies varying amounts of force when flexing and extending the knee. The test can be made simpler and more pleasant for the patient by following a modified technique:

With the patient supine, the examiner supports the foot of the involved extremity with one hand and places the other hand posteriorly over the calf muscles about 10–20 cm distal to the knee joint. First the examiner alternately flexes and extends the knee using slow, gentle movements. This calms the patient's fears and provokes no reflex tensing of the muscles. The hip is abducted, and the foot is held in neutral or external rotation. Then, after three to five flexion-extension cycles, the examiner carefully applies axial compression to the limb while the hand on the back of the lower leg exerts a mild anterior stress. In positive cases the tibia will subluxate softly as the knee approaches extension and will reduce again as the knee is flexed (Fig. 3-34). The forcefulness of the reduction and the subluxation can be accurately controlled by the rate of the flexion-extension movements and the degree of the axial compression and anterior stress. As in the other tests, greater force will causes the reduction to occur with a painful jerking sensation. In this test the examiner literally "feels" his way toward eliciting the target sign.

The soft pivot shift test guarantees a less painful and frequently painless reduction/sub-

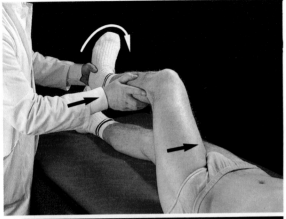

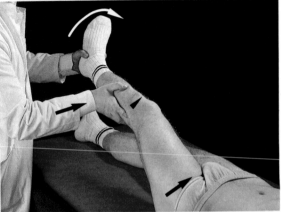

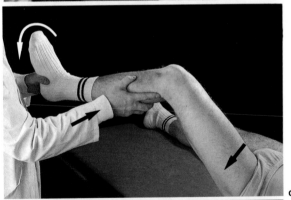

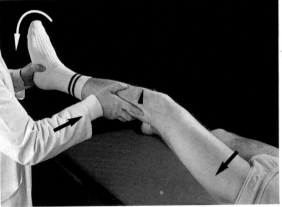

Fig. 3-33 a–d. Modified pivot shift test in adduction of the hip and slight internal tibial rotation (**a, b**) and in abduction and slight external tibial rotation (**c, d**), Marked anterior subluxation of the proximal tibia occurs near extension (**d**)

luxation when ACL insufficiency is present. Carefully performed, the test can be repeated several times without causing objectionable pain.

3.5
Medial Shift Test

The anterior and posterior drawer tests detect pathologic mobility on the transverse plane of the knee joint. But tests are also known that can detect translation on the frontal plane of the joint (see Fig. 3-1c).

Medial and lateral translation are familiar in manual medicine as mobilization exercises and can also serve as diagnostic tests for meniscal injury [706]. We can thus appreciate their potential value as tests for ligamentous injuries.

The examiner begins the test by securing the patient's lower leg between his waist and forearm. To test for medial translation, he places one hand on the lateral side of the tibia just distal to the joint line. He places the other hand on the medial side just proximal to the joint line (Fig. 3-35). He then exerts a varus stress on the tibia with his forearm while simultaneously applying a medially directed stress. The hand on the thigh exerts counterpressure to keep the hip from abducting.

In the case of an ACL rupture, the tibia can be shifted medially. As this occurs, the intercondylar eminence comes into contact with the medial femoral condyle. Because the PCL runs medially to laterally, lesions of the PCL are characterized by a positive lateral translation of the proximal tibia (lateral shift test).

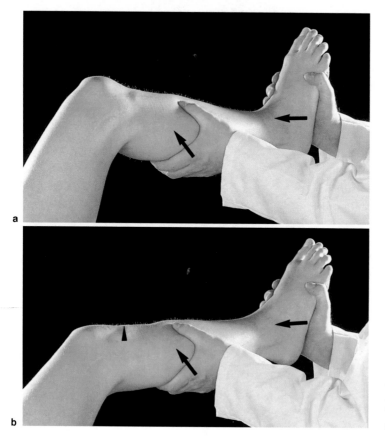

Fig. 3-34a, b. "Soft" pivot shift test. Initial position (**a**). With ACL insufficiency, the tibia will undergo a soft anterior subluxation when a mild anterior stress and axial compression are applied (**b**)

Rarely, in injuries involving the ACL, the AP radiograph will demonstrate medial translation of the tibia with resultant contact between the intercondylar eminence and the medial femoral condyle (Fig. 3-36).

We know of no landmark scientific studies that deal with translational movements on the frontal plane (medial/lateral).

3.6 Function Tests

Function tests are designed to reproduce the subluxating process that patients with ACL insufficiency generally experience several times weekly or even daily, or to provoke typical "avoidance behavior" to guard against subluxation, which likewise is interpreted as a positive sign. The subluxation is elicited not by the examiner but by the patient himself through voluntary or involuntary quadriceps contraction.

Patients with ACL insufficiency who refuse operative treatment despite frequent or occasional episodes of pivot shift subluxation should be informed about the potential adverse effects of their condition. They should understand that each episode causes intraarticular damage that predominantly affects the cartilage and menisci. Losee [406] advises his patients to behave in ways that will minimize subluxation of the knee. The patient can decompress the lateral joint compartment by adducting the leg at the hip. This significantly decreases the extent of the anterior subluxation, a circumstance that is also utilized diagnostically [23] (see Fig. 3-33 a,b). Moreover, the patient should avoid twisting movements and should not change direction suddenly or come to a sudden stop. Instead, he is advised to decelerate slowly and to break direction changes down into several steps. Especially when decelerating, the patient should avoid abducting the hip and externally rotating the tibia as this might cause a gross amount of subluxation [23, 406]. The increase of subluxation by hip ab-

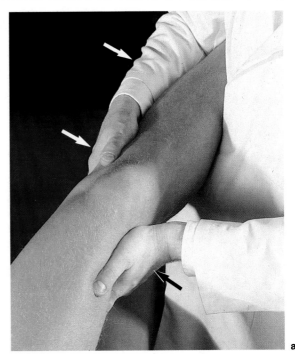

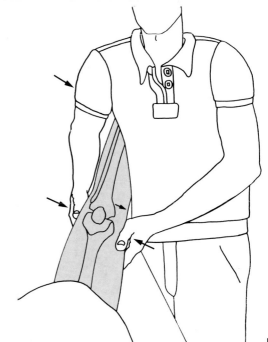

Fig. 3-35 a, b. The medial shift test (after Bryant [73])

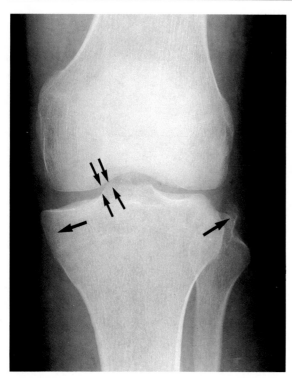

Fig. 3-36. Spontaneous medial shift of the tibia. The intercondylar eminence abuts against the medial femoral condyle *(arrows)*. Additionally there is a Segond fracture *(arrow)* signifying an ACL lesion, and there is widening of the medial joint space signifying damage to the medial capsule

duction can, however, be utilized by the examiner (see Fig. 3-33).

3.6.1
Deceleration Test

The patient is asked to run at full speed and to stop suddenly upon command. The test is positive if the patient, upon stopping, avoids quadriceps contraction, which would subluxate the knee at 10°–20° of flexion. The test is also positive if the patient decelerates in a crouched position to avoid the unstable range of flexion.

3.6.2
"Disco" Test of Losee

In this test the patient assumes a one-legged stance on the injured side with the knee flexed 10°–20°, and he is asked to twist the body alternately to the left and right as if performing a "disco" or jazz dance. Apprehension during the test or refusal to perform the maneuver is interpreted as a positive test [405].

3.6.3
Leaning Hop Test of Larson

The patient hops up and down on the injured leg while abducting the opposite leg. This increases the compression on the lateral compartment of the knee, and a painful subluxation can occur if the ACL is deficient. Apprehension, refusal, or minimal performance of the hopping indicates a positive test [405].

3.6.4
Crossover Test of Arnold

With the patient standing, the examiner steps on the foot of the injured leg. The patient is then asked to cross the healthy leg over the fixed foot, rotating the pelvis and upper body toward the affected side (Fig. 3-37). Quadriceps contraction will cause the lateral tibial plateau to subluxate anteriorly (active dynamic subluxation). Besides the pivoting, a positive test (ACL insufficiency) is indicated by apprehension, refusal, and discomfort [20].

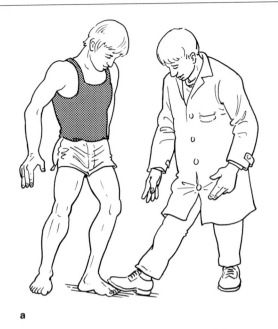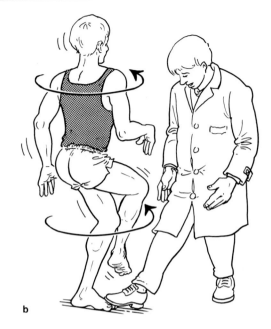

Fig. 3-37. Crossover test of Arnold (from [396 a])

3.6.5
Giving Way Test of Jakob

The patient leans with his sound side against the wall and is told to distribute his weight equally on both legs. The examiner places his hands proximal and distal to the injured knee and exerts a valgus stress while the patient initiates flexion (Fig. 3-38). If the test is positive, this will elicit a palpable jerk (reduction) and the knee will give way [317].

Healthy individuals as well as patients with confirmed ACL insufficiency will show increased laxity after certain forms of exercise (e. g., cycling) [221]. Perhaps exercise tests of this kind can be used to screen patients with ACL insufficiency and identify those who are at greatest risk for entering the stage of the "ACL-deficient knee" without surgical reconstruction. The following three performance tests can also be used to monitor rehabilitation and evaluate the patient's condition [649].

3.6.6
One-Leg Hop Test

From a standing position, the patient does a modified "long jump" by pushing off with one leg and landing on the the same leg. This is done alternately for each leg, and the test is repeated three times. The longest jump on the affected leg is measured and compared with the longest jump on the unaffected leg.

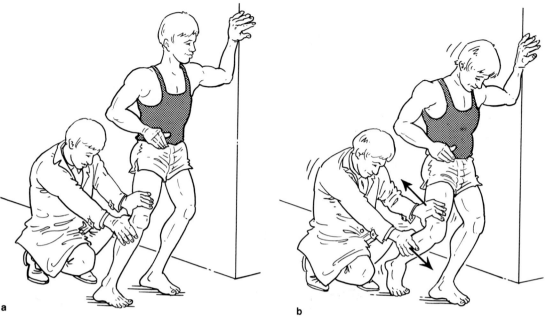

Fig. 3-38 a, b. Giving way test of Jakob (from [396 a])

3.6.7
Running in a Figure of Eight

In this test, two landmarks are positioned 10 m apart. The patient is told to run around the landmarks in a figure-of-eight pattern, so that one lap covers about 20 m [649]. The patient runs two laps in all, and the elapsed time is measured with the aid of two photoelectric cells placed at the level of the turns. Thus the times required to run the straightaways and the turns can be individually measured.

3.6.8
Running Up and Down Stairs

The patient runs up and down a given number of stairs (say, 25), and the elapsed time is measured with a stopwatch.

3.7
Posterior Drawer Test

Like the anterior drawer test (see Sect. 3.3), the "classic" posterior drawer test is performed with the knee flexed 90° and with the tibia in internal, neutral, and external rotation [282, 285, 345, 470]. Again, the examiner sits on the patient's foot to secure it in the desired rotational position (see Fig. 3-10). Testing in 60° flexion is additionally recommended [466, 471].

Hughston [299] calls attention to the fact that a negative posterior drawer test may be obtained following an acute rupture of the PCL. In cases where a positive test is not elicited despite a PCL rupture, there is usually a co-existing rupture of the medial and posteromedial structures. It is believed that an intact arcuate complex prevents posterior displacement [299]. A PCL rupture can be recognized in these cases by pronounced medial opening of the joint in extension or hyperextension. On the other hand, with a chronic PCL insufficiency there will invariably be stretching of the arcuate complex, leading to a positive posterior drawer test and usually a positive spontaneous posterior drawer (positive sag sign) (see Fig. 2-26).

3.7.1
"Soft" Posterolateral Drawer Test

Feagin [159] performs the "soft" posterolateral drawer test with the patient sitting and the knee flexed to about 60°. Because gravity causes the tibia to sag downward, the examiner can easily perceive the posterior translation of the lateral tibial plateau when posterolateral instability is present. The thumbs are placed over the femoral condyles while the balls of the thumbs apply the drawer stress (Fig. 3-39).

3.7.2
Reversed Lachman Test

The posterior counterpart to the Lachman test (anterior drawer test in slight flexion) is the "reversed" Lachman test. But unlike the Lachman test, which is specific for ACL rupture, the reversed Lachman test is not specific for an isolated PCL rupture. The greatest posterior displacement in PCL insufficiency is observed in 90° flexion [65, 189, 421, 447, 504] and not in the slightly flexed knee, as our own studies confirm (see Fig. 3-59). Usually the reversed Lachman test is mildly positive in chronic posterior instabilities; markedly positive tests are less common [120].

As practiced by Feagin [159], the reversed Lachman test is performed with the patient prone, just as in the prone anterior Lachman test (see Fig. 3-17). The examiner places his thumbs on the posteromedial and posterolateral corners of the joint with his index fingers on the anterior aspect of the femoral condyles. At this time the examiner uses the thumbs to check for guarding of the hamstrings. If tension is noted, he tells the patient to relax the muscles. When relaxation is confirmed, and with the knee slightly flexed, the examiner

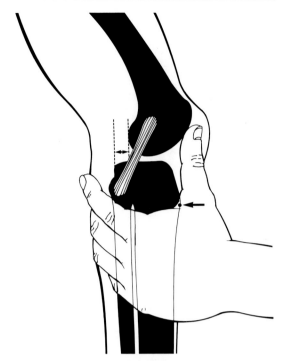

Fig. 3-39. "Soft" posterolateral drawer test in the sitting position to demonstrate posterolateral instability (after Feagin [159])

presses the upper end of the tibia posteriorly and watches for posterior displacement of the tibia. A modified technique is to grasp the proximal tibia with one hand while fixing the distal femur with the other hand. The quality of the end point is more easily evaluated by this method (Fig. 3-40).

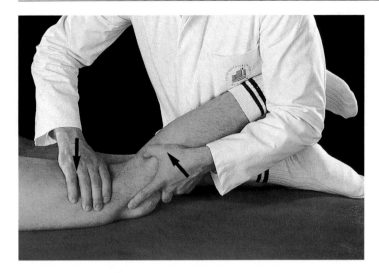

Fig. 3-40. Reversed Lachman test (modified from Feagin)

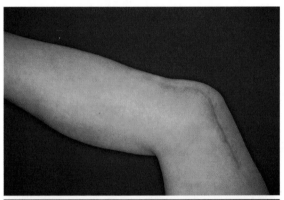

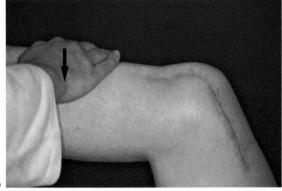

Fig. 3-41a, b. Godfrey test. Even in the initial position (**a**) the slightly dropped position of the proximal tibia is apparent. Manual downward pressure on the tibia elicits marked posterior displacement as an expression of PCL insufficiency (**b**)

3.7.3
Godfrey Test

With the patient supine, the examiner holds and supports the lower legs with both knees and hips flexed to 90°. He then applies manual pressure to the tibial tuberosity of each extremity. A posterior instability with involvement of the PCL is mostly manifested by an increased posterior displacement of the tuberosity (Fig. 3-41) [118].

3.8
Reversed Pivot Shift Test

In the test described by Jakob et al. [317], the patient is supine and the examiner stands on the side of the injured leg. One hand grasps the foot and rotates the tibia externally, causing a posterior subluxation of the lateral tibial plateau when posterolateral instability is present. The other hand is placed on the lateral aspect of the knee, with the thumb positioned on the fibular head and exerting a valgus pressure. Starting from a flexed position, the knee is gradually extended while the valgus stress is maintained. In a positive test the lateral tibial

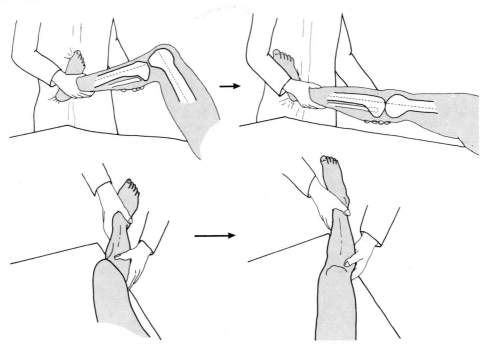

Fig. 3-42. Reversed pivot shift of Jakob (schematic) [317]

plateau palpably reduces to its initial position when about 20° of flexion is reached (Figs. 3-42 and 3-43).

While this test is the functional counterpart to the dynamic anterior subluxation test, it may be positive in individuals with increased constitutional laxity. The test is clinically significant only when it is positive on one side and also reproduces the painful subluxation phenomenon that has been described by the patient. According to Jakob [317], an adequate trauma must exist along with a posterolateral instability manifested by a positive posterior drawer test with the tibia in external rotation.

3.8.1
Dynamic Posterior Shift Test

In this test the patient is supine and the examiner flexes the hip and knee to about 90°. The femur is in a position of neutral rotation. The examiner places one hand on the anterior side of the thigh to steady it, and with the other he slowly extends the knee. With a rupture of the PCL, the tibia will abruptly reduce anteriorly from its subluxated position with a palpable "clunk" when extension is reached (Fig. 3-44). This test is positive with a straight posterior instability and in posterolateral instabilities [590].

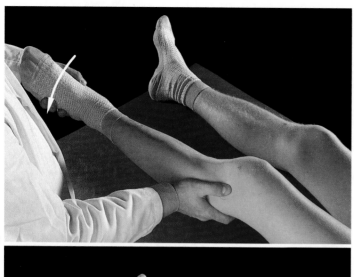

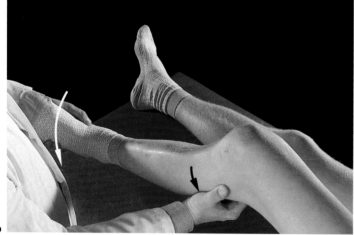

Fig. 3-43a, b. Positive reversed pivot shift test in posterolateral instability. Initial position (**a**). Posterior subluxation of the lateral tibia plateau with further flexion (**b**)

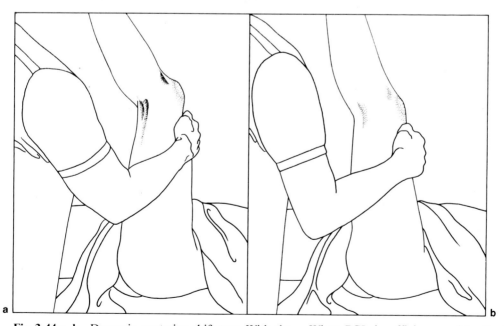

Fig. 3-44a, b. Dynamic posterior shift test. With the knee slightly flexed, the upper tibia subluxates posteriorly due to the pull of the ischiocrural muscles (**a**). When PCL insufficiency exists, the tibia will reduce with a palpable snap as the knee is extended further (**b**) (after [590])

3.9
Active Laxity Tests

Active laxity tests differ from the traditional passive tests but are like the function tests (Sect. 3.6) in that the patient himself elicits the tibial displacement through voluntary muscular contraction. The examiner observes the contours of the tibial tuberosity, the patellar ligament, and proximal tibia to detect their movements.

Besides their technical simplicity, active laxity tests are advantageous in that they cause minimal pain and can effectively differentiate between the anterior and posterior components of tibial displacement.

To understand how the active drawer tests work, it is helpful to know how the alignment of the net force vector (the "resultant" Fx) of the pull of the quadriceps muscle changes with the flexion angle of the knee. In the uninjured knee, the resultant is directed anteriorly when

the knee is near full extension (Fig. 3-45a), but it is directed posteriorly when the knee is strongly flexed (e.g., to 90°) (Fig. 3-45b). Accordingly, contraction of the quadriceps muscle leads to a slight anterior displacement of the proximal tibia when the knee is near extension and to a slight posterior displacement of the tibia in higher degrees of flexion.

3.9.1
Active Quadriceps Test in 30° Flexion (Active Lachman Test)

As early as 1975, Wirth and Artmann [708] described the roentgenographic features of the active anterior drawer test in slight flexion in patients with ACL insufficiency.

The patient is asked to extend his leg by raising his foot from the examining table. The examiner positions his eyes at the level of the patient's knee. The examiner flexes the knee slightly by placing one hand on the contralat-

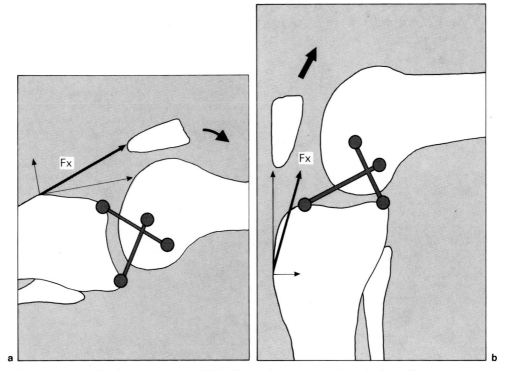

Fig. 3-45a, b. The force resultant *(Fx)* is directed anteriorly when the knee is near extension (**a**) and posteriorly when the knee is flexed 90° (**b**)

eral knee to elevate and support the patient's thigh with his forearm. The foot may be held down on the table to increase the force of the quadriceps pull *(maximum quadriceps test)* (Fig. 3-46). When the ACL is intact, slight anterior motion of the proximal tibia will be observed. But when the ligament is torn, there will be a more pronounced anterior displacement of the tibia relative to the unaffected side due to loss of the restraining action of the ACL.

Daniel et al. [111] report that the "physiologic" active anterior displacement in the healthy knee averages 4 mm in the slightly flexed position. When the ACL is torn, an additional anterior tibial displacement of 3-6 mm is observed.

This test is performed only after a PCL injury has been excluded. A torn PCL will allow "spontaneous" posterior sagging of the tibia, causing the force resultant to acquire a more anterior orientation. This would lead to a conspicuous but false-positive active anterior drawer test in the slightly flexed knee (see Fig. 3-49).

In cases where insufficiency of the medial ligaments and ACL coexists with laxity of the posterior suspension of the medial meniscus, quadriceps contraction can lead to meniscal entrapment *(positive active Finochietto test)*. This locking can be relieved by relaxing the quadriceps muscle or by manually pushing the tibia posteriorly (posterior drawer).

The active Lachman test differs from the passive Lachman test in that the tibia can easily be fixed in various positions of rotation to evaluate the integrity of the medial and lateral stabilizers. If global anterior instability exists (with insufficiency of the ACL and of the medial, posteromedial, lateral, and posterolateral structures), a marked active anterior shift of the proximal tibia will be noted in internal and

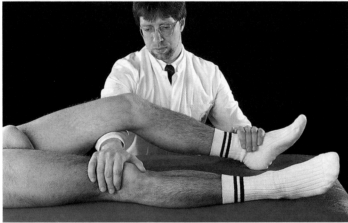

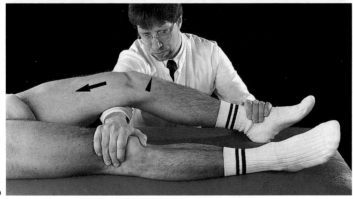

Fig. 3-46a, b. Active Lachman test (Active quadriceps test in 30° flexion). When the muscles are relaxed, the knee presents a normal contour (**a**). With ACL insufficiency, voluntary contraction of the quadriceps muscle produces a marked anterior shift of the proximal tibia (**b**), effacing the normal knee contour. The foot is fixed against the table to increase the force of the quadriceps pull

neutral rotation and especially in external rotation.

Patients with ACL insufficiency commonly practice internal rotation of the tibia in their daily activities as a means of stabilizing the knee. To steady the joint and avoid painful "pivoting," the patients walk and run with slight external rotation of the tibia and internal rotation of the femur [405].

3.9.2
No-Touch Lachman Test
(Active Quadriceps Test in 30° Flexion)

In patients who are anxious or in pain, the examination can be initiated with an active quadriceps test (active Lachman test) in which the examiner does not need to manipulate the patient's leg (no-touch test) [101].

The patient lies supine and is told to grasp his leg above the knee with both hands and elevate it so that the knee is slightly flexed. Alternatively, the knee may be flexed over the examiner's forearm (Fig. 3-47). The patient is then asked to raise his foot from the examining table. By placing his eyes at the level of the knee joint, the examiner can observe any contour change produced by the quadriceps contraction. When the ligaments are intact, little or no contour change will be seen (Fig. 3-48 a).

But if there is an acute or chronic ligamentous lesion involving the ACL and the medial structures, the examiner will observe anterior subluxation of the tibia with an appreciable contour change in the area of the patellar ligament (Fig. 3-48 b).

With this simple test it is possible to exclude relatively complex ligamentous injuries (ACL and medial, posteromedial, and/or lateral, posterolateral structures) without touching the patient or causing him pain.

One difficulty in this test is to define correctly the starting position of the tibia. For example, a significant spontaneous posterior drawer (tibial posterior sag) will be present in the slightly flexed knee when there is a tear of the PCL combined with an insufficiency of medial and lateral capsuloligamentous structures [101, 504].

When the patient is asked to extend his leg from the slightly flexed position by active quadriceps contraction, anterior displacement of the proximal tibia will be seen when there is a rupture of the ACL and/or the PCL (Fig. 3-49). On finding this anterior displacement, then, the examiner should not be content to diagnose an ACL rupture. He should always exclude a PCL lesion by additionally testing for posterior translation of the tibia (reversed Lachman test, soft posterolateral drawer test, spontaneous posterior drawer).

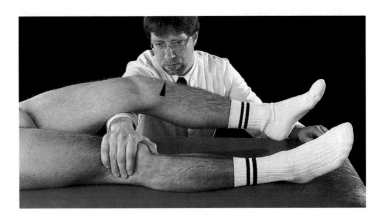

Fig. 3-47. No-touch Lachman test (Active quadriceps test in 30° flexion). The examiner observes the contour of the patella, patellar ligament, and tibial tuberosity during quadriceps contraction

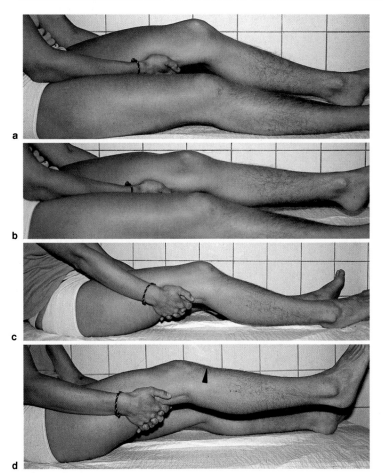

Fig. 3-48a–b. No-touch Lachman test (No touch active quadriceps test in 30° flexion). The test was performed in a very anxious 24-year-old woman with a 3-day-old rotational injury of the right knee. Quadriceps contraction on the uninvolved side does not significantly change the knee contour (**a** intact knee at rest, **b** intact knee on quadriceps contraction), but quadriceps contraction on the injured side produces a marked anterior displacement (**c** rest, **d** quadriceps contraction). The diagnosis of an ACL rupture was made without manual examination of the patient. The test gives no information on the integrity of the medial and lateral capsuloligamentous structures, which can be determined, for example, by examination under anesthesia

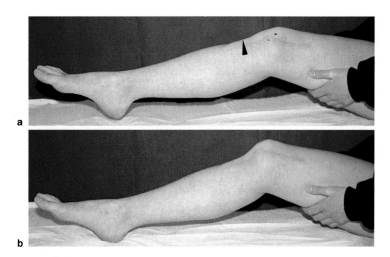

Fig. 3-49a, b. Positive active quadriceps test in 30° flexion (active Lachman test). On contraction of the quadriceps, anterior displacement of the tibia is observed (**a**). Initial position (**b**). However, there is a marked coexisting insufficiency of the PCL in this patient (positive posterior sag sign)

3.9.3
Active Quadriceps Test in 90° Flexion

The patient lies supine with the hip flexed 45°, the knee flexed 90°, and the foot flat on the examining table. The examiner holds the patient's foot down on the table, then tells the patient to attempt to raise the foot. As the quadriceps muscle contracts, the examiner observes the change in the anterior contour of the knee.

If the knee ligaments are intact, quadriceps contraction will cause the proximal end of the tibia to move posteriorly by 0–2 mm [111, 116]. If the PCL is torn, the tibia will sag posteriorly when the initial test position is assumed (spontaneous posterior drawer), and the force resultant will be directed anteriorly (Fig. 3-50). Then, when the patient attempts to extend the knee against a fixed resistance, there will be a conspicuous anterior displacement of the proximal tibia [111, 116, 470]. That is the real advantage of this test in evaluating the PCL.

Daniel [116] states that the 90° active quadriceps test is superior to the classic posterior drawer test in 90° flexion for determining the integrity of the PCL. The major reason for this is that an unequivocally positive posterior drawer sign cannot be demonstrated in all knees with a torn PCL. Another difficulty with the classic test is that patients with an acute knee injury often are unable to flex the knee past 40°–50°.

In the 90° active quadriceps test, the examiner must see to it that only the quadriceps is contracted. The appropriate instruction for the patient is: "Please raise your foot from the examining table." Simultaneous contraction of the hamstrings would prevent or significantly restrict anterior displacement of the tibia.

Thus, the resulting "anterior displacement of the proximal tibia" should not be interpreted as signifying insufficiency of the ACL. It is, rather, an expression of PCL insufficiency.

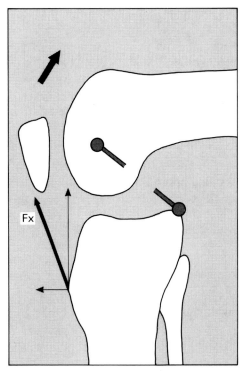

Fig. 3-50. Anteriorly directed force resultant *(Fx)* due to rupture of the PCL

3.9.4
Modified Active Drawer Test in 90° Flexion

Because the 90° active quadriceps test is often difficult to interpret, we conduct the test in a modified form [634].

The patient lies supine with the knees flexed 90° and the feet flat on the table. The examiner positions his eyes level with the knees to check for spontaneous sagging of one of the tibial tuberosities. If a spontaneous posterior drawer is noted, an injury of the PCL should be suspected. But even if a relative posterior sag is not seen, it cannot be automatically assumed that the PCL is intact. For example, there may be a compensated PCL insufficiency that is not manifested by a spontaneous posterior drawer.

The active part of this test consists of two phases. In the *first phase* the patient is told to press his heel against the examining table or to draw his foot up toward the buttock. The examiner checks to see that the hamstrings are tense. With the foot fixed and the knee flexed, these muscles do not function as flexors or rotators of the knee, but merely pull the upper end of the tibia posteriorly. Contraction of the muscles may accentuate a preexisting posterior sag or may provoke a posterior displacement where none was evident before.

In the *second phase* of the test, the patient attempts to raise his foot from the table while the examiner holds it down. In a positive test, quadriceps contraction will actively pull the proximal tibia forward from its posteriorly subluxated position (Figs. 3-51 and 3-52).

The advantage of the modified test is that it elicits a more conspicuous anterior displacement of the tibia from a position of maximum posterior displacement. Compensated posterior instabilities show an increase of posterior displacement in the initial test phase, while in decompensated posterior instabilities the tibia tends to maintain its posterior position.

As in all active tests, the result is influenced by the willingness and ability of the patient to

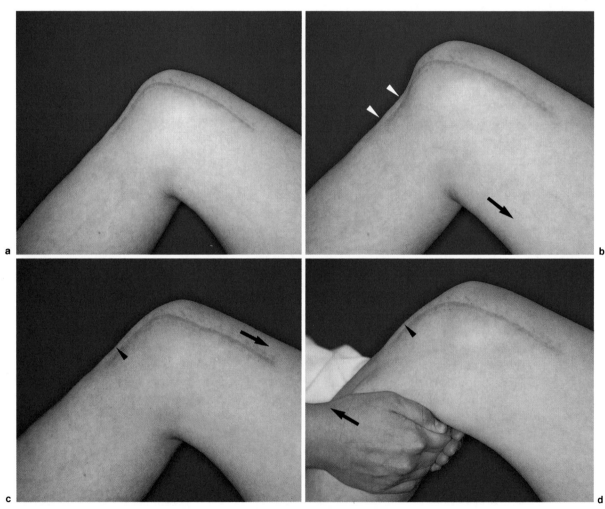

Fig. 3-51a-d. Modified 90° active drawer test. Simple inspection reveals a slight posterior sag of the proximal tibia (**a**). Contraction of the ischiocrural muscles with the foot fixed and the knee flexed 90° (patient is asked to pull the foot toward the buttock) markedly increases the posterior tibial displacement (1st phase of test, **b**). From that position the tibia is drawn forward by quadriceps contraction in the 2nd phase of the test (**c**). Marked anterior tibial displacement indicates PCL insufficiency. Subsequent anterior drawer testing causes further anterior tibial displacement signifying a coexisting ACL insufficiency (**d**)

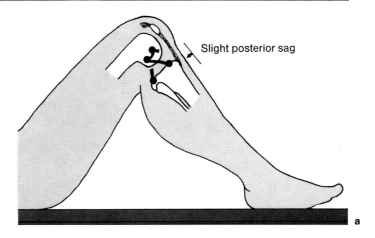

Slight posterior sag

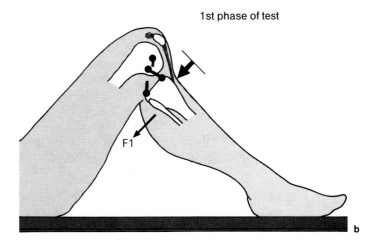

1st phase of test

F1

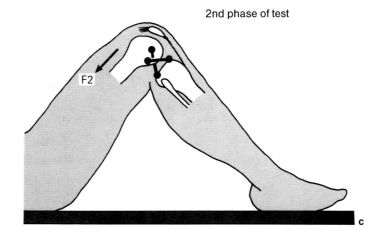

2nd phase of test

F2

Fig. 3-52a–c. Modified 90° active drawer test. Inspection of the PCL-deficient knee shows a slight spontaneous posterior drawer (**a**), which is increased by contraction of the ischiocrural muscles *(F1)* (**b**). Subsequent contraction of the quadriceps *(F2)* produces an active anterior displacement of the tibia and eliminates the posterior sag (**c**) [371]

cooperate with the examiner. A positive test implies insufficiency of the PCL.

1. *Positive active Lachman test:* implies ACL insufficiency.
2. *Positive active quadriceps test in 90° flexion:* implies PCL insufficiency.

3.9.5
Quadriceps Neutral Angle Test of Daniel

All active and passive drawer tests in 90° illustrates the difficulty of distinguishing between an anterior and posterior drawer component. This led Daniel [117] to develop the quadriceps neutral-angle test. The purpose of this test is to determine the "neutral position" of the knee joint, i.e., the position in which quadriceps contraction produces neither an anterior nor posterior excursion of the proximal tibia.

The healthy extremity is tested first. The hip is flexed 45°, the knee is flexed 90°, and the foot is placed flat on the examining table. The examiner asks the patient to raise his foot from the table and watches for associated posterior motion of the proximal tibia (force vector directed posteriorly, see Fig. 3-45b). If posterior displacement is noted, the knee is positioned at a somewhat smaller flexion angle, and the patient is again told to extend the knee. If anterior displacement is now observed (force vector directed anteriorly, see Fig. 3-45a), the test is repeated at a slightly greater flexion angle. This process is continued until the neutral position is identified. Daniel [117] found that the average quadriceps neutral angle was 71° (range of 60°–90°) (Fig. 3-53).

Next the injured knee is examined. It is placed in the position corresponding to the quadriceps neutral angle found for the healthy knee. Starting from that neutral position, the patient is asked to extend the knee (contract the quadriceps muscle). Any anterior displacement of the proximal tibia noted at this time signifies PCL insufficiency (Fig. 3-53).

Determination of the quadriceps neutral angle is also important for the machine testing of laxity (see Chap. 9).

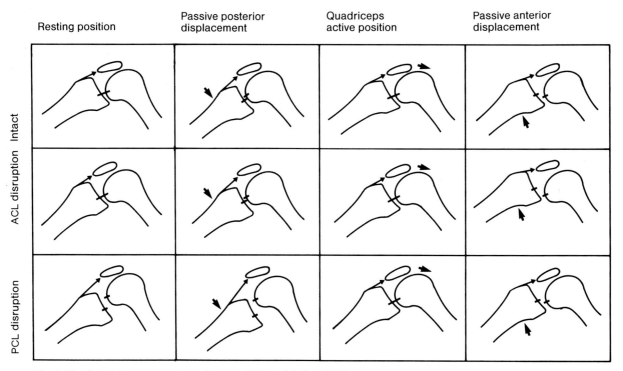

Fig. 3-53. Quadriceps neutral angle test of Daniel (after [117])

3.9.6
Active Pivot Shift Test

Some patients with ACL insufficiency can produce anterior subluxation of the lateral tibial plateau by contraction of the muscles with the knee flexed between 80° and 90° (Fig. 3-54). Peterson [523] showed that this subluxation could be reproduced by electrical stimulation of the popliteus muscle. These claims are plausible, for the author himself has an ACL insufficiency and has observed this active pivot shift maneuver in his own knee.

3.9.7
Active Posterolateral Drawer Sign

Sixty percent of patients with a posterolateral instability can produce a voluntary positive posterolateral drawer test by muscular contraction (Fig. 3-55) [594]. These patients apparently have the ability to contract the popliteus and biceps femoris muscles voluntarily and selectively. The reason for this assumption is that these patients can perform the same voluntary drawer test, though minimally, in the contralateral normal knee [594].

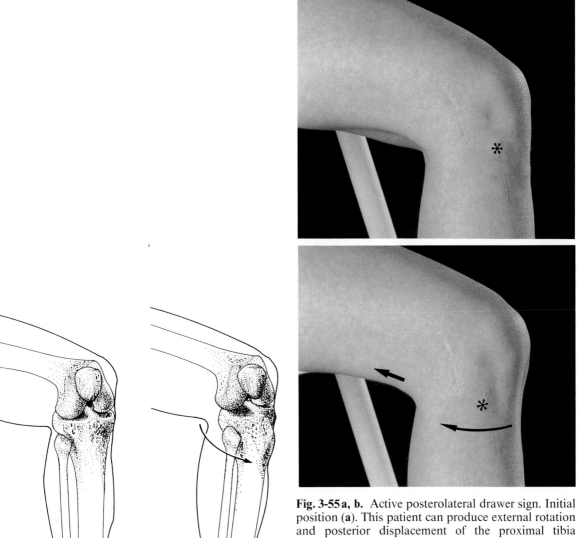

Fig. 3-54. Active pivot shift test (after [523])

Fig. 3-55a, b. Active posterolateral drawer sign. Initial position (a). This patient can produce external rotation and posterior displacement of the proximal tibia through active muscular contraction (b). The external rotation is recognized by the altered position of the tubercle of Gerdy

3.10
External Rotation Recurvatum Test

This test, initially described by Hughston [297], is used to detect posterolateral instability. With the patient supine, both feet are picked up from the table. A positive test, signifying posterolateral instability, is indicated by external rotation of the proximal tibia and hyperextension (recurvatum) with a slight varus deformity (Fig. 3-56).

The test can also be performed unilaterally by moving the injured knee from slight flexion to maximum extension. The examiner places

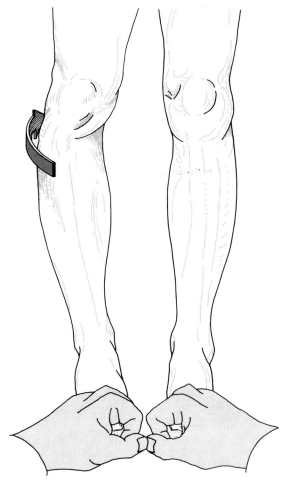

Fig. 3-56. External rotation recurvatum test of Hughston [297]

one hand on the posterolateral aspect of the knee to detect the sagging and slight external rotation of the proximal tibia (Fig. 3-37).

3.11
Classification of Knee Instabilities

There is probably no other joint for which so many systems for classifying and grading capsuloligamentous lesions have been devised as for the knee.

Here we shall not attempt to distill existing classifications into a single scheme. We are concerned, rather, with examining the basic principles that underlie the various classifications. Often the same name is applied to different concepts. To avoid confusion, therefore, we shall make it a point to define exactly what is meant by a particular instability, i.e., to name the structures that are damaged and indicate which laxity tests will be positive or negative [486].

The degree of ligamentous laxity cannot be accurately quantified by clinical examination, so the goal is simply to make the best estimate. We grade abnormal laxity as mild, moderate, or severe (Table 3-10).

The classification of Muhr [466], which is very useful in terms of treatment planning, distinguishes between acute and chronic ligamentous injuries (Table 3-11).

In 1966 Slocum and Larson [605] reported on an injury caused by a flexion-abduction-external rotation mechanism and producing injury of the medial capsular ligament. Observing an increase of external rotation, they described the condition as a "rotatory instability." With additional disruption of the medial collateral ligament and ACL, the severity of the rotatory

Table 3-10. Clinical classification of laxity

Mild	= 1+	3– 5 mm	+
Moderate	= 2+	5–10 mm	+ +
Severe	= 3+	>10 mm	+ + +

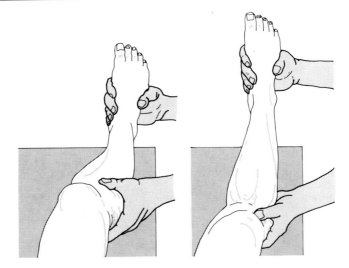

Fig. 3-57. Modified external rotation recurvatum test

Table 3-11. Clinical instability classification of Muhr and Wagner [466]

1. Acute capsuloligamentous injury without instability
2. Acute capsuloligamentous injury with mild instability (on one plane)
3. Acute capsuloligamentous injury with severe instability (on two or more planes)
4. Chronic compensatable instability
5. Chronic decompensated instability

Table 3-12. Classification of knee instabilities

I.   Straight, one-plane, instabilities
   - Medial
   - Lateral
   - Anterior
   - Posterior

II. Rotatory instabilities, complex instabilities
   - Anteromedial
   - Anterolateral
   - Posterolateral
   - Posteromedial

III. Combined instabilities
   - Anterolateral-posterolateral
   - Anterolateral-anteromedial
   - Anteromedial-posteromedial

instability is increased. This pattern of injury causes the axis of rotation in the knee joint to shift toward the lateral side where the capsule and ligaments are still intact. On valgus testing, the authors observed medial opening of the joint in flexion. The anterior drawer test was performed in 90° flexion with the tibia fixed in 30° internal rotation and 15° external rotation. While the test was negative in internal rotation, marked anterior displacement of the medial tibial plateau was observed in external rotation. Building on these observations, Nicholas [479] expanded the classification to include the remaining quadrants of the knee (Table 3-12).

Three different principles have been applied to the classification of knee instabilities within the framework of the above scheme (Table 3-12):

I. *Nicholas* [479] classifies an instability as simple when there is abnormal motion on only one plane and complex when there is abnormal motion on two or more planes.

Nicholas [479] describes four subcategories of complex instability that may occur singly or in combination: anteromedial, anterolateral, posterolateral, and posteromedial. He assigns particular structural deficits to each of the instabilities. Thus, an anteromedial complex instability implies disruption of the ACL ("antero-") and the medial complex ("-medial") while a posterolateral complex instability implies disruption of the PCL ("postero-") and the lateral complex ("-lateral") (see Table 3-1). In all complex instabilities, the axis of rotation is shifted into the intact portion of the joint. For example, in anteromedial instability the axis is shifted anterolaterally, and in posterolateral instability the axis is shifted posteromedially.

Nicholas, then, envisions a rotatory instability as existing on one plane or about one axis. If this is accompanied by further abnormal motion on one or more planes, the instability is classified as complex.

II. The classification of *Hughston* et al. [296] is based on the condition of the PCL, the "keystone of the knee joint." Hughston recognizes two major categories of instability: straight instabilities and rotatory instabilities. If the PCL is ruptured, Hughston claims that a rotatory instability cannot exist because loss of the PCL is tantamount to loss of the rotational center. Only a straight instability can exist in this situation, regardless of what associated structural lesions are present.

Hughston recognizes three types of rotatory instability: anteromedial, anterolateral, and posterolateral. He disputes the existence of posteromedial rotatory instability as a separate entity.

III. The classification of the French groups of *Trillat* (quoted in [470]) and *Bousquet* [60] is based on the loss of stability that is caused by the transection of specific ligaments (see Tables 3-17 through 3-32). Twenty (!) different instabilities – straight and complex – are identified according to the severity of the ligamentous injury [470]. For example, five different patterns of injury are each recognized for anteromedial and posterolateral instability (Tables 3-24 and 3-28).

We classify complex instabilities as anteromedial, anterolateral, posterolateral, or posteromedial and list the associated structures that are damaged:

I. *Anteromedial instability:* medial collateral ligament, medial capsular ligament, posteromedial capsule, ACL.
II. *Anterolateral instability:* arcuate complex, iliotibial tract, ACL.

III. *Posterolateral instability:* arcuate complex, PCL (ACL).
IV. *Posteromedial instability:* medial collateral ligament, medial capsular ligament, posteromedial capsule, PCL (ACL).

Tables 3-17 through 3-31 list the various patterns of injury, by author, that are associated with the four major categories of complex knee instability. This is not intended to create confusion or uncertainty, but to make the reader aware of current viewpoints and their diversity.

3.12
Isolated Ligament Ruptures

Given the close functional and anatomic ties that exist among the capsuloligamentous structures of the knee, the majority of injuries produce complex disruptions in which complete and partial ruptures coexist with stretch injuries of the capsule and ligaments.

Nevertheless, there continue to be reports of isolated ligamentous injuries (Table 3-13). This is especially true of the ACL, which deserves special attention owing to the significant pathomechanical consequences of its disruption [52, 318, 720].

3.12.1
Isolated ACL Rupture

Although the existence of this lesion was doubted for many years [388], today there is no longer any question that the ACL can be torn without concomitant injury to other structures. Numerous authors, including König in 1889 [369], have reported on isolated tears of this ligament [20, 52, 156, 157, 256, 257, 355, 445, 686, 709, 713].

Reportedly, isolated ruptures constitute from 7% [20] to 47% [8] of all ACL tears. Arnold et al. [20] reported a 65% incidence of ACL tears associated with damage to one or

Table 3-13. Knee ligaments in which isolated rupture is known to occur

1. Anterior cruciate ligament (ACL)
2. Posterior cruciate ligament (PCL)
3. Lateral collateral ligament
4. Medial collateral ligament
5. Posteromedial capsule

Table 3-14. Typical history of an ACL rupture

1. Loud pop in the knee joint at the time of injury.
2. Inability to continue previous activity.
3. Rapid development of posttraumatic effusion during the first 12 hours.
4. Mechanism of injury usually involves a direction change.

both menisci, although, strictly speaking, this cannot be classified as an isolated injury.

Bilateral ruptures of the ACLs has a reported overall incidence of 4%. The average interval between the initial and contralateral rupture is approximately four years. A cutting maneuver in noncontact sports is described as the most common mechanism of injury [615].

Patients with an ACL rupture frequently give a typical history (Table 3-14). Often a loud pop in the knee is heard and felt at the time of injury, although this is not specific for a tear of the ACL [159]. A pop may also be caused by a meniscal tear, patellar dislocation, entrapment of a loose body, or rupture of the patellar ligament. The patient cannot always relate the pop specifically to their injury.

If the examiner relies on the "typical" history of an ACL rupture, he is likely to miss some of these lesions. Thus, while an intraarticular effusion (hemarthrosis) is very often present during the first 24h, it need not be, as in the case where the rupture is covered and contained by synovium [256]. Neither do ruptures always result from a massive, "adequate" trauma, for even a "trivial" injury can produce an ACL tear [202]. The question of preexisting degenerative changes of the ACL can be an important one in cases of this kind [257]. Even patients with minimal trauma should be taken seriously, and they should not be excluded from conscientious laxity testing.

Even a "trivial" injury can cause rupture of the ACL.

In children or adolescents who have a positive Lachman test but have not sustained significant trauma, a congenital absence of the ACL should be considered (see Fig. 1-48). Most of these patients will have a positive anterior drawer test in 90° flexion [652].

Since the advent of arthroscopy, it is possible to diagnose even partial ruptures with complete confidence [13, 155, 202, 212]. Reports on the incidence of incomplete tears of the ACL range from 10% [158] to 28% [202, 492]. While these lesions are associated with hemarthrosis, like complete tears, a firm end point is felt in the Lachman test. Partial ruptures may occur in the posterolateral or anteromedial fibers of the ligament, each of which may be completely or partially involved.

The individual fibers of the ACL show opposite behaviors during drawer testing. When the posterolateral fibers are ruptured, the anterior drawer test will be negative at a large flexion angle but will become positive as the knee approaches extension. The pivot shift test likewise will be positive in that position. When the anteromedial fibers are torn, according to Müller [471], increased laxity is seen at large flexion angles, but stability is good at small flexion angles and in the pivot shift test. Other authors report that an isolated rupture of the posterolateral bundle is associated with a negative Lachman test and a positive anterior drawer test in 90° flexion [155]. Given the lack of consensus in this area, we feel that diagnostic arthroscopy should be performed in doubtful cases.

Table 3-15. Anterior displacement in mm (anterior drawer test in 90° flexion) resulting from isolated division of the ACL

2–6 mm	Hertel [278]
3.6 mm	Hertel [279]
1.9 mm	Furmann [191]
2.5 mm	Markolf [424]
1–3 mm	Bargar [28]
1.8 mm	Our investigations

By contrast, there is general agreement concerning the diagnosis of a complete rupture of the ACL. Little or no anterior displacement is elicited in 90° flexion, as shown by numerous experimental studies involving the selective division of the ACL (Table 3-15).

We have plotted our own experimental results in the form of a three-dimensional graph or "landscape" showing the characteristic displacement values produced by isolated transection of the ACL (Fig. 3-58).

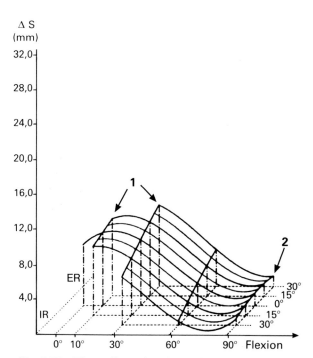

Fig. 3-58. Three-dimensional "landscape" caused by isolated division of the ACL (n = 9). Anterior drawer test was performed in 19 designated joint positions. Anterior displacement is maximal near extension *(1)* and is minimal (no more than 1.8 mm) in the traditional drawer test in 90° flexion *(2)*

1. Isolated complete or partial tears of the ACL are common.
2. The Lachman test is the most important test for evaluating the integrity of the ACL.

Remarkably, some ACL ruptures heal relatively well even when treated inadequately (e. g., by prolonged immobilization) or not at all. Feagin [158] suggests a possible explanation for this by noting that the torn ACL may fall down upon the PCL, where it gains a blood supply and a secondary point of attachment (see also Sect. 1.8.2.1).

An equivocal diagnosis in an apparently stable joint, followed by inadequate therapy such as plaster immobilization or a "well-intended" medial meniscectomy, can lead to complex joint pathology with serious functional consequences.

One important sequel to an isolated ACL rupture is stretching of the secondary ligamentous restraints, which must take over the stabilizing function of the torn ligament. Gradually, depending on the stresses imposed on the knee, a higher grade of pivot shift develops (grade III pivot shift), and a reversed pivot shift may eventually appear. This development poses a particular threat to the posterior horns of the menisci, with frequent anterior translations near extension leading to recurrent entrapment (positive Finochietto sign). If the ongoing trauma causes the meniscus to become nonfunctional or necessitates a meniscectomy, the extent of the anterior subluxation will increase, leading to cartilage erosion in both joint compartments. These developments are promoted by varus deformity, which also leads to global stretching of the lateral and posterolateral capsule and ligaments. The isolated ACL rupture can initiate a true syndrome of anterior and/or posterior complex knee instability [158, 244, 318, 405, 491, 492].

The foregoing sequence of events can vary greatly among different individuals and depends on the factors mentioned. The period in which a complex ligamentous lesion becomes manifest depends on knee loading, axial limb alignment (genu varum is unfavorable), and on the functional expectations and cooperativeness of the patient. If the posterior meniscal horns are destroyed and the patient continues to participate in sports without activity modification, it is imperative that he be counseled regarding the dismal prognosis for his knee joint.

3.12.2
Isolated PCL Rupture

Isolated PCL ruptures have a much lower incidence than the frequently reported isolated ACL tears [30, 402, 446, 515]. The resultant posterior displacement is maximal in 90° of flexion and becomes minimal as the knee approaches extension (Fig. 3-59; Table 3-16) [65, 189, 421, 493]. Again, this underscores the contrasting behaviors of the ACL and PCL. The relative stability of the joint at small flexion angles accounts for the remarkably mild complaints reported by patients with an isolated PCL injury. These patients rarely experience unsteadiness when walking, can easily perform their normal daily activities, and can even participate in sports without restriction [100, 515, 654]. Dejour [120] identifies three stages following an isolated lesion of the PCL.

The first stage, that of *"functional adaptation,"* lasts from 3 to 18 months. The patient experiences functional disability with pain and a feeling of instability that is especially noticeable during stair climbing. Younger patients and athletes with good muscular conditioning experience less instability and can resume their former activities within a relatively short time.

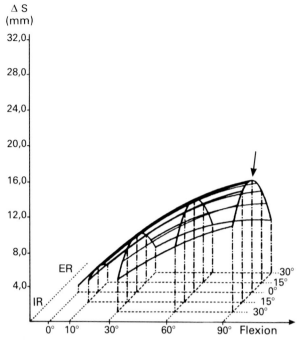

Fig. 3-59. Three-dimensional "landscape" caused by isolated division of the PCL (n = 6). Posterior drawer testing was performed in 19 designated joint positions. Posterior displacement is maximal in 90° flexion with the tibia in neutral rotation *(arrow)* and is not increased by internal or external rotation

In the second stage of *"functional tolerance,"* athletic participation is possible even at a very high level of performance. More than 80% of patients are subjectively satisfied with their knees, and 75% can perform the same kind of athletic activity as before their injury. However, about 50% of patients develop symptoms such as anterior knee pain (caused by excessive femoropatellar pressure with quadriceps contraction) during and after exercise, swelling of the joint, and a feeling of instability [120].

The third stage of *"arthrotic decompensation"* appears to be inevitable, although there is disagreement as to its time of onset and qualitative expression. Within 10 years approximately 30% of patients develop radiographic signs of osteoarthritis, especially in the medial, femorotibial, and femoropatellar compartments. The progression of this stage varies greatly among different individuals.

Table 3-16. Posterior displacement in mm (posterior drawer test in 90° flexion) following isolated division of the PCL

17 mm	McPhee [463]
18 mm	Fukubajashi et al. [189]
13–15 mm	Hertel and Schweiberer [278]
11 mm	Noyes [493]
10–15 mm	Dexel [126]
9.6 mm	Ogata [504]
10.0 mm	Nielsen [484]
15.0 mm	Gollehon [216]
11.4 mm	Grood [225]
10–13 mm	Our investigations

If the PCL lesion coexists with ACL insufficiency, a very pronounced feeling of instability will be experienced when the knee joint approaches extension.

The isolated PCL rupture has been described in the literature as a "simple posterior" instability [126], a "straight posterior" instability [296], and a "one-plane" instability [356, 470, 480].

3.12.3
Isolated Ruptures of the Collateral Ligaments

Isolated tears of the medial and lateral collateral ligaments do occur, but for anatomic and biomechanical reasons they are often combined with tears of the capsular ligaments and of posteromedial or posterolateral structures.

These injuries are easy to detect because the lateral collateral ligament can be easily palpated, and the continuity of the medial collateral ligament is evaluated in acute cases by valgus stress testing in slight flexion.

3.13
Straight Instabilities

3.13.1
Medial and Lateral Instability
(Tables 3-17 and 3-18)

Medial and lateral instability are diagnosed by determining the amount of medial and lateral joint opening, respectively. Hughston [296] states that a medial (or lateral) instability is present only if opening of the joint can be demonstrated with the knee in full extension. Andrews [13] states that varus-valgus testing should be performed in hyperextension, with more than 5 mm of opening on the medial side and more than 10 mm of lateral opening signifying a medial or lateral instability.

Table 3-17. Patterns of injury in medial instability

ACL	PCL	MCL	MCaL	PMC	PCa	Grade	Author
+		+	+	+	+		Nicholas [479]
	+	+	+	+			Hughston [296]
+		+	+	+	+1		
+	+	+	+	+	+1		Kennedy [356]
(+)	+	+					Andrews [13]
		+		+		I	
	(+)	+		+	+1	II	Müller [470]
		+	+			I	
(+)	(+)	+	+	+	2	II	Hackenbruch [234]

Note:
1 = Medial half of posterior capsule; 2 = oblique popliteal ligament

Legend:
ACL = anterior cruciate ligament; PCL = posterior cruciate ligament; MCL = medial collateral ligament; MCaL = medial capsular ligament; MMe = medial meniscus; PMC = posteromedial capsule (semimembranosus corner); Pop = popliteus muscle; ITT = iliotibial tract (iliotibial band, lateral femorotibial ligament); PCa = posterior capsule (oblique popliteal ligament); LCL = lateral collateral ligament; LCaL = lateral capsular ligament; APL = arcuate popliteal ligament; LMe = lateral meniscus; Bic = biceps femoris muscle

+ = injured/ruptured; (+) = possibly injured

Table 3-18. Patterns of injury in lateral instability (Legend see Table 3-17)

ACL	PCL	LCL	LCaL	APL	Pop	LMe	ITT	Bic	PCa	Grade	Author
		+				+					
+	(+)	+	+	+	+	+	+				Nicholas [479]
	+	(+)	+	+	+						Hughston [296]
+	(+)		+	+	+			+			Kennedy [356]
+	+		+	+	+						Andrews [13]
			+	+	+	+		+		I	
(+)	+		+	+	+	+	+	+	+	II	Müller [470]
		+	+			+				I	
(+)	(+)		+	+	+		+			II	Hackenbruch [234]

3.13.2
Anterior Instability (Tables 3-19 and 3-20)

The possible difficulties of accurately distinguishing between anterior and posterior drawer components are illustrated by classification of straight anterior instability [296]. With a rupture of the PCL, there should be equal anterior displacement of both tibial condyles with no rotation. In reality an "anterior drawer" is detected in this situation, but one should be careful about calling it such for actually it represents anterior displacement of the tibia from an initially posterior sagging position (spontaneous posterior drawer).

Table 3-19. Patterns of injury in anterior instability. (Legend see Table 3-17)

ACL	PCL	MCL	MCaL	PMC	LCL	LCaL	APL	Pop	LMe	ITT	PCa	Grade	Author
+												I	
	+	+		+								II	
+	+	+		+								III	Nicholas [479]
		+											Hughston [296]
+		+		+									Kennedy [356]
+		+	+	+								I	
+		+	+	+			(+)	(+)		+	(+)	II	Müller [470]
+			+						+				
+			+			+	+	+	+				
+	+		+		+								Andrews [13]
+		+	+		+		+				+		Hackenbruch [234]

Table 3-20. Diagnosis of anterior instability

ADT			LMT	PST	PDT	VGT		VRT		RCT	Author
IR	NR	ER			ER	Ex	Fl	Ex	Fl	C/T	
	×										Hughston [296]
	×										Kennedy [356]
		+									
+	++	+++	+			+		(+)		+	
++	++	+++	+	+			(+)		(+)	+	Müller [470]
×1	×	×									Andrews [13]
	×			×	×						Hackenbruch [234]

Note:
1. Characteristic test for straight anterior instability (13)

Legend:
ADT = anterior drawer test   PDT = posterior drawer test
LMT = Lachman test   PST = pivot shift test
VGT = valgus test   VRT = varus test
RCT = recurvatum test
IR = internal, NR = neutral, ER = external rotation
+ ++ +++ = 1+, 2+, 3+ instability
( ) = may be positive
− = negative test mandatory
× = positive

3.13.3 Posterior Instability
(Tables 3-21 and 3-22)

3.14 Complex Instabilities (Rotatory Instabilities)

The definition of rotatory instabilities requires some clarification due to inconsistencies in the literature. The initial description of Slocum and Larsen [605, 606] characterizes rotatory instability as an excessive ability of the tibia to rotate in relation to the femur (abnormally increased mobility about a vertical axis) when the joint is tested in 90° flexion and external

Table 3-21. Patterns of injury in posterior instability. (Legend see Table 3-17)

ACL	PCL	MCL	MCaL	LCL	LCaL	APL	Pop	LMe	PCa	Author
+										
	+									
+	+									Nicholas [479]
	+		(+)	(+)	(+)	(+)	(+)			Hughston [296]
(+)			+	+	+	+	+			Kennedy [356]
	+									
	+				+	+	+	+		Müller [470]
	+									Andrews [13]
+	+	+			+	+				Hackenbruch [234]

Table 3-22. Diagnosis of posterior instability. (Legend see Table 3-20)

ADT	PDT			VGT		VRT		RCT	Author
ER	IR	NR	ER	Ex	Fl	Ex	Fl	C/T	
		×							Hughston [296]
		×							Kennedy [356]
		+	+				(+)		
(+)	++	+++	+++		(+)		(+)	+	Müller [470]
		×							Andrews [13]
		×							Hackenbruch [234]

rotation. But injuries that produce rotatory instability can not only change the magnitude of the rotation but can also shift its axis, as Nicholas [479], Müller [470], and others have pointed out. It should be added, however, that both the range of rotation and the location of the rotational axis depend on the angle of knee flexion in the intact knee and especially in the injured joint. Accordingly, the flexion angle should be taken into account when a rotatory instability is defined.

If we combine the rotational behavior of the knee (movements around the degrees of rotational freedom, see Fig. 3-1) in the intact knee with the movements on the translational planes, *three* types of motion are possible in theory:

1. *Increased rotation (= rotatory instability).* This refers to increased mobility about the three axes of rotation. There is no associated translation of the tibia (see Fig. 12-2).

2. *Increased translation (= translatory instability).* This implies equal anterior or posterior translation of the medial and lateral tibial condyles on the plane of translation (see Figs. 12-3 and 12-4). We question the existence of a pure translational instability in the knee, because the primary stabilizers against translation, the ACL and PCL, also play a significant role in rotational stabilization. A cruciate ligament rupture, then, will lead to unequal translations of the tibial condyles.

3. *Combination of increased translation and increased rotation (complex instability).* In this case the medial tibial plateau undergoes a greater or less anterior displacement than the lateral plateau (see Figs. 12-5 and 12-6). This condition always combines at least one translational movement with at least one movement in rotation.

It should be emphasized that the extent of the rotation and translation depend on the condition of the capsule and ligaments, the angle of knee flexion, the rotational position of the tibia, and the applied force. In view of the complex function of each ligamentous structure,

which varies with the position of flexion and tibial rotation, it is conceivable that, even clinically, an injury may behave as an anterior translation with a external or internal rotation (coupled displacement) (see Figs. 12-5, 12-6 and 12-7) depending on the position (flexion, rotation) in which the examination is performed. Our own experience confirms this [636].

Our definition of rotatory, translatory, and complex instabilities, see Table 3-23.

A complex instability is defined as one in which joint motion is abnormally increased on at least two planes or axes. This is illustrated by the isolated ACL rupture, which produces anterior displacement in the slightly flexed knee (Lachman test) and also a positive pivot shift in which the lateral tibial plateau undergoes a greater anterior displacement than the medial plateau (anterior translation of the lateral compartment greater than anterior translation of the medial compartment). Our own studies of anteromedial instability confirm this, indicating that a complex anteromedial instability is demonstrated at large flexion angles whereas a complex anterolateral instability is demonstrated in the slightly flexed knee (with the lateral tibial plateau moving farther anteriorly than the medial plateau) [636].

While the various classifications and definitions have pathomechanical importance and are of great scientific interest, they are difficult to apply clinically because manual methods of examination do not permit a sufficiently differentiated evaluation of the complex biologic system in all joint positions with the laxity parameters satisfactorily defined (see Table 3-3). This could be accomplished only by applying costly machine methods of evaluation. We therefore prefer to classify complex instabilities on the basis of anatomic criteria.

Table 3-23. Definition of rotatory, translatory and complex instabilities

I.   *Rotatory instability*
      Increased rotation with no increase in translation
      (Instability on one axis)
      Medial instability
            positive valgus test
      Lateral instability
            positive varus test
      Internal rotatory instability
            increased internal rotation
      External rotatory instability
            increased external rotation

II.   *Translatory instability*
      Increased translation with no increase of rotation
      (Instability on one plane)
      Anterior instability
            positive anterior translation
      Posterior instability
            positive posterior translation
      Medial instability
            positive medial translation
      Lateral instability
            positive lateral translation

III. *Complex instability*
      Increased translation and increased rotation
      (Instability on one or more planes and one or more axis)
      Anteromedial instability
            positive anterior translation and
            positive valgus test
            increased external rotation possible
      Anterolateral instability
            positive anterior translation and
            positive varus test
            increased internal rotation possible
      Posterolateral instability
            positive posterior translation and
            positive varus test
            increased external rotation possible
      Posteromedial instability
            positive posterior translation and
            positive valgus test
            increased internal rotation possible

3.14.1
Anteromedial Instability
(Tables 3-24 and 3-25)

Valgus testing demonstrates positive medial opening of the joint in 30° flexion and little or no medial opening in extension. The characteristic features of the anterior drawer test are revealed by our experimental studies involving selective division of the anatomic structures (Fig. 3-60).

O'Donoghue [502, 503] coined the term "unhappy triad" to describe a combined injury to the medial meniscus, medial collateral liga-

Table 3-24. Patterns of injury in anteromedial instability. (Legend see Table 3-17)

ACL	MCL	MCaL	MMe	PMC	ITT	PCa	Grade	Author
+	+	+	+	+		+		Nicholas [479]
(+)	+	+		+				Hughston [296]
+	+	+		+				Kennedy [356]
				+			Monad	
	+			+			Duad A	
+	+						Duad B	
+	+			+			Triad	
+	+			+	+		Tetrad	Müller [470]
	+	+		+				
+	+	+		+				Andrews [13]
+	+	+	+	+		+1		Hackenbruch [234]

Note:
1 = Oblique popliteal ligament

Table 3-25. Diagnosis of anteromedial instability (Legend see Table 3-20)

ADT			LMT	PST	VGT		RCT	Grade	Author
IR	NR	ER			Ex	Fl			
		×				×			Hughston [296]
		+						Monad	
		+				+		Duad A	
	+	+ +				(+)		Duad B	
	+ +	+ + +				+ +		Triad	
+	+ +	+ + +		×		+ +	(+)	Tetrad	Müller [470]
−		×			−	×			Andrews [13]
		×	×	×					Hackenbruch [234]

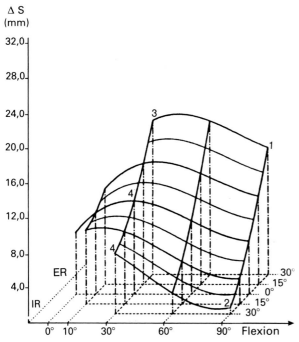

Fig. 3-60. "Landscape" of anteromedial instability on anterior drawer testing. The medial capsular ligament, medial collateral ligament, posteromedial capsule, and ACL were divided (n = 9),

Anterior displacement: *1* Markedly positive in 90° flexion and external rotation. *2* Minimal in 90° flexion and internal rotation (pronounced compensation of laxity in 90° flexion). *3* Most strongly positive in 30° flexion and external rotation. *4* Markedly positive in 30° flexion in neutral and internal rotation

Table 3-26. Patterns of injury in anterolateral instability. (Legend see Table 3-17)

A C L	L C L	L Ca L	A P L	P o p	L M e	I T T	Grade	Author
+	+	+	+	+	(+)	+		Nicholas [479]
(+)	+							Hughston [296]
+	+	+	+	+			I	
+	+						II	Kennedy [356]
						+	Monad	
+						+	Duad	
+	+					+	Triad	Müller [470]
+	+	+				+		Andrews [13]
+	+	+	+	+		+		Hackenbruch [234]

Table 3-27. Diagnosis of anterolateral instability (Legend see Table 3-20)

ADT			VRT			
IR	NR	PST	Ex	Fl	Grade	Author
	+		(+)			Hughston [296]
+	+					Kennedy [356]
+					Monad	
+	+	×			Duad	
+ +	+	×		+	Triad	Müller [470]
−		×				Andrews [13]
×		×		×		Hackenbruch [234]

ment, and ACL. This injury forms a subgroup of the complete anteromedial instability (Fig. 3-60). However, this term disregards the posteromedial capsule with the posterior oblique ligament, one of the most important stabilizing structures of the medial and posteromedial side and one that is frequently involved in this type of injury.

3.14.2
Anterolateral Instability
(Tables 3-26 and 3-27)

Laxity testing demonstrates a positive pivot shift as long as the iliotibial tract (iliotibial band) is intact, a positive Lachman test, and sometimes a positive anterior drawer test in 90° flexion and neutral rotation if the ACL is

damaged. If the iliotibial band and PCL are intact, the anterior drawer test will be negative in internal rotation due to the restraining action of the twisted PCL [13]. If the lateral structures are injured, the varus test (lateral opening) will be positive in 30° flexion and also in extension if the posterolateral structures are ruptured. Marked lateral opening in extension can occur only if the PCL is also torn.

Some authors distinguish anterolateral rotatory instability detected in slight flexion from that detected in higher degrees of flexion [178, 466].

3.14.3
Posterolateral Instability
(Tables 3-28 and 3-29)

Our three-dimensional graph of posterolateral instability (Fig. 3-61) indicates drawer features similar to those seen in anteromedial instabili-

Table 3-28. Patterns of injury in posterolateral instability. (Legend see Table 3-17)

A C L	P C L	L Ca L	L L L	A P L	PL o p	L M e	I T T	P C a	Grade	Author
	+ +		+	+		+				Nicholas [479]
		+	+	+	+					Hughston [296]
+	(+)+		+	+	+					Kennedy [356]
			+		+	+			Monad	
	+		+		+	+			Duad A	
	+		+		+	+			Duad B	
	+ +		+		+	+			Triad	
+	+		+	+		+		+	Tetrad	Müller [470]
(+)	+	+	+	+				+		Holz [288]
	+	+	+	+	(+)		(+)			Hackenbruch [234]

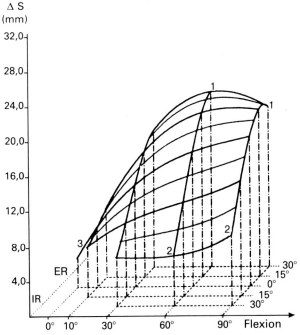

Fig. 3-61. "Landscape" of posterolateral instability on posterior drawer testing. The arcuate complex and PCL were divided (n = 7),
Posterior displacement: *1* Marked in 60° and 90° flexion and external rotation. *2* Less marked in 60° and 90° flexion and internal rotation (compensation of displacement not complete as in anteromedial instability; see Fig. 3-60), *3* Minimal in slight flexion

ty (Fig. 3-60). The greatest posterior displacement is found in external tibial rotation, while displacement becomes minimal in internal rotation. Thus, on superficial examination without differentiated drawer testing, it is quite possible to confuse posterolateral and anteromedial instability. Similar displacement values were demonstrated by Gollehon [216], Grood [225], and Nielsen [484] following division of the PCL and the posterolateral structures.

3.14.4
Posteromedial Instability
(Tables 3-30 and 3-31) (Fig. 3-62)

Posterolateral and especially posteromedial instability are special forms caused by damage to the PCL. The resulting, gross posterior displacement (15–30 mm) prompted Hughston et al. [296] to describe the injury as a "dislocated knee." Müller [470] also gives attention to this phenomenon, referring to posterolateral and posteromedial instability as a "special entity among the rotatory instabilities."

Combined instabilities also occur, but they are not discussed separately because of their com-

Table 3-29. Diagnosis of posterolateral instability (Legend see Table 3-20)

ADT	PDT			VGT	VRT				
ER	IR	NR	ER	Ex Fl	Ex Fl	RCT	Grade	Author
				×		ERT		Hughston [296]
			+				Monad	
			+ +		+		Duad A	
		+	+ +		+		Duad B	
		+ +	+ + +		+ +		Triad	
(+)	+ +	+ + +	+ + +	(+)	+ + +	+	Tetrad	Müller [470]
			(1)		+	+		Hackenbruch [234]

Note:
ERT = External rotation recurvatum test; 1 = Reversed pivot shift possible

Table 3-30. Patterns of injury in posteromedial instability. (Legend see Table 3-17)

ACL	PCL	MCL	MCaL	PMC	PCa	Author
	+	+	+	+	+	Nicholas [479]
+		+	+	+	+	Kennedy [356]
+	+	+		+		Müller [470]
(+)	+	+	+	+	+	Holz [288]
	+	+	+	+	+	Hackenbruch [234]

Table 3-31. Diagnosis of posteromedial instability

ADT	PDT			VGT		
ER	IR	NR	ER	Ex	Fl	Author
+	+	+		+		Dexel [126]
+	+	+		+	+	Müller [470]
		×		×		Hackenbruch [234]

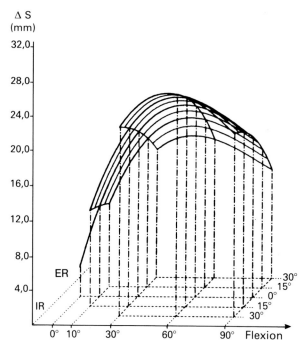

Fig. 3-62. "Landscape" of posteromedial instability on posterior drawer testing. The medial collateral ligament, medial capsular ligament, posteromedial capsule, and PCL were divided (n = 7),
Posterior displacement: Very marked in 30°, 60°, and 90° flexion and internal rotation. Slightly less marked in 30°, 60°, and 90° flexion and external rotation (no compensation of displacement, see Figs. 3-60 and 3-61)

plexity (Table 3-12). They represent combinations of the injury patterns associated with their constituent instabilities.

3.15 Conclusion

Diagnostic evaluation of the injured knee should not be directed primarily toward classification of the type of instability.

The primary goal of the examination of the capsule and ligaments is to identify the structures that are injured or deficient.

For example, we do not believe that "anteromedial instability of the knee" is an acceptable diagnosis. Instead, the structural lesions pro-

Table 3-32. Recommended procedures for the clinical evaluation of acute and chronic ligamentous injuries

Acute injury (painful)
1. Radiographic examination (no bony injury)
2. Exclude PCL lesion (posterior sag?)
   90° active quadriceps test (positive = PCL lesion)
3. Lachman test (ACL lesion)
4. Active tests (active Lachman test, 90° active quadriceps test, etc.)
5. Pivot shift test often false-negative without anesthesia (due to pain)
6. Anterior drawer test often false-negative in 90° flexion (due to pain)
7. Medial and lateral opening (in extension and 20° flexion)
8. Effusion? (Aspirate if Lachman test is equivocal)

Chronic or acute injury (nonpainful)
1. Radiographic examination (in acute injuries)
2. Active laxity tests (have patient demonstrate subluxation?)
3. Check for posterior sag in 60°–90° flexion (exclude PCL lesion)
4. Lachman test
5. Pivot shift test (e.g., soft pivot shift test)
6. Medial and lateral opening (in extension and 20° flexion)
7. 90° anterior drawer test in internal, neutral, and external rotation
8. 90° posterior drawer test in internal, neutral, and external rotation
9. Function tests (deceleration test, giving way test, hop test)

duced by the injury should be identified as accurately as possible, as illustrated by this example: "Fresh complete rupture of the ACL with rupture of the medial and posteromedial capsule, peripheral detachment of the medial meniscus (anteromedial instability), and a suspected lesion of the lateral meniscus."

In chronic instabilities, correspondingly greater time and effort are needed to formulate an accurate diagnosis specifying the anatomic structures that are injured or deficient [235].

The procedures outlined in Table 3-32 are recommended for the diagnostic evaluation of acute and chronic ligamentous knee injuries.

4
Evaluation of the Menisci

Lesions of the menisci can have numerous causes and rank among the most common injuries of the knee joint.

Meniscal lesions are not a product of the industrial age, as indicated by the fact that lay practitioners in England ("bone setters") were reducing displaced menisci as early as 1630 [673].

In 1731, Bass, in his publication "Cartilago tibiae semilunaris elongata locoque sua paulum emota," described the reduction of two displaced menisci. The swollen and softened lateral meniscus, which protruded from the lateral joint space, was reduced by digital pressure (after [72]).

William Bromfield (1773) was the first to publish a detailed account of the therapeutic reduction of displaced menisci [673]. In one case he reduced the meniscus more or less incidentally as he examined the joint while his assistant simultaneously pulled on the foot and slightly flexed the knee. This maneuver caused the meniscus to slip back to its original position. The patient, who had sought treatment for severe knee pain and swelling, experienced immediate relief.

Hey (1803), who introduced the term "internal derangement of the knee," accurately described the clinical features of meniscal entrapment and recounted a reduction maneuver consisting of forced extension and subsequent flexion of the knee joint.

The surgical treatment of meniscal lesions was first attempted by Bradhurst in 1867. By 1885, Annadale was able to report on five successfully performed meniscal operations (after [724]). The first comprehensive treatise on meniscal problems was published in 1892 by Bruns, who summarized contemporary knowledge and also reported on 24 of his own meniscal operations.

Meniscal lesions can result from minor trauma such as stumbles, slips and slight falls, but they are more typically caused by a rotational stress on the weight-bearing knee. Tears in degenerative menisci are most common in older patients and individuals who engage in certain types of occupational or athletic activity. Axial limb deformities can also cause premature tissue degeneration that predisposes to meniscal tears [570, 376, 724].

In all meniscal injuries it should be determined whether the lesion has been caused by a specific, adequate trauma or is a result of chronic stress. For example, if the patient has worked mostly in a crouched position for a long period of time (e. g., a mine worker), the lesion may result from sustained pressure on the meniscal tissue (occupational disease).

The only way to positively differentiate between a traumatic and degenerative etiology is by direct histologic examination. Thus, a meniscal specimen should be obtained for histologic study whenever an open or arthroscopic partial meniscectomy is performed. If the meniscal lesion results from an inadequate trauma, such as rising from a squatting position, degenerative changes are usually present.

Meniscal tears commonly occur in association with capsuloligamentous injuries and especially with chronic and acute ACL lesions [86]. These patients require a particularly careful and thorough diagnostic workup, and if at all possible they should be managed by a meniscus-conserving therapy. If this is not possible, only the injured or degenerated portion of the meniscus should be removed arthroscopically (partial meniscectomy). Even a small peripheral remnant, especially in the posterior horn area of the medial meniscus, will provide an important stabilizing factor against anterior tibial displacement. The lateral meniscus is considered to be of less importance as a purely mechanical stabilizer [392]. The posterior horns of the menisci have also been found to contain a high concentration of proprioceptors, giving them an additional role in the mediation of protective muscular reflexes (see Sect. 1.8).

4.1
Classification

Tears of the menisci are classified according to their shape (longitudinal, bucket handle, horizontal, radial, etc.) and their location (anterior horn, central, peripheral, etc.). The type, location, and extent of the tear should be accurately defined as a prelude to further treatment planning.

The following three main types of tear are recognized:

1. *Longitudinal tear:* This tear runs parallel to the longitudinal fiber structure of the meniscus and may be oriented at right angles or obliquely to the meniscal plane. Complete longitudinal tears involve the full thickness of the meniscus, while incomplete tears are visible only from the superior or inferior surface.

   The exact location of a longitudinal tear is important in terms of treatment selection. For example, a fresh (no more than four weeks old) peripheral longitudinal tear can be arthroscopically repaired owing to the excellent healing potential in the vascular zone [19]. A small, peripheral, posterior longitudinal tear (smaller than 1 cm) can heal well with conservative treatment once the exact nature of the lesion has been established by arthroscopy; four to six weeks' immobilization should be sufficient for healing to occur [465]. A tear on the lateral side extending forward through the popliteal hiatus or a medial tear extending past the central portion of the meniscus cannot be adequately managed by conservative therapy alone. In these cases immobilization should be combined with arthroscopic repair involving the placement of two or three U-sutures to ensure accurate reapproximation of the torn edges.

   For older degenerative tears, partial meniscectomy is the procedure of choice and is preferred, where feasible, over a total or subtotal excision.

2. *Horizontal tear:* This consists of a horizontal split on the plane of the meniscus. The extent of the tear is often difficult to ascertain.

3. *Radial tear:* This lesion extends from the free edge of the meniscus toward the periphery, either reaching it or terminating a variable distance from the convex margin.

Almost all meniscal lesions develop from these three main types and are encountered with varying frequency (Table 4-1). A longitudinal tear developing in the critical load-bearing zone (Fig. 4-1) and extending anteriorly can progress to a bucket handle tear, which in time can progress to a pedunculated tear as the midportion of the bucket handle wears through [668]. Whether the pedunculated flap has an anterior or posterior attachment depends on the point at which the longitudinal tear becomes disrupted (Fig. 4-2). Meniscal flaps can also result from the posterior longitudinal extension of a radial tear along the course of the meniscal fibers.

Given the many functions of the menisci, the indication for meniscectomy should be weighed with caution. Numerous studies have documented the significant role of meniscecto-

Table 4-1. Distribution of arthroscopically diagnosed meniscal lesions (n = 1650) in percent (after Löhnert [400])

Lesion	Medial	Lateral	Total
Bucket handle/vertical tear	19.6	3.7	23.3
Radial tear	8.7	7.0	15.5
Horizontal tear	1.6	0.8	2.4
Flap tear	27.1	6.1	33.2
Complex tears	2.9	1.0	3.9
Degenerative lesions	13.0	8.5	21.5
Discoid meniscus	–	0.2	0.2
	72.7	27.3	100.0

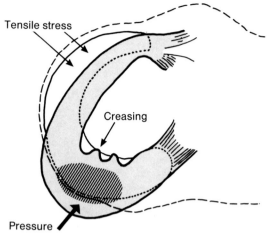

Fig. 4-1. Posterior displacement of the medial meniscus and critical stress zones during flexion of the knee. Peripheral detachment of the meniscus can occur in its anterior portions, and a flap tear may be initiated in the posterior horn (after Zippel [724])

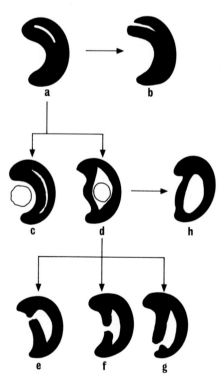

Fig. 4-2a–h. Patterns of progression of a posterior longitudinal meniscal tear *(a)*. The tear may reach the posterior edge of the meniscus, forming a flap *(b)*, or it may extend anteriorly to form a large longitudinal tear *(c)* or a bucket handle *(d)*. The latter may separate at various sites to produce an anteriorly based flap *(e)*, two flaps *(f)*, or a posteriorly based flap *(g)*. In other cases the inner fragment may not rupture and will persist as a bucket handle tear *(h)* (after Trillat [668]),

my in the promotion of osteoarthritic changes (Table 4-2) [27, 175, 263, 333, 470, 549, 685, 724].

Experimental studies prove that meniscectomy decreases the area of tibiofemoral contact and thus aggravates the lack of congruity between the articular surfaces. Hehne [263] measured a 12% decrease in contact area after partial meniscectomy and a 46% decrease after subtotal meniscectomy. Numerous studies and clinical observations confirm the significantly lower incidence of osteoarthritis after partial meniscectomy [263, 579], which therefore has become the preferred operation.

A number of authors have called attention to the eminently important stabilizing function of the posterior horn of the medial meniscus in patients with ACL insufficiency [27, 234, 466, 470]. As a result of meniscectomy, the instability can easily progress from a compensated to a decompensated stage. This is demonstrated by the stress experiments of Wang [685] in cadaver specimens showing the potentiating effect of double meniscectomy and ACL section on knee laxity. In patients with ACL insufficiency, this provides a new rationale for considering ACL reconstruction following a necessary meniscectomy [657].

Post-meniscectomy degenerative changes can occur in older as well as younger patients [7, 333]. Schultz et al. [582] and Abdon et al. [2] found clinical and radiologic evidence of pronounced degenerative changes in patients who had undergone a total meniscectomy in childhood or adolescence (Fig. 4-3).

Table 4-2. Factors promoting osteoarthritis after meniscectomy

1. Long interval between injury and operation
2. Coexisting ligament instabilities
3. Preexisting chondromalacia and osteoarthritis
4. Postoperative hemarthrosis
5. Total meniscectomy
6. Recurrent effusion
7. Axial deformity (e.g., genu valgum, genu varum)

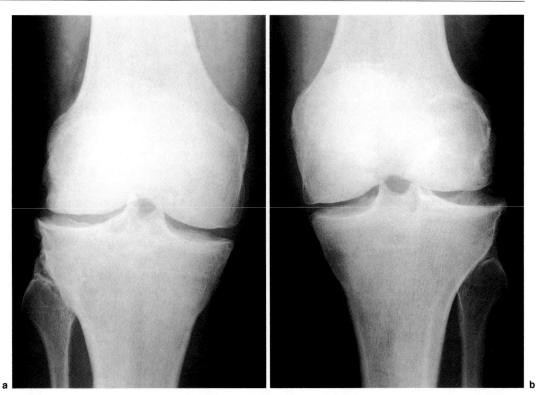

Fig. 4-3a, b. Radiographic findings in a 34-year-old woman with moderate clinical complaints (periodic swelling, pain after walking 1h) who had undergone total lateral meniscectomies in both knees *(!)* 17 years earlier. Marked degenerative changes are apparent in the lateral portions of the joints

4.2 Symptoms

One of the most common symptoms of a meniscal injury is a painful loss of extension, which may develop immediately after the trauma or may occur intermittently at varying intervals.

The blocking effect is usually caused by the entrapment of a torn piece of meniscus (bucket handle or pedunculated flap) between the femoral and tibial articular surfaces, though less frequently it may result from posttraumatic pain and muscle spasm.

The degree of the extension deficit is not proportional to the extent of the tear, so a knee with very little extension loss requires particularly careful examination. A bucket handle tear that extends into the anterior horn allowing displacement of the fragment into the intercondylar fossa will produce very little loss of extension. On the other hand, a profound extension loss (50°–60°) is often seen with a relatively small tear that is confined to the posterior third of the meniscus or extends from the posterior horn of the meniscus to its central portion.

Acute posttraumatic locking can sometimes be relieved by simple passive manipulation of the joint through its range of motion. But if a springy resistance persists, reduction of the entrapped meniscus is required.

All meniscal lesions, whether chronic or acute, require differentiation from various other lesions (Tables 4-3 and 4-4). When an acute extension loss is noted, there are a variety of other diseases and injuries that may be responsible (see Table 2-17).

Table 4-3. Differential diagnosis of an acute meniscal injury

1. Ligamentous injury
2. Sprained or partially ruptured medial collateral ligament
3. Tear of the ACL
4. Patellar dislocation (reduced)
5. Loose body
6. Osteochondral fractures
7. Fractures

Table 4-4. Differential diagnosis of an old meniscal lesion

1. Patellar chondromalacia
2. Chronic ligamentous instability
3. Femorotibial osteoarthritis
4. Synovitis
5. Loose body
6. Plica syndrome
7. Hypertrophic villus in infrapatellar fat pad
8. Meniscal cyst
9. Medial collateral ligament bursitis
10. Saphenous nerve syndrome
11. Discoid meniscus
12. Reflex sympathetic dystrophy

4.3
Discoid Meniscus and Meniscal Cysts

Discoid menisci and meniscal cysts, though rarely encountered, should be familiar to the examiner.

4.3.1
Discoid Meniscus

Developmental errors involving a disturbance in the formation or subsequent differentiation of the rudimentary menisci with a failure of absorption of the central part of the disc can lead to the persistence of a discoid meniscus in postnatal life. This condition is sometimes associated with other anomalies such as elevation of the fibular head, muscular defects, or peroneal tendon displacement (after [724]).

The lateral meniscus is more commonly affected [130, 277, 693, 708]. The reported incidence of discoid lateral meniscus ranges from 1.5 to 2.5% [724] (see Fig. 11-64).

Watanabe [693] distinguishes a complete, incomplete, and Wrisberg-ligament type (WLT) of discoid meniscus. The WLT meniscus lacks adequate posterior fixation, the posterior horn of the lateral meniscus being attached only to the posterior meniscofemoral ligament (Wrisberg ligament). The discoid meniscus does not displace during flexion of the knee, but during extension the Wrisberg ligament tightens and pulls the meniscus posteromedially toward the cruciate ligaments. This is accompanied by the snapping sound that is characteristic of this type of discoid meniscus. In cases where the anterior and posterior meniscotibial attachments are present, tensile and shear stresses develop in the posterior part of the discoid meniscus, just anterior to the popliteal hiatus, resulting in an increased risk of tearing in that zone. The characteristic snapping sound is believed to be less common with this "complete" type of discoid meniscus [130]. The treatment of choice is partial meniscectomy which leaves behind a stable residual base [37, 130, 277]. With a WLT meniscus, there is a danger that partial meniscectomy will leave a hypermobile posterior remnant, so total meniscectomy has been recommended for that type [130]. However, we would still advise a primary partial resection even for a WLT discoid meniscus. If complaints persist after this procedure, a total meniscectomy or saucerization with refixation can be performed arthroscopically at a later time.

4.3.2
Meniscal Cysts

Meniscal cysts result from a mucoid degeneration of the meniscal tissue. Masses detected on the joint line of the knee require differentiation from tumors such as synovial hemangiomas, gout tophi (see Fig. 2-12b), or even malignant neoplasms [670]. Cysts of the lateral meniscus are more common than those of the medial meniscus, predominating by about a 7:1 ratio. Most occur in or on the base of the meniscus. Approximately 50% of cysts coexist with a meniscal tear, which not infrequently is responsible for the clinical symptoms (lateral meniscal symptoms). In addition to pain and local swelling over the lateral joint line (see Fig. 2-12), radiographic changes may also be apparent with meniscal cysts. The cyst may erode a small depression on the lateral aspect of the lateral or medial tibial plateau just distal to the joint space (see Fig. 6-10a).

4.4
Meniscus Tests

The many tests that have been described for the diagnosis of meniscal pathology (Table 4-5) aid the examiner in differentiating these lesions from other types of knee injury. Positive tests confirm the suspicion of a meniscal lesion. However, negative tests do not rule out a tear with absolute confidence. According to Zippel [724], the accuracy rate of the clinical examination in the diagnosis of meniscal lesions is 60%–95%.

Studies on the diagnostic value of meniscus tests show that the major clinical signs are not very helpful when considered in isolation (sensitivity: medial joint line tenderness 74%, Apley grinding test 46%, painful hyperextension 43%, Steinmann I sign 42%, McMurray test 35% [627]). These rates are improved, however, when multiple signs are considered. According to studies by Steinbrück [627], tests with a high sensitivity for detecting lesions of

Table 4-5. Meniscus tests

1. Joint line tenderness
2. Hyperflexion and hyperextension
3. Medial and lateral tibial translation
4. Steinmann I sign
5. Steinmann II sign
6. Payr's sign
7. Böhler's sign
8. Krömer's sign
9. Bragard's sign
10. Merke's sign
11. McMurray test
12. Fouche's sign
13. Childress' sign
14. Apley grinding test
15. Medial-lateral grinding test
16. Rotational grinding test
17. Cabot's sign
18. Turner's sign
19. Tschaklin's sign
20. Finochietto's sign

the medial meniscus also yield a high rate of false-positive results. This uncertainty is compounded by the fact that symptoms of a lateral meniscal tear or a retropatellar cartilage lesion are often projected to the medial side. We therefore feel that a meniscal repair or meniscectomy should not be performed until the lesion has been definitively confirmed and localized by arthroscopy, even if only arthrotomic treatment is possible. This eliminates arthrotomy of the "wrong" compartment.

The most important principle in the clinical evaluation of the menisci is adherence to a standard battery of well-known tests. This is the best overall strategy for increasing the accuracy of diagnosis [550].

Accordingly, the examiner should select three to five tests from the many that are available (Table 4-5) and practice them routinely in every knee examination. There is no reason to perform all of the tests described in this section. Our routine workup consists of joint line tenderness, a modified McMurray test, and the Steinmann signs.

Some patients will be found to have no meniscal signs despite a positive history. It may be helpful in these cases to have the patient perform several deep knee bends. This exercise loosens the capsule and ligaments a little and makes the menisci somewhat more mobile so that positive tests can be more easily elicited.

To understand the meniscus tests, it is important to know how the menisci move during flexion and extension of the knee. As the knee flexes, the menisci move posteriorly (see Fig. 1-17). Almost all meniscus tests are based on the eliciting of pain or snapping by a force applied to the meniscus. This force may be applied directly by the digital pressure of the examiner, indirectly by external movements leading to compression or entrapment of the meniscus between the femur and tibia, or a combination of these (Fig. 4-4). In localizing the lesion, it is important to note the joint position (degree of flexion) in which the pain or snap is elicited, and at what point over the joint line (e. g., posteromedially) it occurs.

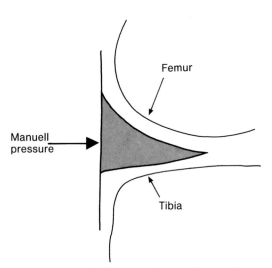

Fig. 4-4. Potential forces acting on the meniscus

4.4.1
Joint Line Tenderness

Tenderness along the joint line is one of the oldest, best-known, and most reliable signs of a meniscal lesion. The examiner tests for this sign by selectively palpating the medial and lateral joint line with the knee in various degrees of flexion. Local tenderness will be noted over the meniscal lesion in 60%–80% of cases.

Krömer [376] describes percussion of the joint line. The examiner places his fingertip over the most painful site and strikes the finger sharply with the middle finger of the other hand, as in percussion of the chest.

It is not unusual to palpate an abnormal resistance in the joint line or even a localized protrusion that may represent a displaced meniscal flap or a meniscus cyst.

4.4.2
Hyperflexion and Hyperextension

In maximum extension the anterior horns of the menisci pass directly between the femur and tibia (see Fig. 1-46). If there is a tear in the anterior horn, the patient will experience pain when maximum extension is attempted. If the resistance to extension feels springy, there may be a bucket handle tear or, less commonly, a pedunculated flap that has become displaced into the intercondylar fossa.

A painful flexion deficit noted on maximum passive flexion of the knee should raise suspicion of a posterior horn lesion.

4.4.3
Medial and Lateral Translation

Medial and lateral translation of the tibia are tested with the patient supine and the knee flexed 90°. To test medial or lateral translation, the examiner pushes the upper end of the tibia medially or laterally while applying resistance with the other hand positioned on the medial or lateral side of the thigh.

Pain during this test is an indication of meniscal pathology. On the other hand, excessive lateral translation of the proximal tibia implies a lesion of the PCL [706].

4.4.4
Steinmann I Sign

In this test pain is provoked by forced rotation of the tibia with the muscles relaxed and the knee in various degrees of flexion. If forced external rotation (internal rotation) evokes pain in the medial (lateral) joint line, an injury to the medial (lateral) meniscus is implied. The forced rotation moves the meniscus in a manner which stretches it anteriorly and compresses it posteriorly. Since tears can occur at various sites, the Steinmann I sign should be tested in various positions of knee flexion (Fig. 4-5).

4.4.5
Steinmann II Sign

Since the meniscus moves posteriorly during flexion, the location of joint line tenderness associated with a meniscal lesion also moves posteriorly with increasing flexion (Fig. 4-6).

When joint line tenderness is present, radiographic examination can exclude small osteoarthritic ridges and osteophytes on the tibial plateau (see Fig. 2-52). Failure of the tender point to move with flexion serves to differentiate this condition from a meniscal tear. It is more difficult to distinguish a meniscal lesion from an injury of the medial capsular ligament and/or medial collateral ligament. On valgus testing of the knee, pressure is removed from the medial meniscus (no pain) while the collateral ligament apparatus is made tense, causing the patient pain. Careful palpation will usually disclose local tenderness slightly proximal or distal to the joint line, corresponding to the origin or insertion of the medial capsular ligament.

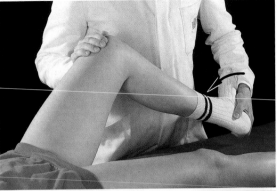
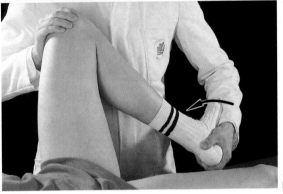

Fig. 4-5a, b. Steinmann I sign. The tibia is forcibly rotated externally with the knee slightly (**a**) and sharply flexed (**b**)

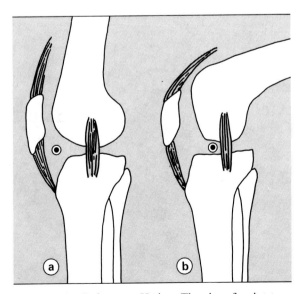

Fig. 4-6a, b. Steinmann II sign. The site of point tenderness (●) moves posteriorly as the knee moves from extension (**a**) to flexion (**b**)

4.4.6
Payr's Sign

With a lesion of the medial meniscus, a patient sitting in a cross-legged posture will experience pain in the medial joint line. The acute knee flexion in this position places considerable pressure on the middle and posterior portions of the meniscus. Pressure on the posterior horn is increased by pressing the knees toward the floor. Payr's test can also be performed with the patient supine (Fig. 4-7).

4.4.7
Böhler's Sign

Varus-valgus stress testing causes pressure to be exerted on the meniscus opposite to the side where the joint space opens. Thus, varus testing loads the medial meniscus while valgus testing loads the lateral meniscus (see Figs. 3-6 and 3-7).

4.4.8
Krömer's Sign

This is an expanded version of Böhler's test in which the knee joint is flexed and extended while a varus or valgus stress is maintained.

4.4.9
Bragard's Sign

This sign reveals tenderness along the anterior joint line. With a lesion of the medial meniscus, the tenderness is accentuated by external rotation and extension of the knee from a flexed position due to compression of the meniscus by the palpating finger. Conversely, internal rotation and increasing flexion of the knee causes the meniscus to recede into the joint, where it is inaccessible to pressure from the examiner's finger, so pain is reduced (Fig. 4-8).

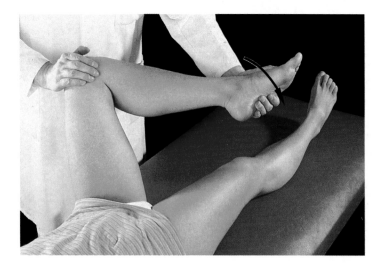

Fig. 4-7. Payr's sign in the supine patient

4.4.10
Merke's Sign

The patient stands on one foot and is told to rotate the knee externally and internally. As in the Steinmann I sign, this maneuver produces rotational movements of the tibia. Because of the increased axial compression imposed by the body weight, this test generally elicits more pain than the non-weight-bearing tests. Pain in the medial joint line on internal rotation of the thigh (=external rotation of the tibia) implies a lesion of the medial meniscus. Conversely, pain caused by external rotation of the thigh (=internal rotation of the tibia) is consistent with a lateral meniscal lesion. Occasionally the Merke sign is positive in patients with collateral ligament injuries.

4.4.11
McMurray Test

The patient lies supine on the examining table with the hip and knee acutely flexed so that the foot is firmly against the buttock. The examiner places one hand around the knee joint and palpates the joint line while securely holding the foot with the other hand. To test the medial meniscus, the examiner externally rotates the foot and, while holding it in that position, slowly extends the knee from maximum flexion. As the femur glides over a tear in the meniscus, there will be a palpable or even audible snap or click that is localized to the area of the joint line (Fig. 4-9). The lateral meniscus is tested analogously, i.e., by internally rotating the foot and then extending the knee. The

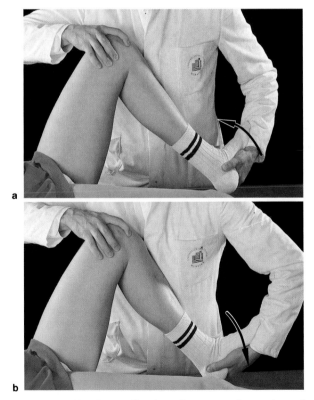
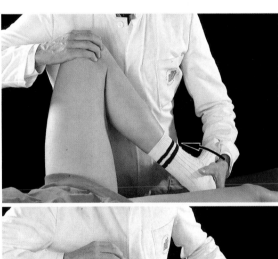
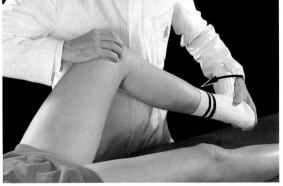

Fig. 4-8a, b. Bragard's sign. On external rotation of the tibia, the medial meniscus is compressed by the examiner's finger (**a**). On internal rotation (**b**) the meniscus can no longer be compressed

Fig. 4-9a, b. McMurray Test. The medial meniscus is tested by starting from a position of maximum flexion and external rotation (**a**) and extending the knee while keeping the tibia rotated (**b**). The "click" of the meniscus can often be amplified by moving the tibia in a circular fashion

location of the lesion can be determined with reasonable accuracy, because a posterior meniscal tear will produce a snap near maximal flexion, while snapping at about 90° suggests a tear of the central portion [724].

The snapping sign can be accentuated by moving the entire lower leg in a circular fashion *(modified McMurray test)*.

The McMurray test appears to be particularly well suited for detecting degenerative or long-standing meniscal lesions whose major symptom is a "snapping or catching sensation" rather than pain.

A positive McMurray test may be obtained in up to 30% of children with healthy knees [684] and in approximately 1% of the healthy population at large [151].

Some patients with a meniscus lesion are able to produce the snap of the McMurray test voluntarily by imitating the typical rotation and extension maneuver that is employed in the test *(active McMurray test)*.

4.4.12
Fouche's Sign

This test is like the McMurray test in that it begins with the patient supine and the hip and knee well flexed, but it is different in that, to test the medial meniscus, the tibia is rotated internally and held in that position while the knee is slowly extended. With a posterior horn lesion, the test will produce a palpable snap in the joint line. This occurs because the meniscus, which is fixed on the tibial plateau, moves anteriorly with increasing extension and almost catches between the femur and tibia before abruptly slipping back posteriorly, producing a snap. The lateral meniscus is tested with the tibia externally rotated. According to Zippel [724], a positive Fouche sign is almost pathognomonic for a meniscal tear.

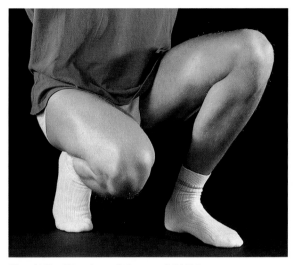

Fig. 4-10. "Duck walk" test of Childress

4.4.13
Childress' Sign

The patient assumes a squatting position with the heels touching the buttocks and is asked to perform a "duck walk" (Fig. 4-10). With a posterior horn lesion, the patient will feel a painful snap or click just before reaching maximum flexion or in the early phase of extension. This is caused by the entrapment of the torn meniscus. Patients experiencing a great deal of pain will be unable to assume a full squatting position.

A positive Childress sign, according to Zippel [724], is diagnostic for a posterior horn tear of the medial meniscus.

4.4.14
Apley Test

The Apley test is unique among the meniscus tests because of its ability to distinguish between ligamentous and meniscal lesions.

The patient lies in the prone position with the hip extended and the knee flexed. Fixing the thigh against the table, the examiner presses the foot and leg downward while rotating the tibia in various degrees of flexion

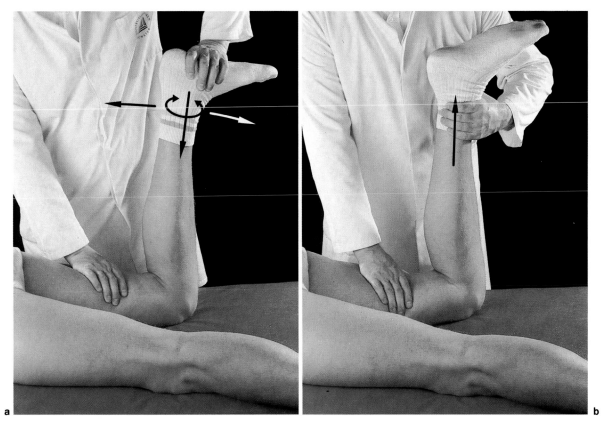

Fig. 4-11a, b. Apley test. Grinding test (**a**) in various positions of flexion. Distraction test (**b**)

(grinding test, Fig. 4-11a), and then pulls the foot and leg upward to distract the joint while again rotating the tibia (distraction test, Fig. 4-11b). Pain noted during axial compression implies a meniscal lesion. Pain in the acutely flexed knee suggests a more posterior tear, while pain in the range of 60°–70° suggests a tear in the central portion of the meniscus.

Wirth et al. [714] describe a modification of the grinding test in which the knee is extended while the tibia is held in a fixed position of rotation. Using this *modified Apley test,* Wirth obtained a true-positive result in more than 85% of patients with meniscal tears.

Pain felt during axial distraction of the joint suggests the presence of a ligamentous lesion, although the extent of the lesion cannot be ascertained.

4.4.15
Medial-Lateral Grinding Test

This test is performed with the patient supine. The examiner holds the lower leg with one hand while fixing the foot between the forearm and waist. The examiner places his free hand over the anterior joint line of the knee. A valgus stress is applied as the knee is flexed to 45°, and a varus stress is applied as it is extended. This maneuver produces a circular motion of the knee (Fig. 4-12) [9].

According to Anderson [9], a longitudinal or flap tear of the menisci produces a grinding sensation at the joint line, whereas a more complex tear produces prolonged grinding. A grinding sensation may also be present in patients with osteoarthritis or previous meniscectomy.

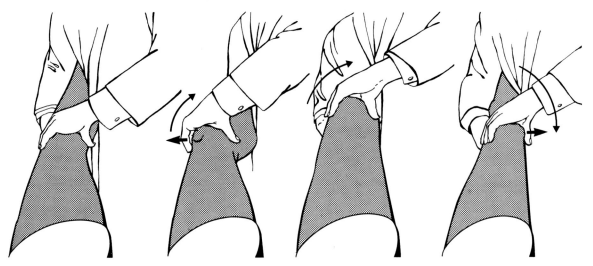

Fig. 4-12. Medial-lateral grinding test of Anderson (after [9])

Because forces are exerted on the knee in positions of slight and moderate flexion, this test frequently produces a pivot shift in the ACL-deficient knee [9].

Anderson reports that this test is positive in 68% of meniscal tears, questionably positive in 3%, and false-positive in 1% [9].

4.4.16
Rotational Grinding Test

With the patient in the sitting position, the examiner fixes the foot of the involved extremity between his legs just proximal to his own knees. To check the medial meniscus, the examiner places both thumbs over the medial joint line and moves the knee in a circular fashion so that the tibia rotates internally and externally and the knee assumes various flexion angles (Fig. 4-13). A varus or valgus stress is simultaneously applied [518].

In a positive test, pain is elicited by the circular movement of the joint. The test is markedly positive if pain is elicited by the maneuver itself, while the examiner's thumbs are not on the joint line [518]. Pain localized to the medial joint line suggests a medial meniscal lesion, while pain in the lateral joint line suggests a lateral meniscal lesion.

4.4.17
Cabot's Sign

The popliteal sign ("signo del popliteo") described by Cabot belongs to a symptom complex which he called the "popliteal hiatus syndrome." This syndrome, caused by a posterior horn lesion of the lateral meniscus, is characterized by:

1. spontaneous pain radiating to the popliteal fossa and calf,
2. tenderness localized to the lateral joint line just anterior to the lateral collateral ligament, and
3. a positive popliteal sign.

The popliteal sign is elicited with the patient supine. The knee is flexed and the lower leg is crossed over the contralateral lower leg. The examiner places his hand on the knee and palpates the lateral joint line with his thumb. The free hand grasps the lower leg just above the ankle joint, and the patient is asked to extend the knee. In positive cases the patient will feel a painful resistance and will be unable to extend the knee further because of the pain. The pain will persist as long as the examiner keeps his thumb on the lateral joint line (Fig. 4-14). Cabot states that concurrent resistance and pain on extension signify a positive test.

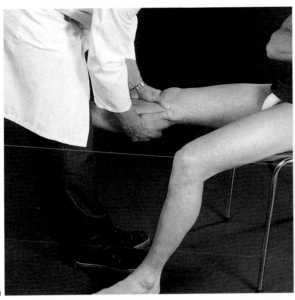
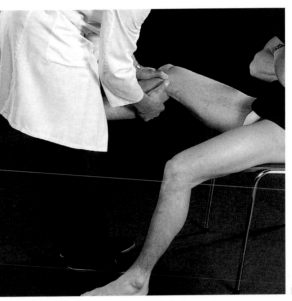

Fig. 4-13a, b. Rotational grinding test of Pässler [518]. Both thumbs are placed over the medial joint line (**a**), and the knee is moved in a circular fashion (**b**). The test is markedly positive if the examiner takes his thumbs from the joint line and the circling maneuver still elicits pain

4.4.18
Finochietto's Sign

When anterior drawer testing is performed with the knee in 90° flexion, a coexisting ACL insufficiency will allow the femur to ride up onto the meniscus, which may produce locking [169, 170] (see Fig. 3-20 and Chap. 3.3.4).

4.4.19
Turner's Sign

Turner in 1931 described a meniscal sign that is caused by chronic irritation of the infrapatellar branch of the saphenous nerve. When the medial meniscus is torn, an irregular area of hyperesthesia about 4-5 cm in size may be

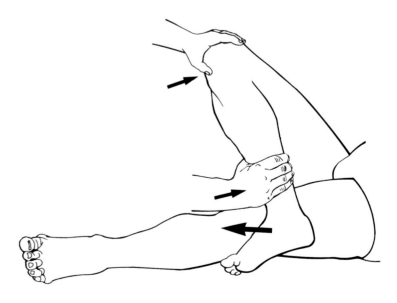

Fig. 4-14. Popliteal sign of Cabot

found over the course of the infrapatellar nerve, level with and slightly proximal to the medial joint line. Local hypersensitivity is tested using thermal and mechanical pain-producing stimuli (needle pricks). Zippel [724] states that, with careful technique, this symptom can be demonstrated with greater frequency than might be assumed. A similar sign is not known to exist for the lateral meniscus.

4.4.20
Tschaklin's Sign

Older meniscal lesions are commonly associated with atrophy of the quadriceps muscle. With a lesion of the medial meniscus, atrophy of the vastus medialis is often combined with a compensatory increase in the sartorius muscle tone. This has become known as Tschaklin's sign [724].

4.5
Reduction of the Menisci

Severe pain and a springy loss of extension are the major complaints produced by an entrapped meniscus. Once bony injuries have been excluded by radiographic examination, reduction of the entrapped meniscal segment should be carried out.

The physician attempting to reduce an entrapped meniscus should proceed with great caution. He must avoid sudden, forceful manipulations, since the resulting pain can provoke reflex muscular contractions. Mild sedation and analgesic medication are helpful in anxious patients.

The basic requirement for a successful reduction is optimum muscular relaxation. Prior to the reduction the leg should be placed in a relatively painless position that is comfortable for the patient. A slightly flexed knee position is recommended. Zippel [724] additionally recommends gentle warming of the femoral muscles. It is especially important that the examiner proceed in a calm, confident manner.

The following reduction maneuvers have proven most effective in practice:

4.5.1
Kulka's Maneuver

The flexed leg is relaxed and allowed to hang over the edge of the table or bed. In many cases this relaxation is sufficient in itself to allow spontaneous reduction of the displaced meniscal segment. Otherwise the examiner applies gentle axial traction to the lower leg while carefully rotating the tibia (Fig. 4-15).

A modification of this technique is to position the patient supine with the hip abducted and externally rotated and the lower leg hanging over the side of the examining table. This opens the medial compartment, an effect that is accentuated by the weight of the unsupported tibia. Slight axial traction combined with careful rotation of the tibia effects reduction of the meniscus.

4.5.2
Popp's Maneuver

For this maneuver the patient is placed in a lateral decubitus position with the affected side up. To reduce an entrapped medial meniscus, the slightly flexed leg is raised to produce a valgus stress which opens the joint medially. In that position the examiner gently rotates and shakes the lower leg and subsequently extends the knee. In a successful reduction the meniscus will slip back into its anatomic position.

4.5.3
Jones' Maneuver

The patient is positioned supine with the hip and knee flexed 90°. To reduce an entrapped medial meniscus, the lower leg is abducted (valgus stress) and externally rotated. The examiner then extends the leg while internally rotating the tibia and maintaining the valgus stress. To reduce a lateral meniscus, the tibia is first internally rotated and then externally rotated as the knee is extended.

4.5.4
Winkel's Maneuver

With the knee relaxed and fully flexed, the examiner alternately rotates the tibia internally and externally while pressing on the medial joint line with his fingers. As he slowly extends the knee, the examiner continues to rotate the tibia while applying increasing valgus pressure as the joint extends. A maximum valgus stress is applied when the knee approaches full extension [706]. However, the knee should not be

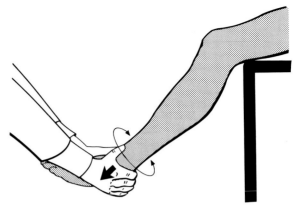

Fig. 4-15. Reduction maneuver of Kulka. The lower leg is relaxed and is flexed over the edge of the table. The examiner pulls downward on the lower leg while carefully rotating the tibia internally and externally

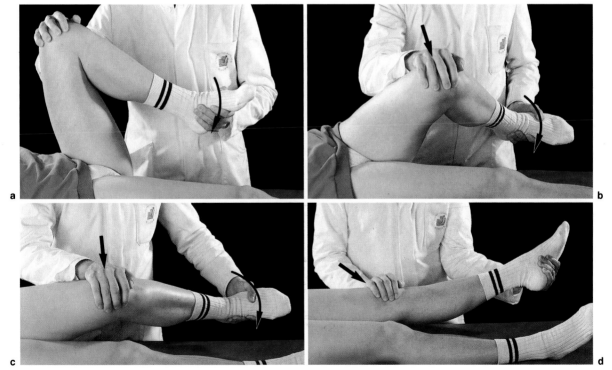

Fig. 4-16a–d. Our maneuver for reducing a trapped medial meniscus. Starting from a position of maximum flexion (**a**), the examiner internally rotates the lower leg (**b**) and slowly extends the knee while exerting a valgus stress (**c**). When extension is reached, the tibia is rotated externally (**d**). An opposite procedure is followed for reducing the lateral meniscus (flexion-varus stress-external rotation-extension-internal rotation)

completely extended in this maneuver, as this would cause pain with reflex tensing of the muscles and would make a second attempt at reduction much more difficult.

Our own technique does not differ significantly from maneuvers 3 and 4 described above (Fig. 4-16).

4.5.5
Follow-up Treatment

With a successful meniscal reduction, the patient will immediately experience substantial or complete relief of pain. This does not mean, however, that further evaluation and treatment are not required. The joint should at least be evaluated by arthroscopy. Sometimes the effect of the reduction will be to relieve painful locking and restore full extension to the knee. As this relief may be due to the anterior extension of a bucket handle tear, for example, we feel that arthroscopy is an essential follow-up to every "successful" meniscal reduction. At the same time the meniscus can be secured in its reduced position with arthroscopic sutures, or it may be found that the torn meniscal segment needs to be resected.

5
Evaluation of the Femoropatellar Joint

Despite its essential contribution to the "well-being of the knee joint," the femoropatellar joint is easily overlooked in diagnosis and treatment. It is common for patients who have undergone major reconstructive knee surgery to obtain relief of the unstable feeling which prompted the operation, but then to start complaining of pain in the anterior knee. Anterior knee pain is a very common sequel to major knee operations, trauma, and even as an "idiopathic" condition in persons who have not sustained trauma.

A further goal of the diagnostic evaluation of the femoropatellar joint is to identify acute injuries (e. g., patellar fracture, patellar dislocation) and recognize conditions predisposing to chronic disease (e. g., angular limb deformity, muscular imbalances).

5.1
Femoropatellar Pain Syndrome (Anterior Knee Pain)

Anterior knee pain is among the most common of all knee problems that lead patients, especially female adolescents and young adults, to consult an orthopedist. Sometimes the complaints are very complex and not easily evaluated. However, their importance should not be trivialized by dismissing the condition as "growing pains" or a response to overexertion. Many young patients with patellofemoral pain experience significant disability and distress.

Conversely, the pronounced pain symptoms mislead many physicians into taking a far too aggressive approach to treatment. The following clinical history is typical:

After a brief period of conservative therapy, which fails to improve symptoms, arthroscopy is performed. This reveals retropatellar chondromalacia grade I or II, which is assumed to be the cause of the pain. At that point either the involved cartilage is arthroscopically pared down to firm cartilage, or some other type of surgical procedure is recommended and performed. The options range from palliative "symptomatic" measures such as arthroscopic cartilage abrasion and drilling to purportedly "causal" treatments such as lateral retinacular release, advancement of the tibial tuberosity, sagittal patellar osteotomies, and tethering operations on the patella.

Unfortunately, many patients who undergo these kinds of surgery do not have their symptoms relieved. The multitude of available treatments reflects a situation of both diagnostic and therapeutic despair. When we consider the high rate of spontaneous recoveries, with many patients becoming pain-free without specific treatment, we can appreciate the need to reflect seriously upon the clinical manifestations, diagnosis, and especially the treatment of femoropatellar joint disorders [473].

It is time to approach the evaluation of anterior knee pain with a new understanding, especially as regards the interpretation of morphologic changes, which show little if any correlation with the patient's symptoms. Thus, while pronounced retropatellar cartilage changes may be found in patients who are virtually asymptomatic, arthroscopy often reveals only a localized grade I or grade II chondromalacia in young patients who are having severe anterior knee pain. These relatively mild cartilage changes are all too often held responsible for the patient's complaints. The subsequent diagnosis of "chondromalacia" or "chondropathy" then focuses all attention on the cartilage pathology that has been identified. However, the term "chondromalacia" merely designates a pathoanatomic and morphologic presentation of the cartilage and should not be used as a diagnosis [473].

A more appropriate term for this complex condition is *femoropatellar pain syndrome,* or simply *anterior knee pain.* Consideration is given not just to cartilage pathology in this condition but to all the structures of the knee and their possible functional disturbances.

Normally active adults are less commonly affected, but the incidence of femoropatellar pain increases again with advancing age. Most cases in older patients reflect degenerative arthritis in the femoropatellar joint. The pain is often exertion-related and tends to progress with the degree of joint loading. Often this is accompanied by the classic signs of osteoarthritis (effusion, limited motion, warmup pain, radiographic changes).

5.1.1
Symptoms

The symptoms of femoropatellar pain syndrome are diverse. Pain is the most common symptom and the most subjectively disabling (Table 5-1). The cause of the femoropatellar pain, however, remains poorly understood. Since cartilage is devoid of nerve fibers and receptors, the pain must originate from tissues that possess corresponding receptors and nerve fibers.

The characteristics of the pain depend largely on the age and activity level of the patient.

In adolescents, the pain often occurs spontaneously or after a single, extreme load on the retropatellar cartilage, e.g., after prolonged mountain climbing or skiing. The pain is frequently bilateral. Limitation of motion and intraarticular effusions are uncommon. The pain often remains constant but may worsen over a period of several weeks or months. Usually improvement is noted within a period of several days or weeks, but in rare cases the pain may persist for months or even years.

Table 5-1. Symptomatology of femoropatellar pain syndrome

1. Pain on retropatellar loading (e.g., stair climbing)
2. Pain after prolonged sitting or at rest
3. Giving way
4. Feeling of instability
5. Proneness to swelling
6. Crepitation

5.1.2
Pathogenic Factors

Since the pain cannot be ascribed to the condition of the cartilage alone, other causes must be sought. According to Munzinger [473], the retropatellar cartilage is a site where disturbances in the balance between stress and stress tolerance are most clearly manifested. On the one hand, the cartilage is exposed to stresses imposed by occupational and athletic activities (e. g., an intermittent rise of retropatellar pressure caused by quadriceps contraction during deceleration). But the cartilage is also vulnerable to direct trauma, as in patellar dislocation or a fall onto the flexed knee. Very strenuous sports that cause excessive loading of the retropatellar cartilage, such as mountain jogging, are becoming increasingly popular (Fig. 5-1).

Excessive loading of the articular cartilage can also result from individual factors such as anatomic variants (patellar dysplasia, dysplasia of the femoral trochlea, patella baja, patella alta, angular limb deformity, foot deformity) and functional variants (ligament instability, ligamentous hyperlaxity, muscular insufficiencies, contractures), which may occur singly but are usually combined. Each of these factors can lead to disproportionate loading of the femoropatellar joint.

The mobility of the patella is an important pathogenetic factor. It is increased in constitutional hyperlaxity and in quadriceps dysplasia, and it is reduced by shortening or tightness of the quadriceps muscle. Taking ligamentous laxity and muscular function as criteria, Munzinger [473] distinguishes between a type I and type II femoropatellar pain syndrome (Table 5-2). He also classifies the syndrome as primary or secondary, the primary form denoting a simple functional disturbance and the secondary form having intraarticular pathology as its cause. Several disorders must be considered in the differential diagnosis of secondary femoropatellar pain (Table 5-3).

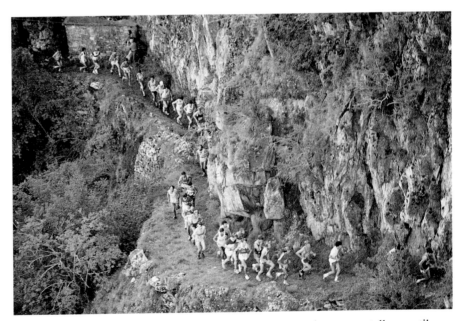

Fig. 5-1. Alpine jogging exerts punishing stresses on the retropatellar cartilage. Extreme retropatellar contact pressures are generated, especially during downhill jogging (photo: S. Simon)

Table 5-2. Classification of femoropatellar pain syndrome by ligamentous laxity and muscular function (modified from [473])

Type I:
Increased ligamentous laxity
Quadriceps dysplasia or atrophy
Other clinical criteria:
    Proneness to swelling
    Patella alta
    Genu valgum
    Normal Q angle
    "Outfacing" of the patella (divergent strabismus)
    Familial occurrence

Type II:
Ligamentous laxity not increased
Quadriceps strong, shortened, or contracted
Hamstring muscles shortened or contracted
Other clinical criteria:
    No proneness to swelling
    Increased Q angle
    No patella alta
    "Infacing" of the patella (convergent strabismus)
    Facet tenderness

Indifferent criteria are:
    Intensity of pain
    Character of pain
    Provocation of pain
    Snapping and grinding sounds

Table 5-3. Potential causes of secondary femoropatellar pain syndrome

- Patellofemoral osteoarthritis
- Ligamentous insufficiency (e. g. old ACL rupture, old PCL rupture)
- Meniscal lesion
- Medial shelf syndrome
- Intraarticular adhesions
- Tumors
- Osteochondritis dissecans
- Arthritis
- Femorotibial osteoarthritis
- Patella baja
- Entrapped synovial plica
- Synovitis

5.1.3
Diagnostic Tests

5.1.3.1
Assessment of Laxity

Individual laxity is assessed by maximum extension of the wrist and phalangeal joints (e. g., hyperextension of the little finger) or by hyperflexion tests (maximum wrist flexion, see Fig. 3-4).

5.1.3.2
Patellar Mobility

The examiner should be alert both for increased patellar mobility in patients with constitutional hyperlaxity and for hypomobility in older patients with osteoarthritic changes or patients who have undergone surgical procedures. Hypomobility of the patella is especially likely to interfere with cartilage nutrition and predisposes to cartilage pathology [470]. The hypermobile patella is prone to recurrent subluxation with repetitive microtraumatization leading to cartilage injury.

Patellar mobility is tested with the knee extended by pushing the patella as far medially and laterally as it will go (Fig. 5-2). A tendency toward subluxation is usually seen in patients with constitutional ligamentous weakness.

Potential causes of patellar hypomobility are:

1. quadriceps tightness and rigidity, most commonly seen in muscular athletes
2. intraarticular adhesions following surgery
3. advanced osteoarthritis of the femoropatellar joint
4. extension deficit (see Table 2-17 and 2-18).

5.1.3.3
Patellar Tracking

Simple inspection will disclose atrophy of the quadriceps muscle or hypertrophy of that muscle in muscular patients. With the patient in a sitting position, the examiner evaluates patellar tracking by holding the patella between the thumb and index finger and having the patient

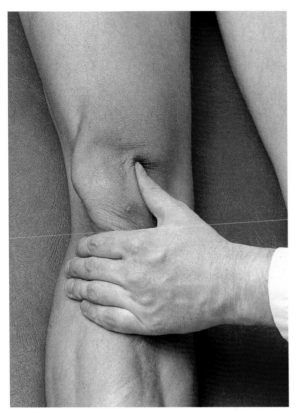

Fig. 5-2. Test of patellar mobility, here demonstrating hypermobility with lateral subluxation

pletely extended during running, walking, or even standing. Especially in the standing posture, the hamstring tightness requires a disproportionately high quadriceps tonus, leading to increased patellofemoral compression.

Hamstring tightness is assessed with the patient lying supine. The uninvolved leg is left extended on the examining table. On the side to be examined, the patient flexes the hip 90° and is told to extend the knee upward as far as he can while keeping his other leg on the table. Patients with shortened hamstrings have a tendency to raise the opposite leg from the table and assume a position of lumbar kyphosis to shorten the distance between the ischial tuberosity and the knee joint (Fig. 5-3 c, d).

5.1.3.5
Hyperpression Test

Compression of the patella against the femur can elicit pain when femoropatellar cartilage damage is present. Tenderness to compression of the superior or inferior pole of the patella against the femur implies cartilage lesions in the proximal or distal retropatellar area, respectively.

5.1.3.6
Facet Tenderness

With the knee extended, the patella is tilted laterally or medially, and the medial or lateral patellar facet is palpated. Patients with chondromalacia will experience and report pain, especially on palpation of the medial facet (Fig. 5-4).

alternately extend and flex the knee. Progressive lateralization of the patella often will be noted with increasing flexion (see Fig. 5-12).

5.1.3.4
Muscle Tightness

As the mass of a muscle increases, the muscle becomes less distensible. A tight, poorly distensible quadriceps muscle can directly increase the contact pressure between the articular surfaces of the femur and patella.

Quadriceps tightness is tested with the patient in the prone position (see Figs. 2-32 and 5-3 a,b). Patellofemoral compression can be increased by quadriceps tightness as well as by hamstring tightness, which opposes full extension of the knee. The knee joint is constantly held in a slightly flexed position. In athletes with powerful but shortened hamstrings, it may be observed that the knee is never com-

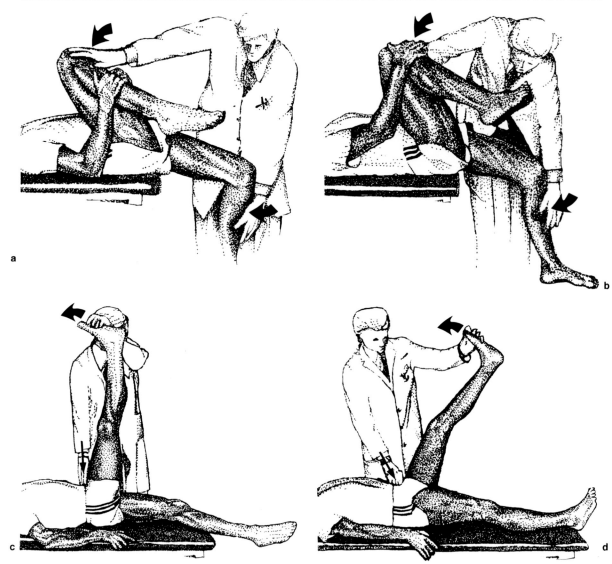

Fig. 5-3a–d. Test for tightness. **a, b** of the *rectus femoris muscle*. The patient lies supine with the leg projecting over the edge of the table; he holds the nonexamined leg in a position of maximum flexion at the hip and knee. The examiner then flexes the knee joint to be examined (**a**), making sure that the hip remains extended and there is no compensatory lumbar lordosis. With normal rectus femoris tightness, the examiner can eas-ily flex the knee to 90° (**a**). If the muscle is shortened, the knee cannot reach 90° (**b**). **c, d** Test for *hamstring* tightness. With normal hamstring tightness, the knee can be fully extended while the hip is completely flexed (**c**). If the muscles are tight, the hip will straighten somewhat from 90° flexion as the knee is extended, or the patient will be unable to extend the knee fully (**d**)

5.1.3.7
Zohlen's Sign

With the knee extended, the examiner pulls downward on the patella and askes the patient to straighten the leg. Contraction of the quadriceps will pull the patella upward over the femoral condyles (Fig. 5-5), eliciting pain when retropatellar cartilage damage is present. However, this test is also positive in a large percentage of the normal population, so it is of minor importance for evaluation of the femoropatellar joint.

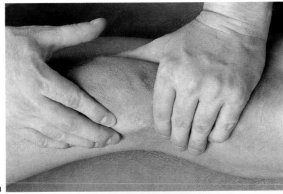

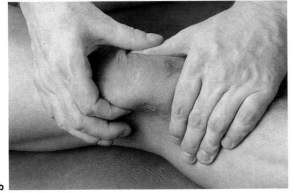

Fig. 5-4 a, b. Palpation of the medial (**a**) and lateral (**b**) patellar facet

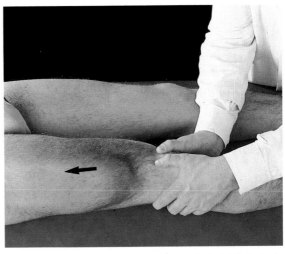

Fig. 5-5. Zohlen's sign. The patella is held inferiorly and then pulled superiorly by contraction of the quadriceps

5.1.3.8
Crepitation Test

The examiner kneels in front of the patient and asks the patient to squat down or perform a deep knee bend. As the patient squats, the examiner listens closely for retropatellar sounds (Fig. 5-6). A crepitus having the quality of a "snowball crunch" implies the presence of grade II or grade III chondromalacia. Snapping sounds like those typically occurring during the first one or two knee bends have no significance [518]. We always have the patient perform several deep squats before the test is begun, as this generally reduces the intensity of inconsequential snaps and clicks.

If retropatellar crepitus is not detected, significant retropatellar chondral damage may be ruled out with very high confidence. We prefer this test over Zohlen's sign and the next two tests described below.

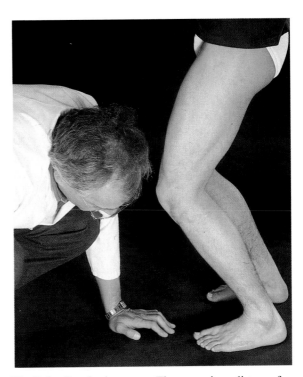

Fig. 5-6. Crepitation test. The examiner listens for retropatellar crepitus as the patient performs a full squat

5.1.3.9
Fründ's Sign

The examiner percusses the patella with the knee in various positions of flexion. Pain may signify retropatellar chondromalacia.

5.1.3.10
Tuning Fork Test

In a knee with stage I chondromalacia, it is reported that the vibrations of a tuning fork touched to the patella are perceived for a shorter time when there is a marked retropatellar cartilage defect that exposes the underlying bone [524].

The tuning fork test, like Fründ's sign, is not considered to be very reliable [26].

5.1.4
Therapeutic Implications

The distinction between primary and secondary patellofemoral pain makes clear the importance of first ruling out intraarticular pathology. Causal therapy may be possible once an accurate differential diagnosis has been made. If intraarticular changes are excluded, treatment should be nonoperative with emphasis placed on physiotherapeutic exercises aimed at stretching or/and strengthening the muscles, depending on the etiology of the femoropatellar pain.

Tight muscles should be stretched, while lax muscles require strengthening.

Operative measures should be limited to diagnostic arthroscopy, especially in young patients, as a means of verifying intraarticular lesions and demonstrating any cartilage damage that may exist. Ordinarily we do not feel that more extensive operative measures are warranted [188], although they may be considered as a last recourse in older patients after all conservative options have been exhausted.

5.2
Patellar Fracture

The clinical picture of a patellar fracture is determined by a combination of definite and equivocal signs. Often the fracture line is palpable and may even be obvious on visual inspection. The patient with a transverse patellar fracture will be unable to extend the knee against a resistance. However, a longitudinal fracture may cause little or no apparent interference with knee extension.

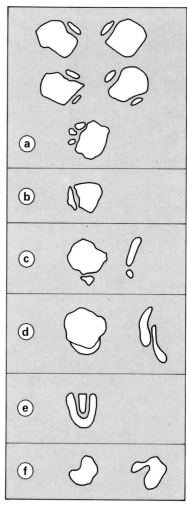

Fig. 5-7. Various forms of bipartite patella, after Pfeil [524]. The line of separation may be diagonal *(a)*, vertical *(b)*, transverse *(c)*, frontal *(d)*, or centrally placed *(e)*, Emargination *(f)* is rare

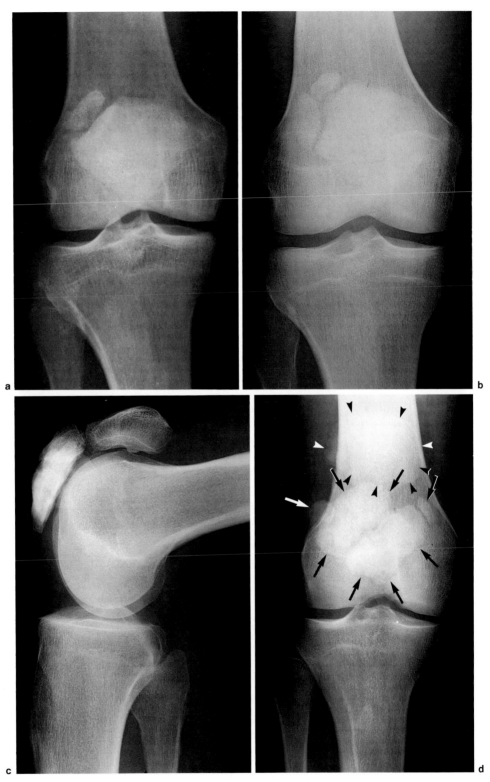

Fig. 5-8a-d. Bipartite patella of the diagonal type (**a**), This is the most common form, accounting for 80% of cases. The tripartite form (**b**) is rare. Congenital uni- lateral double patella is very rare (**c**). Distal patella is of multipartite type (arrows), proximal patella normal *(arrowheads)* (**d**)

The radiographic examination is diagnostic. The main condition requiring differentiation is bipartite patella, which can assume various forms (Figs. 5-7 and 5-8). Duplication of the patella is also known to occur [201].

Since a fracture cannot always be definitely excluded on AP and lateral radiographs, bilateral sunrise views, which plainly demonstrate longitudinal fractures, should be routinely obtained in 30°, 60°, and 90° of flexion (Fig. 5-9).

It is also important to exclude osteochondral fractures on the undersurface of the patella following patellar dislocation or direct trauma (see Fig. 5-15).

5.3
Patellar Dislocation

Patellar dislocation is one of the most common knee injuries (Fig. 5-10). Indeed, its prevalence has led Smillie [610] to recommend that every internal knee injury in young women be treated as a patellar subluxation until proven otherwise.

If the patella is still in the dislocated position when examined, which is the case in approximately 17% [293] to 30% of patients (our material), it will usually be seen and felt alongside the lateral femoral condyle. The patient complains of severe pain and keeps the knee flexed.

The *reduction of a dislocated patella* should be accomplished as gently as possible. We do this by manually fixing the patella on the lateral side of the knee, tilting the patella slightly medially, and slowly extending the leg. As the knee approaches extension, the patella should slip back into place by itself. The goal of the maneuver is to effect the reduction without force. Extensive cartilage lesions can result just as easily from an "iatrogenic" reduction as when the patella reduces spontaneously.

It is far more common for the patella to reduce spontaneously immediately after dislocating and to be in the reduced position when

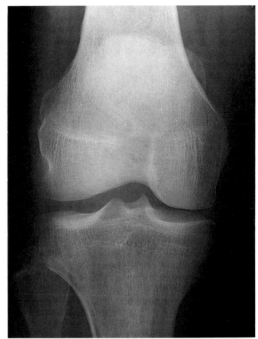

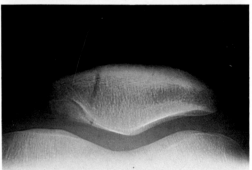

Fig. 5-9a, b. A longitudinal fracture of the patella is poorly demonstrated by the AP projection (**a**) but is seen clearly on the sunrise view (**b**)

examined. The patient may report that something "jumped out" toward the inside of the knee, accompanied by an episode of giving way. While this history may suggest a medial dislocation, the patella almost always dislocates laterally, and it is likely that the patient merely saw his empty femoral trochlea flanked by the prominent medial femoral condyle. The symptoms of a patellar dislocation are variable (Table 5-4).

As in the material of Hughston [293], a review of our own cases (112 patients with 114 dislocations) indicates a preponderance of males affected by patellar dislocation (63%

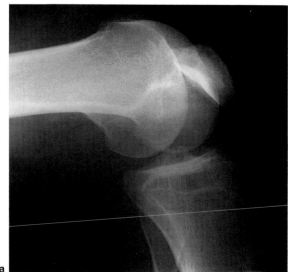

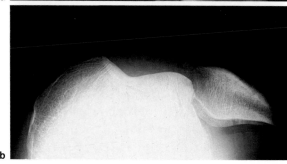

Fig. 5-10a, b. Lateral patellar dislocation. The lateral radiographic view demonstrates tilting of the patella (**a**). However, the effects of the dislocation are seen only in the sunrise view (**b**), which shows flakes of cartilage sheared from the medial patellar facet or lateral femoral condyle

Table 5-4. Symptoms following patellar dislocation. (After [293])

1. Pain	58%
2. Joint swelling	32%
3. Giving way	42%
4. Locking, popping	27%
5. Grating	9%
6. Dislocated position	17%

males vs. 37% females). Except for one case, all the dislocations were lateral. Medial subluxation has been known to occur as a complication of lateral retinacular release [298].

For further diagnosis and management, it is important to understand the mechanics of patellar dislocation and reduction (Fig. 5-11) so

that a selective search can be made for associated injuries [293, 298].

It can be difficult to determine whether the patella has been traumatically dislocated or whether the dislocation occurred during the course of normal activities. Patients frequently report a traumatic incident in which they fell to the ground while their knee cap simultaneously slipped out of place. Establishing the exact sequence of events is difficult and allows room for misinterpretation. The question to be resolved is: Did the patellar dislocation happen first and cause the knee to give way because of pain, or did the fall happen first and cause the patella to dislocate? In most cases, analysis of the mechanism of injury shows that there was no adequate precipitating trauma, and that the patella dislocated during some "ordinary" knee movement.

Thus, in the patient presenting with patellar dislocation, it is important to identify the type of dislocation that has occurred:

1. *Acute traumatic dislocation:* This is rare because it requires direct violence to the medial aspect of the knee (impact mark!). Dysplastic changes are seldom present.
2. *Acute initial (endogenous) dislocation:* A particular movement or action (e. g., forced external rotation, jumping down stairs) leads to an initial dislocation or subluxation to which the knee has been predisposed by a congenital or acquired dysplasia in the femoropatellar system.
3. *Recurrent dislocation:* A particular movement or action (see above) causes the dislocation to recur as a result of dysplastic changes in the femoropatellar system or the inadequate treatment of an acute initial (endogenous) or traumatic dislocation.
4. *Habitual dislocation:* Habitual dislocation of the patella occurs during ordinary activities and usually reduces spontaneously (Fig. 5-12). There need be no particular movement or action that precipitates the dislocation.

In our own case material (114 patellar dislocations), 14% of the dislocations were traumatic in origin, 42% were initial dislocations, and another 42% were of the recurrent type.

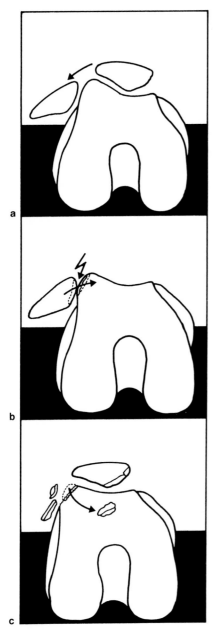

Fig. 5-11a–c. Patellar dislocation. The patella dislocates laterally (**a**), so reduction requires bringing it back over the lateral femoral condyle. As the patella relocates, it may cause cartilage contusions, cartilage flaking, or osteochondral fractures to occur at the site of contact between the medial patellar facet and the outer aspect of the lateral femoral condyle (**b**, see also Fig. 5-13). That is why chondral or osteochondral fragments may be found near the lateral femoral condyle after the patella reduces to its original position. Fragments sheared from the lateral femoral condyle may lodge in the superior recess (**c**) (after [470])

To make an accurate diagnosis and identify cases where causal treatment is feasible, it is helpful to know the factors which promote or predispose to patellar dislocation (Table 5-5). Histologic studies of muscle biopsy specimens from patients with recurrent patellar dislocation indicate an increased proportion of abnormal type 2C fibers in the muscle tissue [176].

Pain on the medial side of the joint can be difficult to distinguish from a medial meniscal lesion. It should be noted, however, that meniscal tears are not known to coexist with patellar dislocation due to the different etiologic mechanisms for each disorder [470].

In every patient with an acute knee injury, the examiner should consider the possibility of a patellar dislocation and be alert for clinical signs (Table 5-6).

It is mandatory that patellar sunrise views be obtained to check for osteochondral fractures of the medial patellar facet and lateral femoral condyle and to exclude patellar subluxation (Figs. 5-13 to 5-15).

If the diagnosis is still unclear following a careful clinical examination in the presence of hemarthrosis, arthroscopy is indicated. Arthroscopy following patellar dislocation may reveal tearing of or hemorrhage below the medial retinaculum as well as cartilage contusions or chondral fragments sheared from the medial patellar facet and/or the lateral aspect of the lateral femoral condyle. Larger osteochondral fragments may be found in the superior or lateral recess.

Table 5-5. Factors predisposing to patellar dislocation

1. Femoropatellar dysplasias
2. Patella alta
3. Altered direction of pull by extensor muscles
   - Q angle > 15°
   - Imbalance between vastus medialis obliquus and vastus lateralis
   - Lateral attachment of tibial tuberosity
   - Increased internal rotation of femur
   - Increased femoral antetorsion
   - Genu valgum
4. Constitutional
5. Hyperlaxity (e.g., in Ehlers-Danlos syndrome)

Fig. 5-12 a, b. Habitual patellar dislocation (left knee) (a) in a patient with constitutional hyperlaxity and marked dysplasia of the patella and femoral trochlea (b)

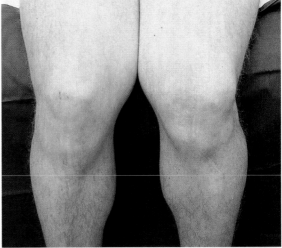

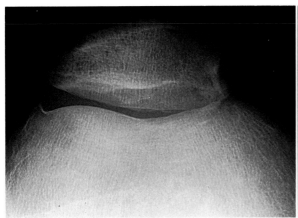 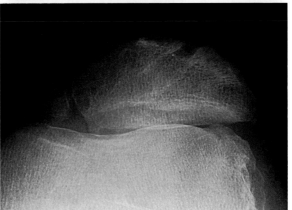

Table 5-6. Clinical signs of patellar dislocation

1. Tenderness over the medial retinaculum (torn during dislocation)
2. Tenderness over the medial patellar facet (cartilage injury during reduction)
3. Tenderness over the lateral femoral condyle (cartilage injury during reduction)
4. Fairbank's apprehension test (attempt to reproduce dislocation)
5. Bloody effusion frequently but not invariably present

5.3.1
Fairbank's Apprehension Test

This procedure, often referred to as Smillie's test, was described by Fairbank in 1935 (in [610]). With the patient supine, the knee extended, and the thigh muscles relaxed, the examiner attempts to reproduce the dislocation by pushing the patella laterally. The patient is then asked to flex the knee. If patellar dislocation has occurred, the patient will experience significant pain and anxiety over the impending redislocation. This may occur while the knee is extended or, at the latest, after flexion is initiated (Fig. 5-16). If the apprehension test is positive, patella dislocation is evident.

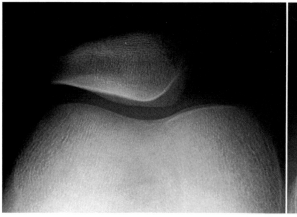

Fig. 5-13. Radiographic signs of an old patellar dislocation with a fragment from the medial patellar facet and calcifications in the medial retinaculum *(arrow),* The small, lateral osteochondral fragment *(arrows)* is from a more recent dislocation

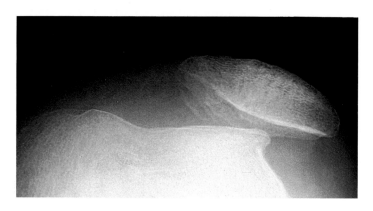

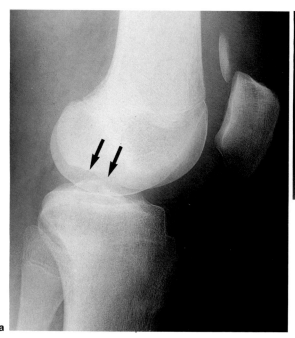

Fig. 5-14. Patellar subluxation

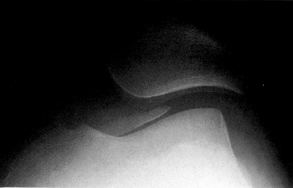

a

b

Fig. 5-15 a, b. Osteochondral fracture following patellar dislocation. The lateral view demonstrates a large osteochondral fragment in the superior recess (**a**). The sunrise view confirms that the posterior surface of the patella is intact (**b**). Close scrutiny reveals a defect in the lateral femoral condyle (**a,** *arrows*)

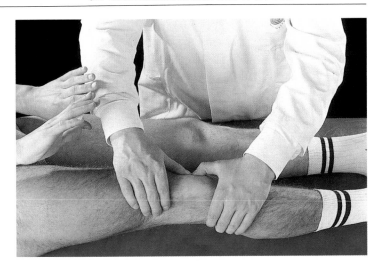

Fig. 5-16. Fairbank's apprehension test. With the leg extended, the examiner attempts to lateralize the patella. Patients with a recent patellar dislocation will experience pain and anxiety, especially when flexion is initiated, and often will resist the procedure

5.4
Osteochondritis dissecans of the Patella

Osteochondritis dissecans of the patella, first described by Rombold in 1936 [557], is a very rare disorder (Fig. 5-17). Schwarz and Blazina [586] report on the most comprehensive study to date involving 31 operatively treated cases

Table 5-7. Findings on preoperative examination of patients with osteochondritis dissecans of the patella. (After [586])

Patellofemoral crepitus	74%
Effusion	45%
Subpatellar pain on compression	41%
Hypermobile patella	32%
Quadriceps atrophy	29%
Decreased range of motion	25%

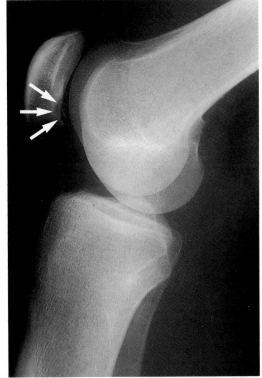

a

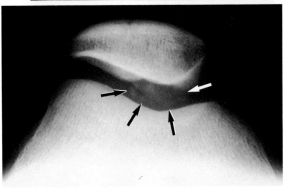

b

►
Fig. 5-17. Osteochondritis dissecans of the patellae *(arrows)*

in 25 patients. The symptoms include pain (87%), swelling, accompanying trauma, locking, patellar subluxation, and giving way (22%) [586]. The clinical findings (Table 5-7) are very similar to those of femoropatellar pain syndrome.

Lateral radiographs will very often demonstrate a localized lucency on the undersurface of the patella, corresponding to the osteochondritic area (Fig. 5-17). The major sites of occurrence are the middle and distal thirds of the patellar ridge [586].

Special Diagnostic Procedures

6
Radiographic Examination

Radiography cannot replace the clinical examination of the knee, nor should it attempt to do so. It is, however, an essential part of a complete workup and is indispensible for the exclusion of fresh fractures, old bony injuries, degenerative changes, congenital dysplasias, and neoplasms of bone. Even when complaints are nonspecific, such as retropatellar pain suggesting an immediate diagnosis of "chondromalacia," it would be a mistake to omit radiographs, which may well disclose degenerative changes or, less commonly, a bone tumor (Fig. 6-1), old fracture, intraarticular

loose body, or foreign body (Fig. 6-2) that could account for the patient's symptoms.

In acute injuries and before every initial knee-joint aspiration, standard radiographic views should be obtained to exclude bony injuries before the special clinical examination of the capsule and ligaments is begun.

The routine views to be obtained on initial examination are the *anteroposterior (AP)* and *lateral* projections of the affected knee and patellar *sunrise views* in both knees. Only a comparison of both sides can furnish adequate diagnostic information in patients with knee

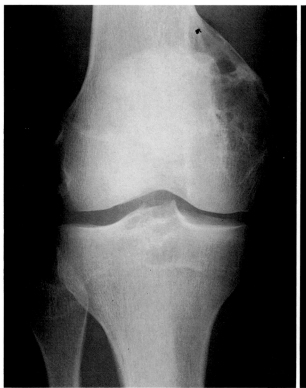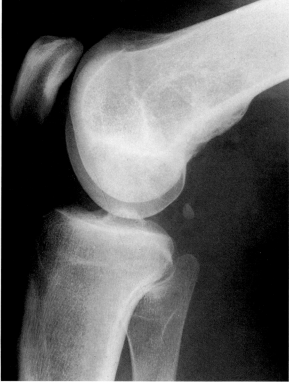

a   b

Fig. 6-1a, b. Aneurysmatic bone cyst of the medial femoral condyle found incidentally during a standard radiographic examination. The 26-year-old male complained of vague anterior knee pain after prolonged running and inquired about the possibility of a pharmacologic chondroprotective therapy

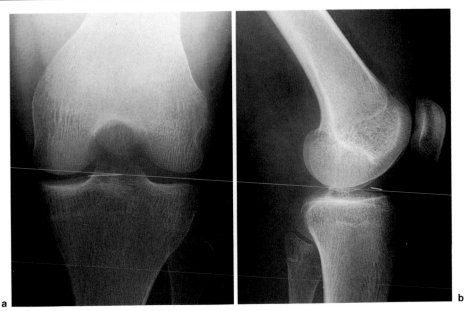

a   b

Fig. 6-2 a, b. Foreign body of metallic density in the knee joint (broken-off pin)

pain of uncertain etiology. In patients with acute injuries, there are only a few cases in which bilateral radiographs will be necessary, but they should always be obtained in children or adolescents whose epiphyseal growth plates are still open. If bony or intraarticular lesions are suspected, further special views should be obtained.

In evaluating and classifying radiographic findings, it is helpful to know the potential sources of error in the preparation of X-ray films, normal anatomic variants about the knee, and borderline pathologic findings. It is not unusual to encounter anatomic variants in the knee as well as accessory sites of ossification (see Fig. 6-10), bone islands and tubercula in the intercondylar region, and the various forms of bipartite patella (see Fig. 5-7).

Radiography has become a mainstay in postoperative follow-up, and biplane views should always be taken following internal fixations of the proximal tibia, patella, or femoral condyles and after the repair of bony ligament avulsions using internal fixation material.

The drill channels made for ligament reconstructions or repairs are visible on standard postoperative radiographs only if they are larger than 5-6 mm in diameter. If some time has passed since the operation, MR imaging is the only noninvasive study that can clearly demonstrate the original drill channels and enable the course of the repaired or reconstructed ligament to be evaluated. Of course if staples, screws, or wire sutures were used in the original repair, they can provide radiographic landmarks for identifying the site of ligament reattachment. They can also serve as reference points for the subsequent analysis of faulty repairs (Fig. 6-3).

In joints with an old ACL tear, radiographs will demonstrate stenosis of the intercondylar notch and, in about 40% of cases, a thickening and elevation of the intercondylar tubercles [10, 22, 565] (see Fig. 6-30).

A scoring scale has been devised for determining the rate of posttraumatic osteoarthritis occurring after ligamentous injuries [340]. This scale is based on the presence of osteophytes, subchondral sclerosis, flattening of the femoral condyles, subchondral cysts, ligament calcifications, joint-space narrowing, and angular deformity.

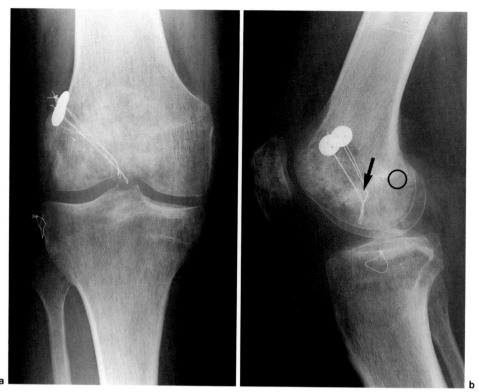

a   b

Fig. 6-3a, b. A proximal tear of the ACL and a small Segond fracture were repaired with wire sutures. The following errors are apparent: *1.* Extra-anatomic insertion of the ACL on the lateral femoral condyle *(arrow)*. The insertion site should be placed more posterosuperiorly *(circle)* to ensure isometry. *2.* The use of metal washers is not advised, because tearing of the sutures will allow the washers to "migrate." *3.* Wire sutures should not be used. If the initial repair is deemed inadequate and revisionary surgery (e. g., an arthroscopic ACL reconstruction) is proposed, the wire sutures can be difficult to remove. There is patchy decalcification as evidence of reflex sympathetic dystrophy

6.1
Standard Radiographic Examination

In acute injuries a search is made for bone fractures, bony ligament avulsions, and osteochondral fractures. If the patient has a severe, possibly open injury and his general condition is poor, the examiner may elect to omit lateral projections in cases where severe bone injuries are plainly visible on the AP view.

Besides fresh bony injuries, the examiner should be alert for degenerative changes such as joint-space narrowing, marginal osteophytes, subchondral sclerosis, subchondral cysts, and aseptic necrosis of bone (osteochondritis dissecans) (Figs. 6-4 through 6-6). Old bony avulsions or a Stieda-Pelligrini shadow may provide evidence of earlier injuries (Fig. 6-7 and 6-10a).

Three types of Stieda-Pelligrini shadow may be seen:

Type I: Fibroostosis or ossified avulsion at the insertion of the adductor magnus muscle. X-rays show a conspicuous adductor tubercle or a bone shadow that is demarcated from the tubercle.

Type II: Paraosseous metaplastic new bone formation showing no relation to the medial collateral ligament (may occur in tendinous tissue or directly on the femur.)

Type III: Ossified collateral ligament avulsion at the origin of the medial collateral ligament.

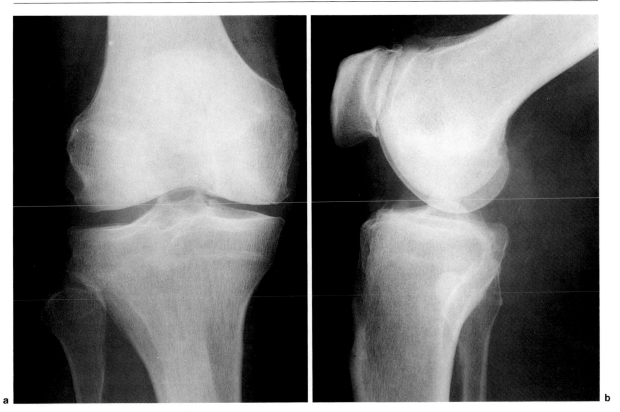

Fig. 6-4a, b. Moderate degenerative changes

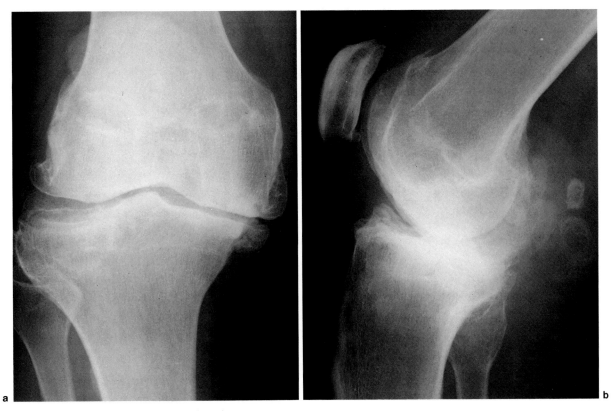

Fig. 6-5a, b. Very severe degenerative changes

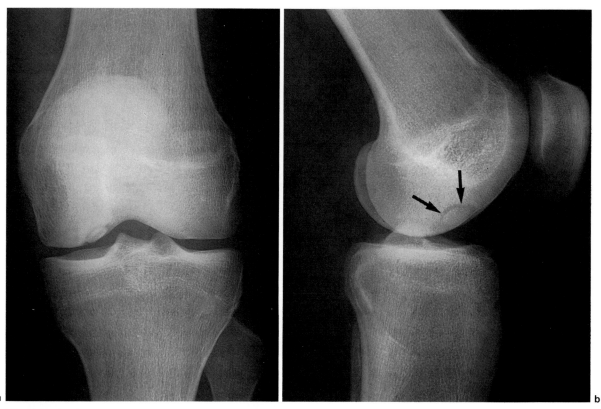

Fig. 6-6a, b. Osteochondritis dissecans (medial femoral condyle)

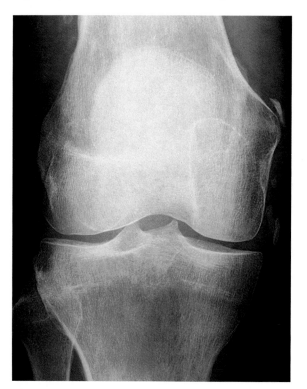

Fig. 6-7. Type II Stieda-Pelligrini shadow and post-traumatic calcifications in the medial capsuloligamentous apparatus

Calcium deposits may be found in the lateral collateral ligament, popliteus tendon, infrapatellar fat pad, infrapatellar bursa, both cruciate ligaments, the patellar ligament, or the oblique popliteal ligament (Fig. 6-8) [137]. Meniscal calcifications are noted as an incidental finding in 0.1% to 0.3% of patients over 50 years of age [553]. Patients run the gamut from a complete absence of symptoms to the typical symptoms of meniscal lesions (Fig. 6-9).

The development of soft-tissue calcifications can result from the secondary ossification of a hematoma, new bone formation in scarred portions of the ligament or joint capsule, trauma-induced metaplastic tissue changes, ossified tears and avulsions of muscle, or ossification of neurogenic origin [329, 724].

Extensive bony injuries such as mono-, bi- and supracondylar fractures of the femur and proximal tibia are usually obvious on standard radiographic views. Accurate evaluation of the extent of the fracture may require the procurement of additional special views (45° oblique views, tomograms, CT scans).

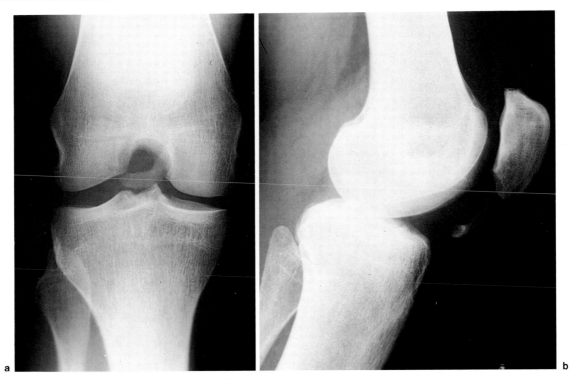

Fig. 6-8 a, b. Ossification in the patellar ligament

A deepened lateral condylopatellar groove (lateral notch sign) [22] is commonly found in patients with an old ACL tear. It can also be produced by marked hyperextension of the knee (see Fig. 1-46). Depressed fractures in the area of the limiting groove, known as "lateral notch fractures," may be seen in the wake of hyperextension injuries (see Fig. 2-3).

Hemarthrosis of the knee is a common occurrence in the life of hemophiliacs. Intraarticular hemorrhages that recur more frequently than three times per year almost invariably lead to osteoarthropathy [150]. This led Patterson to develop a scoring scale for hemophiliac osteoarthropathy based on the presence of osteoporosis, epiphyseal enlargement, subchondral surface irregularities, joint-space narrowing, subchondral cysts, erosive changes in the articular margins, incongruities, and joint deformities (after [150]).

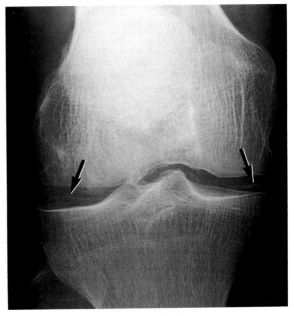

Fig. 6-9. Calcification *(arrows)* of the medial and lateral meniscus (incidental finding)

6.1.1
Bony Ligament Avulsions and Ossifications

Ligamentous avulsion-fractures, indentations, impressions, and ossifications can occur at numerous sites about the knee joint (Table 6-1, Figs. 6-10 through 6-14) [142, 163, 329, 433].

Meyers and McKeever devised the following system for classifying avulsions of the intercondylar eminence and isolated bony avulsions of the ACL:

Table 6-1. Sites of occurrence of bony ligament avulsions

1. Fibular head (lateral collateral ligament)
2. Margin of lateral tibial plateau = Segond fragment (lateral capusloligamentous apparatus)
3. Tubercle of Gerdy (iliotibial tract)
4. Anterior intercondyle eminence (ACL)
5. Posterior intercondylar area (PCL)
6. Posteromedial tibial border (posteromedial capsule)
7. Margin of medial tibial plateau (medial capsular ligament)
8. Lateral femoral condyle (lateral capsular ligament)
9. Medial aspect of lateral femoral condyle (ACL)
10. Medial aspect of medial femoral condyle (PCL)

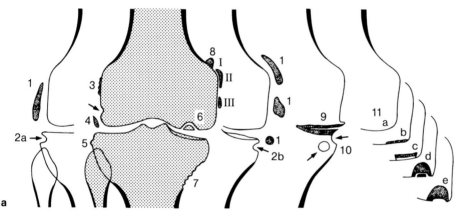

Fig. 6-10a. Possible sites of occurrence of bone changes in the anteroposterior projection (modified from Dihlmann [131]). *1*. Heterotopic ossifications (e. g., after extensive burns or in neurogenic disorders), *2*. Erosion with a sharp, sclerotic border on the lateral *(2a)* or medial *(2b)* tibial plateau due to pressure from a lateral or medial (rare) meniscal cyst. *3*. Fibroostosis at the origin of the lateral collateral ligament. *4*. Calcification in the popliteus tendon or lateral collateral ligament. The lateral femoral condyle shows variable indentation *(arrow)* for passage of the popliteus tendon (normal variant). *5*. Tubercle of Gerdy (normal variant). *6*. Osteochondritis dissecans of the medial femoral condyle. *7*. Localized subperiosteal bone resorption in the medial tibial plateau due to hyperparathyroidism. (Requires differentiation from malignant bone tumor.) *8*. Stieda-Pelligrini shadow type I-III (after Volkmann). *9*. Joint-space narrowing, subchondral sclerosis, and osteophytes *(arrow)* in an osteoarthritic knee. *10*. Marginal erosion with fine serrations *(arrow)* and sharply marginated bone defects in chronic gout. These defects represent marginal and intraosseous

gouty tophi. Pleomorphic calcifications (tophi) may occur simultaneously at other sites, such as proximal to the tibial tuberosity. The combination of erosive changes and circumscribed foci of decalcification should direct suspicion toward rheumatoid arthritis and other arthritides. *11*. Spontaneous osteonecrosis of the medial femoral condyle. *a*. Normal radiographic finding. Though patients may complain of severe pain, radiographs remain negative for up to 6-8 weeks. Only bone scans are positive at this stage, showing a local increase in radionuclide uptake. *b*. Slight flattening of the medial femoral condyle with a slight increase in subchondral density (early radiographic finding). *c*. Increased subchondral lucency (appearing no earlier than 8-12 weeks) with variable, perifocal increase in cancellous bone density. *d*. Local defect surrounded by area of increased cancellous bone density. The flat bony plate in the area of the defect is a typical radiographic finding. *e*. Resorption of the flat bony plate. At this stage there is usually a pronounced increase in cancellous bone density in the affected portion of the tibia.

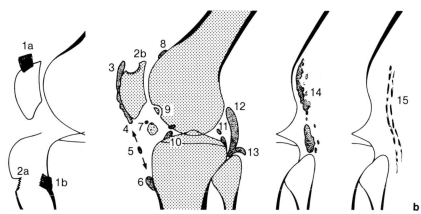

Fig. 6-10 b. Possible sites of occurrence of bone changes in the lateral projection (modified from Dihlmann [131]). *1.* Fibroostitis (productive form) at the attachment of the quadriceps tendon *(a)* and patellar ligament *(b)*. *2.* Fibroostitis (rarefying form) at the attachment of the quadriceps tendon *(a)* and patellar ligament *(b)*. Both forms of fibroostitis occur in ankylosing spondylitis and other seronegative spondyloarthropathies. *3.* Fibroostosis at the attachment of the rectus femoris muscle (superior patellar spur). *4.* Fibroostosis at the origin of the patellar ligament (inferior patellar spur). Irregular bony deposits on the patella may also be seen. *5.* Bony metaplasia in the patellar ligament (e. g., after trauma). The ossification may occur at various levels *(arrows)*. *6.* Fibroostosis of the patellar ligament at the tibial tuberosity. *7.* Calcifications (nonhomogeneous) in the infrapatellar fat pad, usually of posttraumatic etiology. (Differentiation from loose bodies is required). *8.* Outerbridge ridge (rare), osteochondral deposit on the medial femoral condyle involving the medial portion of the trochlear groove. *9.* Osteochondritis dissecans. *10.* Tertiary intercondylar tubercle. Calcifications may be seen proximal to the tubercle in the course of the ACL. *11.* Quarternary intercondylar tubercle (probably represents fibroostosis of the PCL). *12.* Calcification in the area of the posterior capsule (oblique popliteal ligament, arcuate ligament). *13.* Persistent portion of the proximal fibular epiphysis. (Requires differentiation from calcified bony avulsion of the lateral collateral ligament). *14.* Heterotopic ossifications. *15.* Vascular calcifications

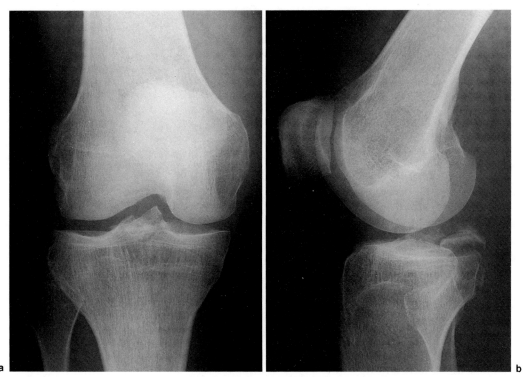

Fig. 6-11 a, b. Fresh ACL avulsion-fracture in the AP projection (**a**). The lateral projection additionally shows a complete avulsion of the posterior intercondylar area (PCL avulsion-fracture) (**b**)

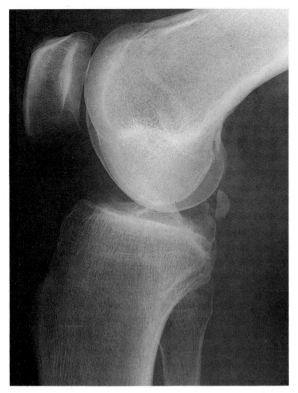

Fig. 6-12. Old bony avulsion of the PCL

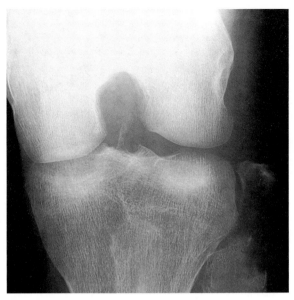

Fig. 6-14. Bony avulsions of the lateral collateral ligament and the tibial insertion of the ACL

Type 1: Anterior edge of fragment is elevated.
Type 2: Fragment is still in contact with the bone.
Type 3: Fragment is completely detached from its bony bed.
Type 3a: Diastasis and rotation of the fragment.

A special type of bony avulsion is the Segond fragment, known also as the lateral capsular sign, for it is interpreted as signifying an associated lesion of the ACL [470, 571, 717] (see Fig. 2-48).

6.1.2
Rauber's Sign

As early as two or three months after a meniscal injury, the rim of the affected tibial plateau may show radiographic changes in the form of periosteal deposits or a projecting "ledge" with a sharp or blunt margin. The ledge may curl upward or downward, or it may appear simply as a thickening of the cortex. These changes, first described by Rauber [534], were demonstrated radiographically by Barucha [31] in more than 80% of patients with old meniscal injuries (Figs. 6-15 and 6-16).

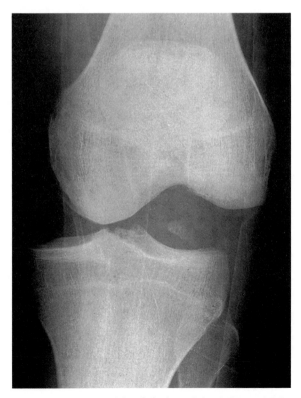

Fig. 6-13. Bony avulsion injuries of the ACL and PCL with subluxation of the knee joint

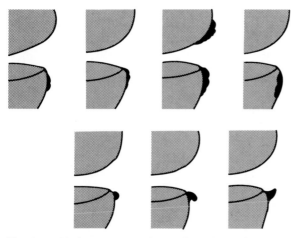

Fig. 6-15. Various presentations of Rauber's sign, after Barucha [31]

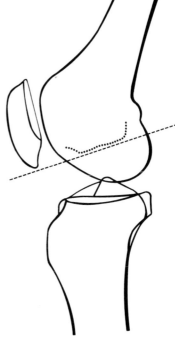

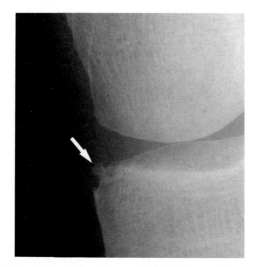

Fig. 6-16. Rauber's sign on the medial tibial condyle

Fig. 6-17. Blumensaat's method of determining patellar height [54]. With the knee flexed 30°, the continuation of the line from the radiodense intercondylar notch (Blumensaat's line) should be level with the patellar apex when patellar height is normal. Bandi [26] prefers to determine patellar height in 50° of flexion, claiming that patella alta is overdiagnosed at 30°

6.1.3
Patellar Position

The patellar position (patellar height) as determined on lateral radiographs is considered to be a significant etiologic factor in retropatellar chondromalacia and patellar dislocation. A basic distinction is drawn between the high-riding patella (patella alta) and the low-riding patella (patella baja).

Of the many methods available for determining patellar height, the most widely used are those of Blumensaat [54], based on a lateral

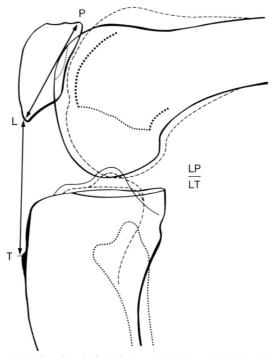

Fig. 6-18. Patellar height index (LP:LT ratio) of Insall and Salvati [301]

radiograph taken with the knee flexed 30° (Fig. 6-17), and that of Insall and Salvati [301], in which the greatest diagonal length of the patella (LP) is divided by the length of the patellar tendon (LT) (Fig. 6-18). Because the ratio of Insall and Salvati has been stated differently by these authors (LT/LP and LP/LT), it is necessary to specify the ratio that is being used.

The advantage of the patellar height index of Insall and Salvati [301] over Blumensaat's method is that the LP/LT ratio can be determined at an arbitrary angle of knee flexion (Fig. 6-18). The major difficulty is determining the exact position of the tibial tuberosity due to its variable prominence [26, 276].

6.1.3.1
Patella alta

An Insall-Salvati patellar height index (LP/LT) less than 0.8 signifies patella alta, a condition which aggravates the stresses on the central and distal portions of the retropatellar cartilage [26]. Because of the greater cartilage load, Haglund's impression, a retropatellar indentation with subchondral sclerosis, has a relatively distal location. Bandi [26] mainly observed this feature in adolescents with a high-riding patella (Fig. 6-19). It can account for the predisposition to chondromalacia and retropatellar osteoarthritis in knees with patella alta. An association with patellar dislocation is also apparent (Fig. 6-20).

6.1.3.2
Patella baja

Patella baja, signified by an Insall-Salvati patellar height index (LP/LT) greater than 1.15, causes greater loading of the proximal portion of the retropatellar cartilage (Fig. 6-21). Bandi [26] notes that the dropping of the patella between the femoral condyles causes the cartilage stresses to become concentrated within a very small area.

Frequently, patella baja is secondary to intraarticular adhesions in the anterior portion of the joint. The adhesions may result from an arthrotomy, hemarthrosis, arthroscopy, or inju-

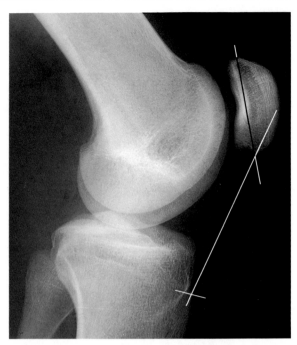

Fig. 6-19. Patella alta in a 17-year-old male. The LP:LT ratio of Insall and Salvati is 0.68

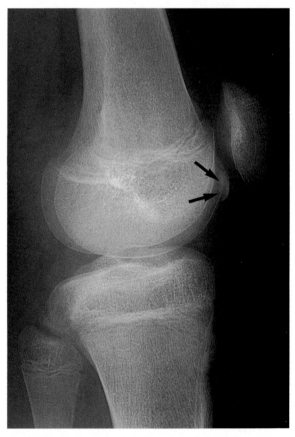

Fig. 6-20. Osteochondral fragment (easily missed, *arrows*) following patellar dislocation. There is coexisting patella alta

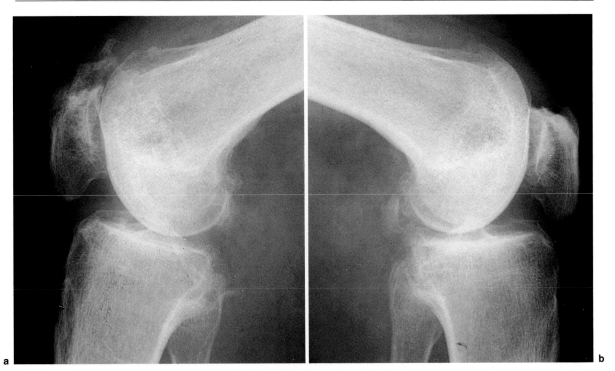

a   b

Fig. 6-21a, b. Patella baja with pronounced bilateral retropatellar osteoarthritis

ry to the infrapatellar fat pad. In this condition, known as infrapatellar contracture syndrome, the patella is fixed in the anterior part of the joint by the connective tissue of the patellar ligament (see Fig. 2-24) [521]. This compromises the extensor function of the quadriceps muscle, resulting often in an extension deficit.

The clinical importance of patellar height determinations has declined in recent years. We know from arthroscopic studies that femoropatellar pain and retropatellar cartilage lesions show little correlation with patellar height. This also explains why tibial tuberosity transfer operations are performed less frequently than before. These procedures should be considered only as a last resort in patients with very pronounced patella alta or patella baja whose pain cannot be controlled by other means.

6.2 Patellar Sunrise Views

Sunrise views taken bilaterally in 30°, 60°, and 90° of flexion provide the best source of information on the status of the femoropatellar joint and patella (Table 6-2). This view will

Table 6-2. Potential findings on patellar sunrise views

- Thick patella
- Thin patella
- Patellar dysplasia (Wiberg types III and IV, hunter's cap)
- Dysplasia of the femoral trochlea
- Lateralization of the patella
- Bipartite patella
- Patellar fractures (especially longitudinal fractures)
- Osteochondritis dissecans of the patella
- Patellar dislocation (fresh)
- Sequelae of patellar dislocation (calcifications, specks of bone in the medial retinaculum)
- Retropatellar osteoarthritis
- Lateral pressure syndrome (narrowing of lateral joint space)

demonstrate patellar and trochlear dysplasias, centering of the patella in the trochlea, the width of the radiographic joint space, and the cancellous and trabecular structure of the patella and femoral condyles (Figs. 6-22 through 6-27).

Wiberg and Baumgartl [416] classified cross-sectional patellar morphologies into types I through IV and a fifth type called the "hunter's cap" (Fig. 6-22). The merits of the Wiberg classification have been questioned, however, because the type I shape is encountered in only about 10% of patients while types II and III predominate very strongly with a prevalence of 70%-80%. Hepp [276] found that 19% of the patellae evaluated in his study could not be fitted into the Wiberg scheme. He therefore proposed the following classification:

1. *Euplasia* (= Wiberg type I)
2. *Medial hypoplasia* (= Wiberg type II–III)
3. *Patellar dysplasia* (hunter's cap, pebble shape, crescent shape, Wiberg type IV, patella magna, patella parva, bipartite patella)

In a functional and biomechanical sense, it matters little whether the bony medial patellar facet has a slightly concave, flat, concave-convex, or convex shape. A far more important factor is the cartilaginous surface, which even in a Wiberg III patella (bony convexity) can show favorable conditions of congruity [276].

Teidtke [648] describes the use of stress radiographs for evaluating femoropatellar instabilities. In this technique the knee is positioned as for a sunrise view of the patella (Merchant technique). With the leg muscles as relaxed as

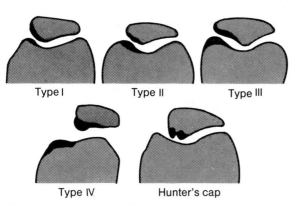

Fig. 6-22. Wiberg classification of patellar morphologies

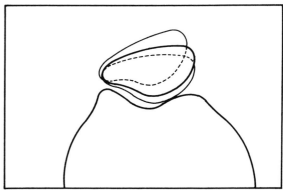

Fig. 6-24. Patellar tilt

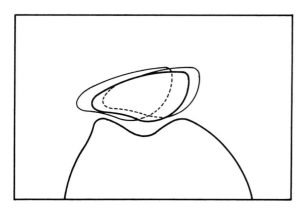

Fig. 6-23. Patellar shift

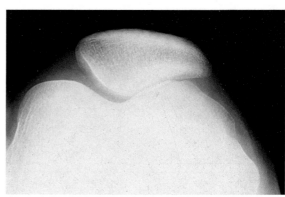

Fig. 6-25. Lateralization of the patella (lateral pressure syndrome)

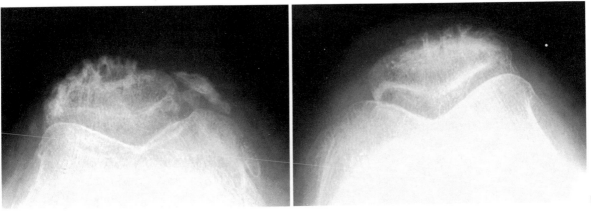

a   b

Fig. 6-26 a, b. Retropatellar osteoarthritis with marginal osteophytes, joint-space narrowing, and subchondral sclerosis

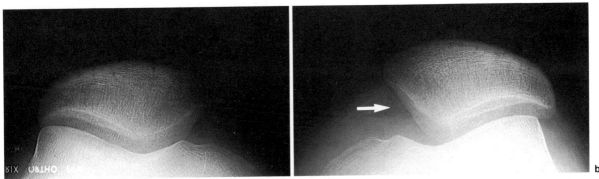

a   b

Fig. 6-27 a, b. Suboptimum sunrise view. The field is too small and the central beam is improperly positioned. The femoropatellar joint space and the profile of the lateral condyle (osteochondral fragment?) can- not be adequately evaluated. On the right side there is evidence of a vacuum sign *(arrow)* and lateral patellar tilt consistent with a previous patellar dislocation

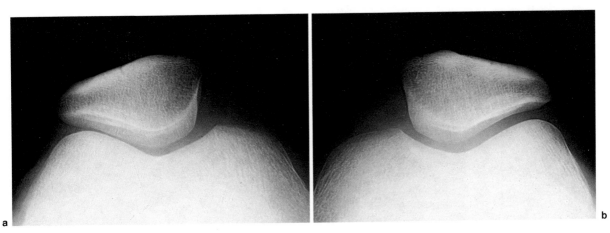

a   b

Fig. 6-28 a, b. Patella with "hunter's cap" shape

possible, the patella is pushed medially and then laterally with the aid of a pushing instrument. The associated patellar tilt (Fig. 6-23) and patellar shift (Fig. 6-24) are evaluated. When femoropatellar instability is present, the applied stress will often produce a pronounced lateral subluxation of the patella and, less frequently, a medial subluxation.

6.3
Tunnel View

The tunnel view through the intercondylar notch, first described by Frick, allows radiographic visualization of the intercondylar fossa and the posterior portions of the femoral condyles [186]. This view should be obtained whenever there is suspicion of an intraarticular loose body, a bony avulsion of the ACL, or osteochondritis dissecans (Fig. 6-29).

With chronic ACL insufficiency, bilateral tunnel views are part of the routine radiographic workup. In many cases the intercondylar eminence cannot be clearly evaluated on the standard AP projection. But the tunnel view demonstrates both the condition of the eminence and the width of the intercondylar notch. ACL insufficiency of long standing leads to a disintegration of joint mechanics which is manifested by stenosis of the intercondylar notch and "peaking" of the intercondylar eminence (Teton's sign) [10, 22, 159] (Fig. 6-30).

Anderson et al. [10] were able to identify five basic types of intercondylar notch shape on CT scans (Fig. 6-30a). Types I and IV are the most common, occurring in 18% and 47% of the normal population. Types IV are less (29%) and especially type V (35%) is more prevalent in patients with an ACL tear. Type V (wave shaped) is found in only 6% of persons with normal knees.

Patients with unilateral or bilateral ACL tears also show a narrowing of the opening notch angle (48.6° versus 54.7° in normal individuals). The ratio of the notch width at two-thirds the notch height to the condylar width was found to be significantly smaller in patients with ACL tears than in normal controls (0.185 versus 0.207) [10].

Souryal et al. [615] describe a different method for determining the intercondylar notch width. They calculate a notch width index by measuring the condyle width and notch width parallel to the joint space at the level of the small lateral groove made by the popliteus tendon (popliteal groove). The ratio of the notch width to the condyle width at that level gives the notch width index [615]. Patients who sustained an ACL tear at a young age through a non-contact maneuver and also have a small notch index are said to be at significant risk for sustaining a rupture of the contralateral ACL [615].

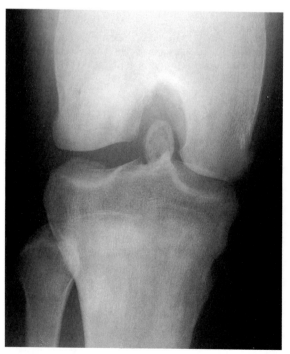

Fig. 6-29. Tunnel view demonstrating a large loose body in the intercondylar fossa

Fig. 6-30 a–c. Various notch shapes identified by Anderson [10] (**a**). Bilateral tunnel views eight years after an ACL tear in the right knee. There is peaking of the intercondylar eminence and stenosis of the intercondylar notch with osteophytosis of the medial femoral condyle. Multiple loose bodies are also present (**b**). The healthy side shows a type IV intercondylar notch of normal width (**c**)

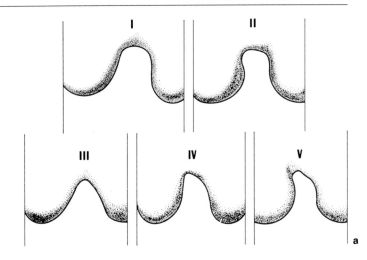

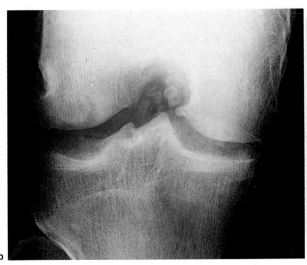

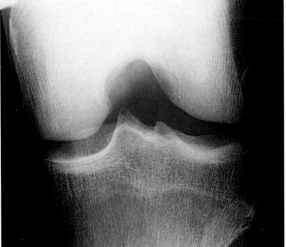

6.4
Oblique Views

If standard radiographic findings are normal but there is reason to suspect an osseous injury, 45° oblique views are indicated to evaluate for a possible fracture of the proximal tibia or femoral condyles and to delineate its extent (Fig. 6-31) [106, 393].

6.5
Functional Views

6.5.1
Weight-Bearing Radiographs

A weight-bearing radiograph is helpful in the evaluation of early osteoarthritis of the femorotibial joint. For this study the patient stands upright with his full body weight distributed equally on both legs. Incipient osteoarthritis is manifested by a narrowing of the joint space, usually on the medial side. The exposure is made of both knees simultaneously to ensure identical imaging conditions for each extremity (Fig. 6-32).

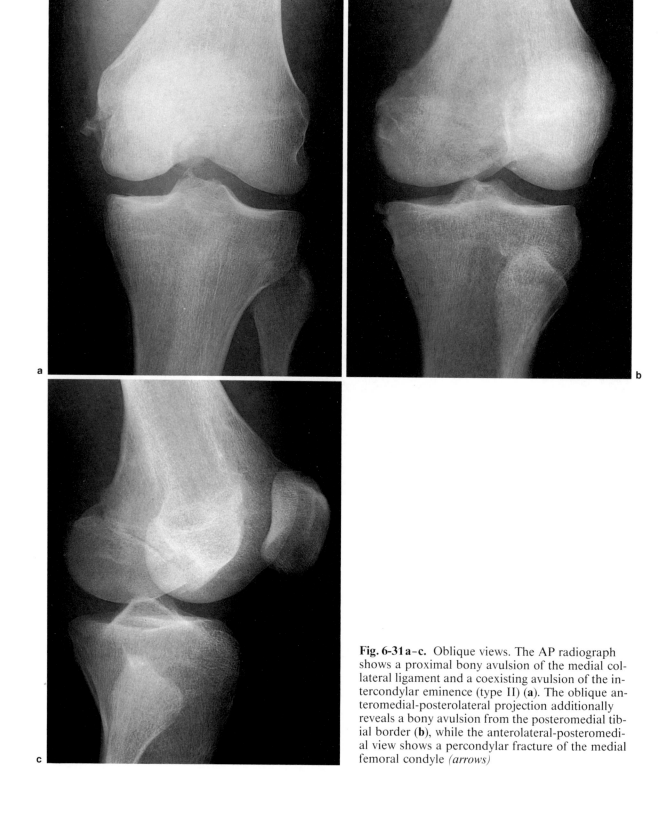

Fig. 6-31 a–c. Oblique views. The AP radiograph shows a proximal bony avulsion of the medial collateral ligament and a coexisting avulsion of the intercondylar eminence (type II) (**a**). The oblique anteromedial-posterolateral projection additionally reveals a bony avulsion from the posteromedial tibial border (**b**), while the anterolateral-posteromedial view shows a percondylar fracture of the medial femoral condyle *(arrows)*

Fig. 6-32 a–c. Weight-bearing radiographs. The standard AP view shows minimal narrowing of the medial joint space (**a**). Somewhat greater narrowing is seen on the conventional extension weight-bearing AP radiograph (**b**).

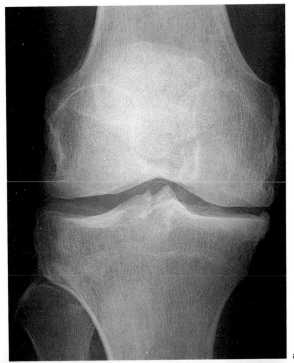

a

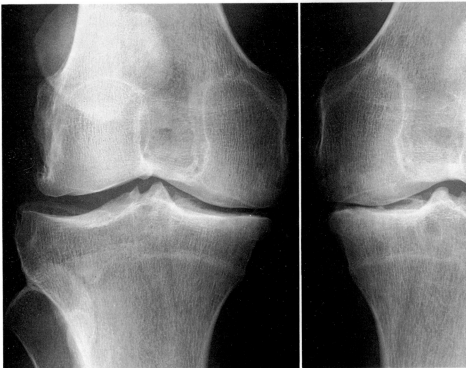

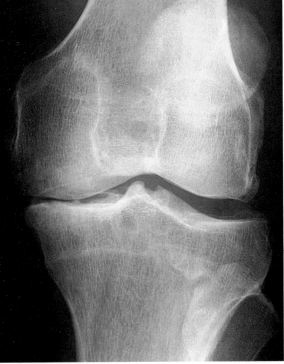

b

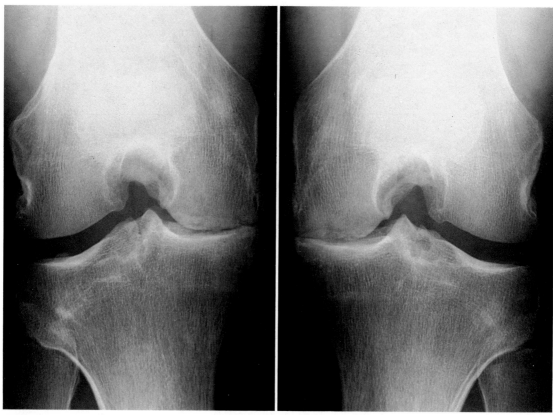

c

Fig. 6-32c. However, the 45° PA flexion weight-bearing radiograph (Rosenberg view) demonstrates profound degeneration of the medial joint compartment in the principal weight-bearing zone (**c**). The medial joint space is almost completely obliterated on this view

6.5.1.1
Rosenberg View

Rosenberg [559] recommends a weight-bearing radiograph made with the knee in 45° of flexion. With this technique, joint-space narrowing of 2 mm or more signifies a relatively high grade of cartilage degeneration (grade III to grade IV chondromalacia), as proven by correlation with arthroscopic findings. Compared with the conventional anteroposterior (AP) extension weight-bearing radiograph, the 45° posteroanterior (PA) flexion weight-bearing radiograph (Rosenberg view) is more specific and more sensitive in the diagnosis of cartilage lesions [559]. Positioning the knee between 30° and 60° of flexion loads the cartilage area which bears the greatest contact loads and makes that area accessible to X-ray visualization (Fig. 6-32c).

6.5.2
Maximum Flexion View

A lateral radiograph made with the knee in maximum flexion is indicated when there is suspicion of loose bodies in the anterior portion of the joint. This view delineates the anterior intercondylar area, and any loose bodies there can be accurately localized. This is not always possible on conventional lateral views taken in the slightly flexed knee (Fig. 6-33).

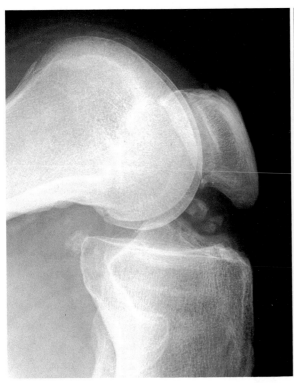
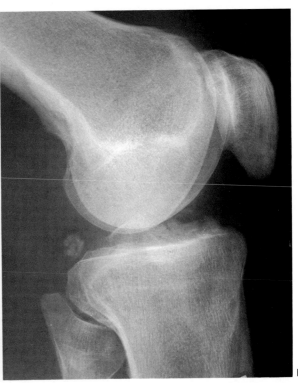
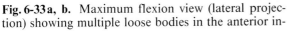

a   b

Fig. 6-33a, b. Maximum flexion view (lateral projection) showing multiple loose bodies in the anterior intercondylar fossa (**a**). Standard lateral radiograph in slight flexion (**b**)

6.6
Arthrography

In years past, the relatively poor image quality provided by arthrography with a negative contrast medium (air) prompted a change to positive media, but this, too, was problematic because it obscured many important features. Finally the desired image quality was obtained by combining air with an opaque contrast material (double-contrast method) [379]. Although arthrography has had its main clinical application in the diagnosis of meniscal tears, it has been reported to miss these lesions in 35% [71] to 40% of cases [207]. The more experienced the radiologist, the higher the diagnostic accuracy. Experienced examiners with more than 200 arthrographies report accuracy rates as high as 85% to 97% [379, 578] (Fig. 6-34). Nevertheless, when we directly compare arthroscopy with arthrography, we must rate arthroscopy as the more reliable procedure. Various indications for arthrography are recognized [50, 379, 595] (Figs. 6-35 and 6-36).

Arthrography may be recommended for selected lesions of the posterior horn of the medial meniscus that sometimes are poorly visualized by arthroscopy [91, 381]. Separations of the meniscal posterior horn from the posterior joint capsule, which in a strict sense are ligamentous rather than meniscal lesions, can also be evaluated [470, 510, 511].

A variant of arthrography called arthrotomography also has been used in the diagnosis of cruciate ligament injuries [338]. However, this technique is associated with a high rate of inaccurate diagnoses [207, 256]. Single-contrast arthrography, when performed by an experienced examiner, has been found to have a high rate of accuracy (78%–88%) [540].

As arthroscopy becomes more widely practiced, there has been a steady, almost universal decline in the use of arthrography. We feel that

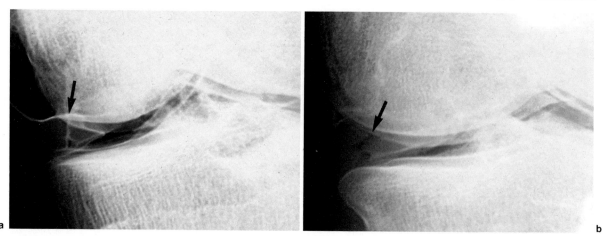

Fig. 6-34a, b. Arthrographic visualization of meniscal lesions. Longitudinal tear (**a,** *arrow*), bucket handle tear (**b**)

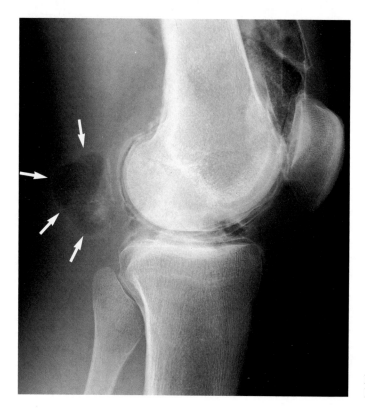

Fig. 6-35. Arthrographic delineation of a Baker's cyst

arthrography is indicated only if the patient refuses arthroscopy and a definitive diagnosis cannot be established by the clinical examination.

6.7
Tomography

In patients with bony ligament avulsions or fractures of the proximal tibia or femoral condyles, tomography is helpful in determining the extent of the fracture and the number of fragments (Fig. 6-37a and b). Detailed visualization is obtained in combination with computed tomography (Fig. 6-37c).

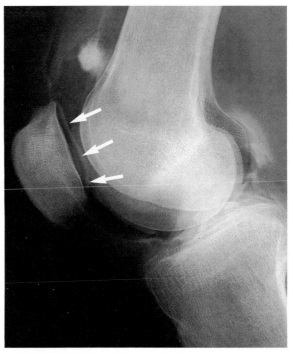

Fig. 6-36. Arthrographic evaluation of the retropatellar cartilage

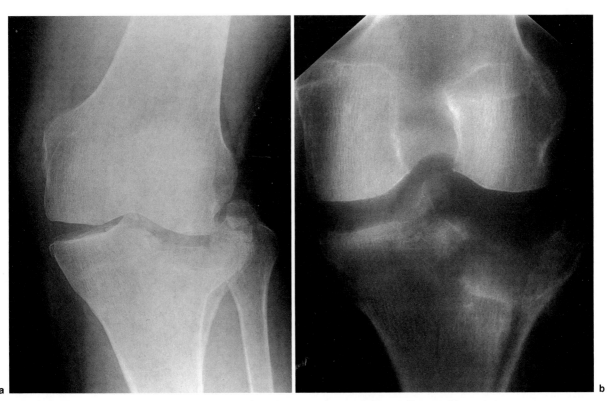

a

b

Fig. 6-37a–c. Lateral fracture of the depression type of the tibia. Initial radiograph shows the distinct dislocation and depression (**a**). Nevertheless, the real extent of the depression is only displayed by tomography (**b**).

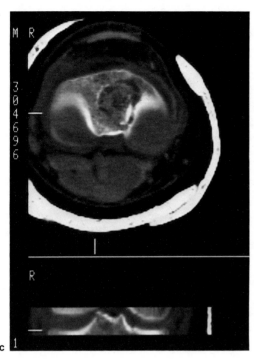

Fig. 6-37 c. Computed tomogramm in avulsion fracture of intercondylar eminence (c)

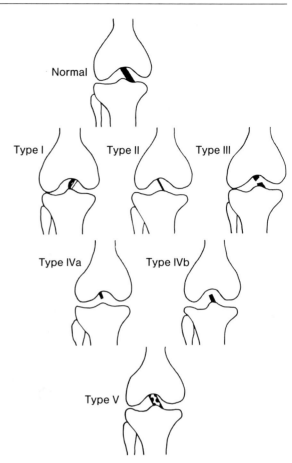

Fig. 6-38. Reiser classification of ACL lesions in CT arthrography [542]: *Type I* (proximal tear, with torn ligament falling upon the PCL, 38%) *Type II* (intraligamentous tear with attenuation of the remaining ligament, 33%) *Type III* (complete rupture with retraction of the torn ends, 6%) *Type IV a* (bony tibial avulsion, 3%) *Type IV b* (bony femoral avulsion, 2%) *Type V* (nonhomogeneous density pattern with hypodense areas, 9%)

6.8 Computed Tomography

Computed tomography (CT) has gained an established place in orthopedic radiology as a means of evaluating the extent of complicated proximal tibial and femoral condyle fractures and determining the number of fragments (Fig. 6-37 c).

CT arthrography can be used to evaluate the morphology of the ACL [522, 542]. However, this study is difficult to perform in acutely injured patients due to the pain caused by flexing the knee joint 90°. It is better suited for older ACL lesions, which are easy to evaluate and classify according to the scheme of Reiser et al. [542] (Fig. 6-38).

CT arthrography is like any imaging procedure in that it permits only a morphologic evaluation. Thus, while CT can detect an attenuation or tear of the ACL, it cannot disclose the functional status of the ligament as clinical tests can.

High-resolution axial CT can detect meniscal lesions with a sensitivity of 96.5%, a specificity of 81.3%, and an accuracy of 91% [417].

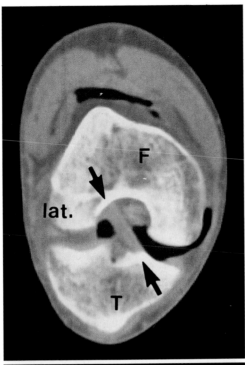

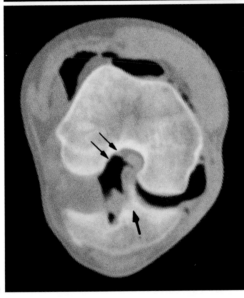

Fig. 6-39 a, b. CT arthrograms demonstrating an intact ACL (**a**) and a Reiser type I tear of the ligament (**b**)

6.9
Xeroradiography

Xeroradiography is a special roentgenographic technique used for the detection of soft-tissue pathology. Besides bony structures, it can portray and differentiate ligaments, fasciae, muscles, and subcutaneous fat.

In the knee, xeroradiography is used chiefly for the diagnosis of popliteal fossa lesions owing to its ability to demonstrate soft-tissue tumors, Baker's cysts, and aneurysms. Even slight contrasts in radiodensities are clearly appreciated, making it possible to evaluate the size and extent of soft-tissue lesions. Because of the edge enhancement inherent in the xerographic technique, marginal structures are well defined even on survey films. Otto [509] claims that this noninvasive technique is superior to conventional arthrography for evaluating the extent of a Baker's cyst.

Xeroradiographic tomography also has been used to evaluate the cruciate ligaments [541], although this application has not become widely practiced.

6.10
Angiography, Digital Subtraction Angiography

Angiography and digital subtraction angiography (DSA) can be used in the diagnosis of posttraumatic, intermittent, and arteriosclerotic vascular changes and occlusions about the knee (Fig. 6-40; see also Figs. 2-34 and 2-35).

6.11
Stress Radiographs

Ligamentous structures are not visualized on conventional X-ray films. Often a ligament injury can be inferred by demonstrating an asso-

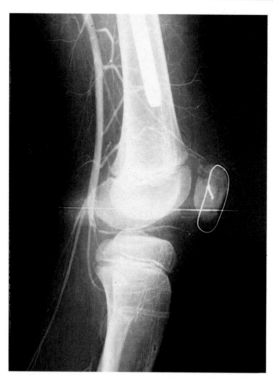

Fig. 6-40. Angiogram demonstrating a posttraumatic occlusion of the popliteal artery at the level of the knee joint. The poorly perfused condition of the extremity was recognized only after emergency treatment had been initiated for obvious orthopedic injuries (fractures of the femur and patella)

ciated bony injury (e. g., a Segond fragment) or foci of calcification. But in capsuloligamentous injuries where there is no osseous involvement, stress radiographs provide a means of documenting the increase of laxity that has been caused by the trauma [77, 160, 238, 527, 528, 620, 632].

As in clinical laxity tests, the varus-valgus or anterior-posterior displacement of the knee can be tested by exerting a force on the knee which causes a relative tilting or shifting of the bony joint members. The direction and amount of the displacement provide information on the underlying capsuloligamentous disruption.

Stress radiography follows the same basic rules that apply to the clinical examination:

1. The patient should be placed in a relaxed position.

2. Pain should be alleviated. The masking of instability by pain-induced muscle spasm accounts for the frequent use of local [227, 327] regional, or general anesthesia [96] to ease or eliminate pain. The laxity increases by approximately 10%–20% when testing is performed under general anesthesia.

3. The uninvolved extremity should be examined first to familiarize the patient with the procedure.

Stress radiographs should be made in both knees under identical conditions. Abnormal laxity can be determined by measuring the difference in the amount of laxity provoked by the applied stress in both knees (Fig. 6-41).

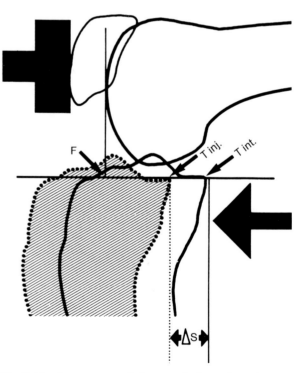

Fig. 6-41. Assessment of the translation of the intact knee *(T intact)* versus the injured knee *(T injured)*. The difference *(ΔS)* represents the increased translation caused by the injury, assuming that both knees are examined under identical conditions (after [623])

6.11.1
Advantages, Disadvantages, and Indications

In the selection of patients for stress radiography, it is important to weigh the advantages (Table 6-3) [77, 125, 234, 291, 309, 319, 329, 428, 469, 527, 662, 665, 700, 715] and disadvantages of the procedure (Table 6-4) [192, 234, 428, 620, 700, 710] and to identify the specific questions that need to be addressed, e. g.:

1. Abnormal laxity?
2. Is there medial or lateral opening? Anterior or posterior drawer ?
3. What is the magnitude of the laxity (quantitative)?
4. What is the magnitude of the laxity in a designated joint position (e. g., 30° flexion)?
5. What is the rotational response of the tibia (internal/external rotation) to the stress?

If questions 1 and 2 need to be addressed, the clinical examination should be repeated. If questions 3 to 5 need to be resolved, machine testing is indicated.

Stress radiographs are made strictly for the purpose of documenting laxity.

Today it is no longer appropriate to use radiographically documented laxity as the criterion for deciding how long to maintain cast immobilization [56, 291, 527, 700].

Müller [470] states that the following stress views are necessary for complete radiographic documentation of instability:

1. Anterior drawer test in 90° flexion with the tibia in internal, neutral, and external rotation.
2. Posterior drawer test in the same positions.
3. Lachman test (anterior drawer in slight flexion).
4. Reversed Lachman test (posterior drawer in slight flexion).

This protocol would require making 10 radiographs, including nonstress views, for each knee. While this would be of considerable scientific interest, it would involve an unacceptably high level of radiation exposure (total of 20 radiographs) for the patient [470].

Table 6-3. Advantages of stress radiography

1. Can differentiate between medial/lateral opening and between anterior/posterior drawer.
2. Can determine degree of laxity.
3. Can determine type of instability.
4. Affords definitive documentation.
5. Demonstrates rotatory components of anterior and posterior drawer.
6. Useful for follow-up.
7. Can differentiate ligament injury from epiphyseal plate separation in children and adolescents.

Table 6-4. Disadvantages of stress radiography

1. Improperly made films are worthless because they cannot be evaluated.
2. Risk of aggravating ligament damage, especially when stress is applied under general, local, or regional anesthesia.
3. Machine-assisted stress views are time-consuming and technically demanding.
4. A negative study does not exclude ligament disruption.
5. Manual and semimanual studies expose the examiner to radiation.
6. The force applied for manual stress views is examiner-dependent.

Accordingly, we recommend that stress radiography be limited to the following indications [632]:

1. Acute capsuloligamentous injury with a suspected ACL tear.
   Anterior drawer test:
   - 30° flexion, neutral rotation (Lachman test),
   - Optional: 60° flexion, 30° internal rotation and 30° external rotation.
   Posterior drawer test:
   - 30° or 60° flexion, neutral rotation.
2. Chronic capsuloligamentous lesion.
   Anterior drawer test:
   - 30° flexion, neutral rotation (Lachman test)
   - 90° flexion, 30° internal rotation and 30° external rotation.

Posterior drawer test:
– 90° flexion, neutral rotation.
With suspected PCL involvement:
– 90° flexion, 30° internal rotation and 30° external rotation.

Two to five radiographs are obtained per knee, depending on clinical findings. We no longer obtain varus-valgus views because of the large intra- and interindividual variations that are encountered. With gross medial and lateral openings, rotation of the femoral condyles relative to the tibial plateau makes a standardized evaluation difficult or impossible.

The follow-up examination to document residual abnormal laxity is performed no earlier than six weeks after operation.

6.11.2
Manual and Semimanual Techniques

Stress radiographs of the knee can be obtained using manual techniques in which the examiner exerts a displacing force on the knee without the use of mechanical aids. As early as 1943, Böhler [56] described a technique for varus-valgus testing in which the knee is flexed over a wooden positioning block of specified dimensions while a varus or valgus stress is manually applied (Fig. 6-42a) [287, 291].

Semimanual techniques of stress radiography have been described by Hohmann [700], Nyga [496], Haffner [238], and Wirth [707]. The wedge-and-strap method is the most familiar (Fig. 6-42b).

Both manual and semimanual techniques are compromised by a lack of standardization in the applied force, the angle of knee flexion, and the position of tibial rotation. The manual techniques, moreover, are patently unacceptable because of the radiation exposure to the examiner (Fig. 6-43).

It should be reemphasized that the purpose of stress radiography is not to exclude or confirm a capsuloligamentous injury but to quantify the amount of laxity that exists in a specified joint position.

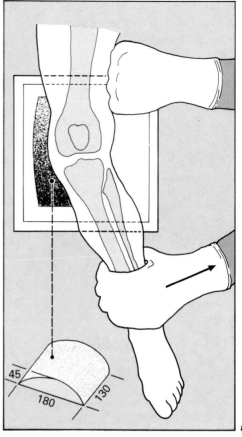

Fig. 6-42a. Böhler's technique for valgus stress radiography of the knee [56]

6.11.3
Machine Techniques

The fundamental drawbacks of manual and semimanual techniques prompted a search for new solutions leading to the development of machine techniques (stress devices, positioning devices) for the radiographic documentation of varus-valgus laxity (Table 6-5) and anterior-posterior displacement (Table 6-6).

The various devices differ in their technical complexity, the types of accessory equipment needed, and the kinds of laxity testing that can be performed. Some devices are relatively simple, being designed purely for varus-valgus or anterior-posterior testing [143, 192, 227, 238, 290, 464, 662]. Devices capable of testing both medial/lateral and sagittal laxities have far

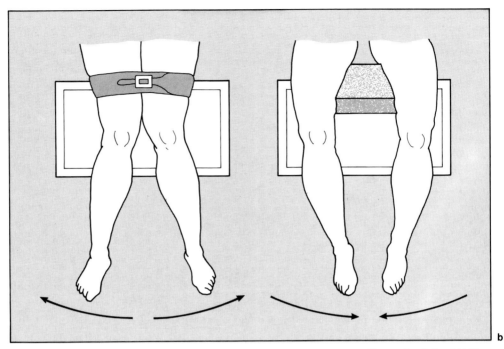

Fig. 6.42 b. Wedge-and-strap technique (**b**) for valgus-varus stress radiography (after [632])

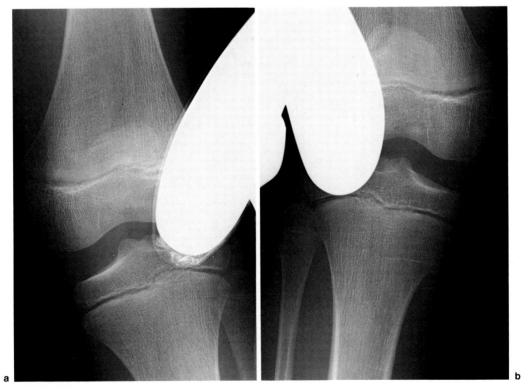

Fig. 6-43 a, b. Manual stress views in a 12-year-old girl. The information content of these radiographs is "nil" because of the nonstandardized technique (un-specified flexion angle) and because portions of the joint spaces are obscured by the lead gloves

Table 6-5. Machine techniques for varus-valgus stress radiography of the knee. (Legend see Table 6-6)

Author	Year	Pos	Ext	20°	Rot	F
Wentzlik	1952	Sup	W			2-4
Quellet I	1969	Sup	x	x		8-12
Kennedy	1971	Sit		x	NR	n.d.
Jäger I	1973	Sup	x	x		8
Grosch	1975	Sup	x	x		Man.
Hafner	1975	Sup	x	x		Man.
Edholm	1976	Sup	x			5
Jacobsen	1976	Sit		x	NR	9
Moore	1976	Sup	x	x		Man.
Scheuba	1978	Sit	x	x		15
Rippstein	1983	Sup	x	x		
Stedtfeld	1983	Sup	x	x	INER	10
Hejgaard	1984	Sit		D	NR	9

more complex designs. In some cases compromises are made in which the design and operation of the device are simplified by omitting means to secure the limb in a specified position of flexion and tibial rotation [551, 574].

As in the clinical examination, it is better to position the knee at a small flexion angle (Lachman test position) than at 90° when stress radiographs are obtained (Table 6-7) [303, 622]. Thus, it is important to check for this capability when a stress device is being considered for purchase. The radiographic Lachman test can be performed using simple apparatus. With the patient lying supine, the lower leg is positioned on a holder so that the knee is slightly flexed and unsupported. Then a weight is suspended from the distal third of the thigh to pull the femur posteriorly. This results in a relative anterior displacement of the proximal tibia (Fig. 6-44) [389].

Pässler [517] has described a simple but reliable technique for radiographic documentation of the Lachman test. He employs the Scheuba apparatus traditionally used for the diagnosis of fibular capsuloligamentous injury. A specified anterior drawer stress is applied to the slightly flexed knee while the patient lies on his side so that the X-ray cassette can be easily positioned beneath the knee (Fig. 6-45). Tibial rotation is disregarded in this technique. The same device can be used for posterior drawer testing in the slightly flexed knee (reversed Lachman test) [517].

Table 6-6. Machine techniques for anterior and posterior stress radiography of the knee

Author	Year	Pos	Anterior drawer					Posterior drawer					F
			90°	60°	30°	10°	Rot	90°	60°	30°	10°	Rot	
Quellet II	1969	Sit	D				NR	D				NR	8-12
Kennedy	1971	Sit	D				NR						n.d.
Volkov	1971	Sit	D				NR						15-20
Jäger II	1973	Sit	D				NR						
Jacobsen	1976	Sit	D				INER	D				INER	20-30
Scheuba	1978	Lat	x					x					15
Stankovic	1979	Sit	D				INER	D				INER	5-10
Gäde	1980	Sit	D	D			INER	D	D			INER	9.5
Torzilli	1981	Sit	D				NR						15
Pavlov	1983	Sit	D	D	D	D		D	D	D	D		n.d.
Rippstein	1983	Lat	x		x			x					n.d.
Stedtfeld	1983	Lat	D	D	D	D	INER	D	D	D	D	INER	15
Hejgaard	1984	Sit	D				INER	D				INER	30
Satku	1984	Sup						x					BW/10
Hooper	1986	Sup			W								3
Latosiewicz	1986	Sit	D				NR	D				NR	14.8
Pässler	1986	Lat			x					x			15

Legend for Tables 6-5 and 6-6:
Position of subject (Pos); tibial rotation (Rot); sitting (Sit); defined neutral rotation (NR); lateral decubitus position (Lat); defined internal, neutral, and external rotation (INER); supine (Sup); extension of knee joint (Ext); applied force (F, in kg); wooden positioning block (W); undefined manual force (Man.); apparent position, not defined (x); body weight (BW); defined position (D); force not defined (n.d.)

Table 6-7. Anterior displacements measured in the radiographic Lachman test

	n	ACL ruptured Ant. displacement	n	ACL intact Ant. displacement
Lerat [389]	125	10.8 mm (+/− 2.7)	180	3.3 mm (+/− 2.0)
Stäubli [622]	85	12.8 mm (+/− 4.1)	53	3.4 mm (+/− 2.0)
Pässler [517]	51	14.7 mm (+/− 3.9)	80	2.5 mm (+/− 1.7)

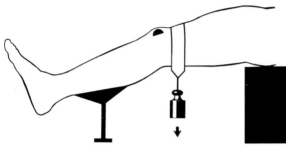

Fig. 6-44. Radiographic Lachman test (after [389])

6.11.4
Standardized Stress Radiographs

Truly standardized stress radiographs cannot be obtained by manual or semimanual techniques, but require a relatively sophisticated mechanical device to position the knee and apply the necessary stress (Table 6-8). Any simplification of the device compromises its ability to provide standard, reproducible examinations.

Table 6-8. Requirements of a device to position the knee for standardized stress radiographs

1. Can hold the limb in a specified position of knee flexion and tibial rotation.
2. Can apply a precisely defined stress.
3. Prevents axial loading and unloading.
4. Allows relaxed positioning of the patient.
5. Easy to store, transport, service, and maintain.
6. Can test anterior-posterior drawer in specified positions of slight flexion and tibial rotation (e. g., Lachman test, reversed Lachman test).

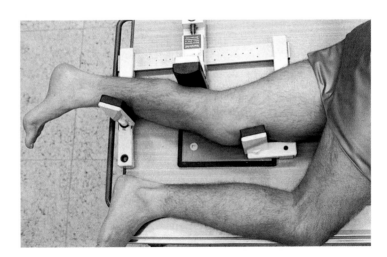

Fig. 6-45. Radiographic Lachman test (after [517])

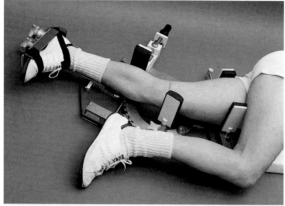

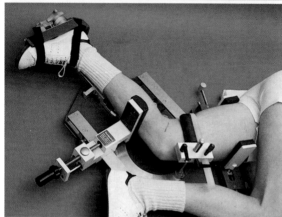

We have developed a positioning device for making standardized stress radiographic views of the knee [623] (Fig. 6-46). The device can test medial and lateral opening in extension and 20° flexion in a specified position of tibial rotation as well as anterior and posterior translation in the range of 0°–90° flexion with the tibia secured in any position between 30° internal rotation and 30° external rotation.

However, the complexity of the device makes it too costly for routine clinical tests, and it should be reserved for special investigations. Stress radiographs should always be made under the supervision of the attending physician, who sees to it that the limb is properly relaxed and positioned. Only in this way can useful, reproducible results be obtained (Figs. 6-47 and 6-48).

Fig. 6-46a, b. Holding device for standardized stress radiography [363], shown applying an anterior drawer stress in 30° of knee flexion (Lachman test) and neutral tibial rotation (**a**), and a posterior drawer test in 60° flexion and neutral rotation (**b**)

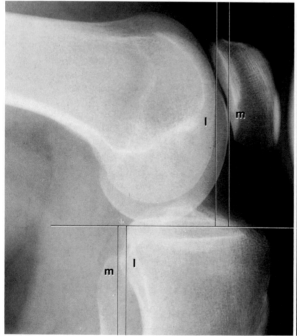

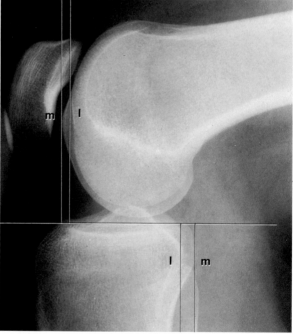

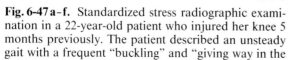

Fig. 6-47a–f. Standardized stress radiographic examination in a 22-year-old patient who injured her knee 5 months previously. The patient described an unsteady gait with a frequent "buckling" and "giving way in the right knee, as if the lower leg wanted to keep moving forward." She was no longer able to walk on uneven ground.

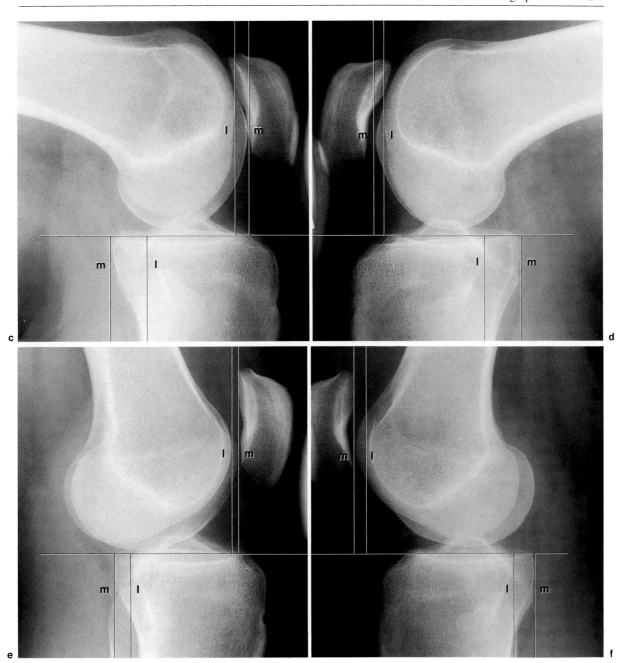

An anterior drawer stress of 15 kg was applied 12 cm distal to the joint line of the knee. Anterior translation *(AT)* was measured for both the medial (med.) and lateral (lat.) condyles using the technique of Jacobsen (see Fig. 6-50).

Position: 90° flexion, 30° external rotation
Right: med. AT: 40.0 mm   lat. AT: 32.0 mm **(a)**
Left: med. AT: 50.0 mm   lat. AT: 42.0 mm **(b)**
Difference: med. AT: 10.0 mm   lat. AT: 10.0 mm

Position: 90° flexion, 30° internal rotation
Right: med. AT: 52.0 mm   lat. AT: 33.0 mm **(c)**
Left: med. AT: 56.0 mm   lat. AT: 38.0 mm **(d)**
Difference: med. AT: 4.0 mm   lat. AT: 5.0 mm

Position: 30° flexion, neutral rotation (Lachman test)
Right: med. AT: 48.0 mm   lat. AT: 39.0 mm **(e)**
Left: med. AT: 71.0 mm   lat. AT: 58.5 mm **(f)**
Difference: med. AT: 23.0 mm   lat. AT: 19.5 mm
Interpretation: Chronic complex anterior instability with insufficiency of the ACL, medial collateral ligament and posteromedial capsule, laxness of the lateral and posterolateral ligamentous structures of the right knee.

The Lachman test demonstrates extreme anterior translation (Fig. 6-47 **e**, **f**). On clinical examination, a positive pivot shift was elicited not just in internal tibial rotation but also in neutral and external rotation

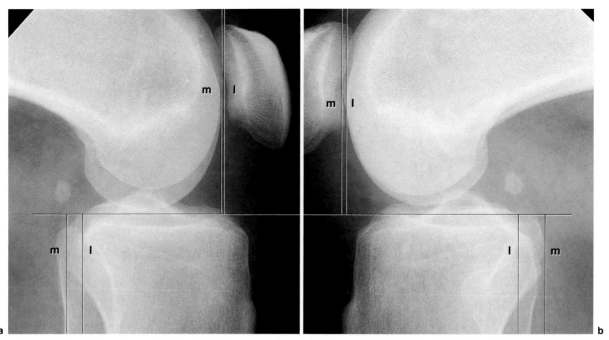

Fig. 6-48a, b. Standardized stress radiographic examination in a 31-year-old woman who sustained an automobile dashboard injury of the left knee 6 weeks previously. A posterior drawer stress of 15 kg was applied 12 cm distal to the joint line of the knee. Posterior translation *(PT)* was measured for both the medial (med.) and lateral (lat.) condyles using the technique of Jacobsen (see Fig. 6-50).

Position: 90° flexion, neutral rotation
Right: med. PT: 60.0 mm   lat. PT: 53.0 mm   **(a)**
Left: med. PT: 78.0 mm   lat. PT: 65.0 mm   **(b)**
Difference:med. PT: 18.0 mm   lat. PT: 12.0 mm
Interpretation: Marked posterior instability with rupture of the PCL of the left knee

The trend toward standardized stability testing has led to the development of "nonradiographic" techniques of machine evaluation, as described in Chap. 9.

6.11.5
Measuring Techniques

Because stress radiographs are made not just in neutral rotation but also with the tibia rotated internally and externally [125, 192, 308, 354, 620, 623], tibial rotation is an important factor to be considered.

Once the anatomic structures have been identified, it is necessary to locate well-defined landmarks that occur consistently on every radiograph and to relate those features to one another through a system of tangential, perpendicular, or parallel lines. Both femoral and tibial reference lines (f, t) and reference points (F, T) are established.

Once the geometric relationship between the reference lines and points has been determined (distance in mm, angles), anterior-posterior translation and varus-valgus displacement can be calculated for the joint in question.

The choice of the measuring technique depends on time requirements, the technical standard of the positioning device, the question to be addressed and the quality of the radiograph [624].

The literature is replete with descriptions of techniques for measuring medial/lateral and sagittal laxities on stress radiographs of the knee joint [624].

Of the techniques for determining varus-valgus displacement [309, 354, 464, 513], we favor that of Palmer [513] owing to its simplicity and practicality (Fig. 6-49). Gross laxity is difficult

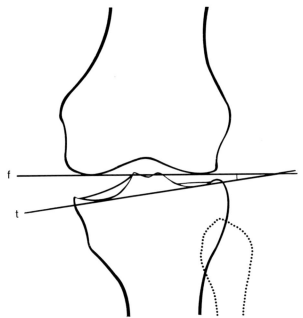

Fig. 6-49. Technique of Palmer [513] for measurement of medial-lateral opening. Line f is tangent to the most distal points on the medial and lateral femoral condyles; line t is tangent to the highest (or lowest) points on the medial and lateral tibial plateaus

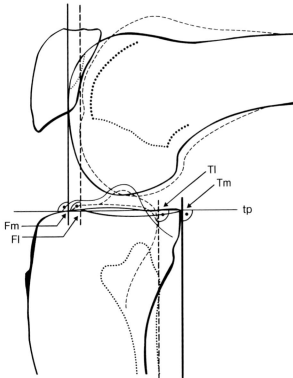

Fig. 6-50. Technique of Jacobsen [308] for measurement of anterior-posterior translation. The tibial-plateau line tp (Jacobsen's "baseline") is drawn through the highest anterior and posterior points of the tibial plateau. Lines perpendicular to tp are then drawn tangent to the most anterior points of the medial *(solid line)* and lateral *(broken line)* femoral condyle and to the most posterior points of the medial *(solid line)* and lateral *(broken line)* tibial condyle. The points where the tangents intersect line tp represent the femoral *(Fm, Fl)* and tibial *(Tm, Tl)* reference points. The difference between the distance *FmTm (FlTl)* in the healthy knee and *FmTm (FlTl)* in the injured knee indicates the degree of the medial (lateral) translation (after [632])

to measure because the varus-valgus stress causes a twisting of the joint components, especially the femur, that cannot be quantified by any known measuring technique.

Of the many techniques available for measuring displacement on the sagittal plane [180, 308, 354, 390, 391, 470, 496, 517, 620, 662], we favor that of Jacobsen [308] because the reference lines and points are easy to define, and displacements can be measured without regard for the angle of knee flexion. Additionally, this method makes allowance for rotational movements of the tibia, i.e., the displacements of the medial and lateral joint compartments can be individually determined (Fig. 6-50) [624].

If it is acceptable to disregard tibial rotatory motion, the technique of Pässler [517] can be recommended. This method employs a template for the measurement of anterior or posterior tibial displacement (Fig. 6-51).

6.12
Radiographic Documentation
of Active Laxity Tests

6.12.1
Active Lachman Test
(Active Quadriceps Test in 30° Flexion)

The anterior displacement of the proximal tibia elicited by contraction of the quadriceps muscle with the knee in slight flexion (active

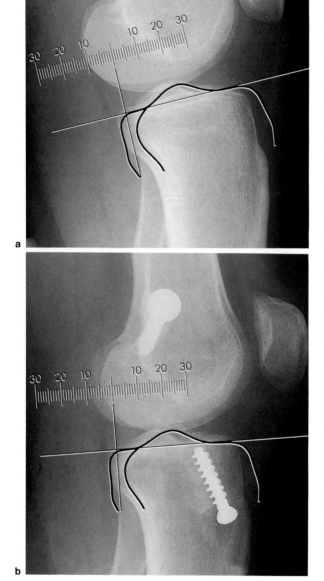

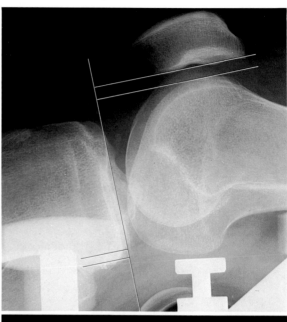

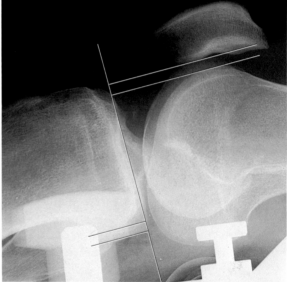

Fig. 6-51a, b. Measuring technique of Pässler [517] with overlay. Preoperative view (**a**) and postoperative view (**b**) following ACL reconstruction

Fig. 6-52a, b. Radiographic 30° active quadriceps test (active Lachman test) with flexion defined by positioning device, initial position (**a**). As the patient performs the maneuver, the proximal tibia subluxates anteriorly by 10 mm due to ACL rupture (measuring technique of Jacobsen) (**b**)

Lachman test) can be documented radiographically [24, 121, 389] (Fig. 6-52).

Dejour [121] and Lerat [389] measured an average anterior displacement of 3.2 mm and 3.3 mm, respectively, in normal populations. This contrasts with values of 11 mm [121] and

10.8 mm [389] measured for anterior displacement in patients with a torn ACL. The correlation with nonradiographic machine measurements (e.g., the KT 1000 arthrometer) confirms the accuracy of radiographic documentation of active laxity tests. Lerat [389] found a

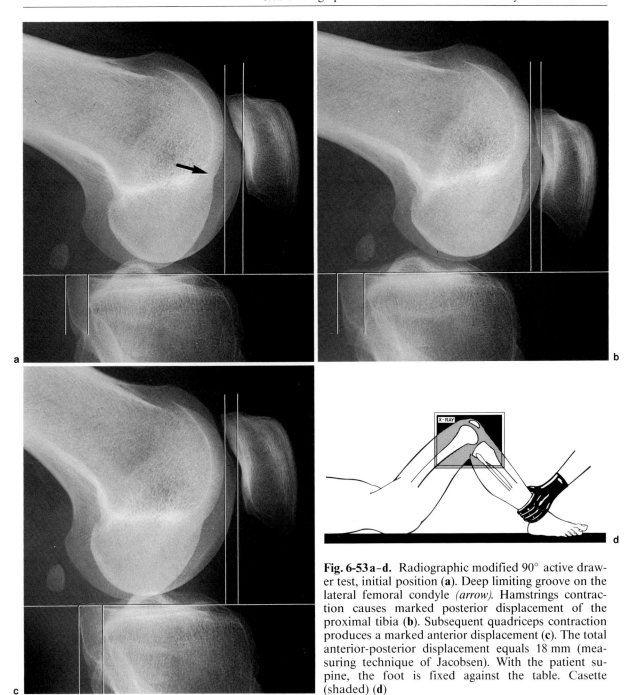

Fig. 6-53a–d. Radiographic modified 90° active drawer test, initial position (**a**). Deep limiting groove on the lateral femoral condyle *(arrow)*. Hamstrings contraction causes marked posterior displacement of the proximal tibia (**b**). Subsequent quadriceps contraction produces a marked anterior displacement (**c**). The total anterior-posterior displacement equals 18 mm (measuring technique of Jacobsen). With the patient supine, the foot is fixed against the table. Casette (shaded) (**d**)

smaller radiographic value of anterior tibial displacement by muscular contraction than was determined by machine laxity testing (with the KT 1000 arthrometer). However, no significant difference was found in patients with ACL tears. In addition, the radiographically documented active Lachman test proved significantly more reliable in demonstrating the diagnostically important difference between the healthy and affected sides [389].

6.12.2
Modified 90° Active Drawer Test

The active laxity tests in 90° flexion are as easy to document radiographically as the Lachman test. Especially in patients with suspected PCL damage, the posterior displacment of the tibia elicited by hamstring contraction can be simply and reliably documented on an X-ray film. The modified active test in 90° flexion (see Fig. 3-52) also can be documented radiographically (Fig. 6-53).

These radiographically documented active test procedures are advantageous in that they use relative simple apparatus and cause little or no pain. For examinations with the knee flexed 90°, the X-ray cassette is mounted on a height-adjustable holder positioned lateral to the knee joint. For a lateral projection the foot is immobilized and the patient is told alternately to straighten the leg (quadriceps) and pull the foot in toward the buttock (hamstrings). By closely observing the limb, the examiner can make the exposure at the exact moment when the corresponding muscle group is maximally tense.

Further studies on these new techniques are required.

7
Magnetic Resonance Imaging

Magnetic resonance imaging (MRI) is the only imaging modality besides sonography that does not utilize ionizing radiation. While the early focus of interest in MRI was on studies of the parenchymatous organs and the detection of brain pathology, in recent years the technique has proved to be well suited for the examination of articular structures. In the knee joint, MRI can demonstrate the bony joint components, the hyaline articular cartilage, the menisci, the cruciate and collateral ligaments, and even the synovium and surrounding soft tissues with a clarity that permits the evaluation of numerous pathologic conditions [4, 124, 194, 233, 242, 250, 305, 334, 351, 371, 529, 537, 543, 580, 602, 614, 716].

Every technique for the diagnostic imaging of joints must meet stringent quality criteria in terms of image contrast and spatial resolution.

7.1
Instrumentation

The use of a high-field magnet operating at a static field strength of 1 tesla or more (e. g., the 1.5-T Magnetom, Siemens, West Germany) yields a very high signal-to-noise ratio that affords excellent anatomic detail (Fig. 7-1). Special coils should be used for examinations of the knee joint. Nonhomogeneous signal patterns can arise when a surface coil is used, leading to image distortions that can hamper diagnosis. It is better to use volume coils having at least two conducting elements which multiply encircle the joint being examined (Helmholtz coil, wrap-around coil). The collected data should be displayed on at least a 256 × 256 image matrix. The patient is positioned supine with the hip fully extended and the knee slightly flexed. The inferior pole of the patella should be positioned at the center of the coil (Fig. 7-1 b).

7.1.1
Pulse Sequences

T1- and T2-weighted spin-echo sequences, the standard pulse sequences used for imaging the abdominal organs, brain, and spinal cord, are also suitable for articular examinations. However, the MRI of joint disorders has been greatly enriched by the use of gradient echo (GE) sequences. These sequences can be optimally tailored to specific investigations by modifying the repetition time (TR), echo time (TE), and flip angle. The system that we currently use (Fig. 7-1) has the capability for imaging in FLASH (high proton density, flip angle determines T1 or T2 weighting) as well as FISP sequences (image contrast defined by the T1/T2 ratio).

A major advantage of the gradient echo sequences is their suitability for the 3-D imaging technique, in which the entire volume of interest is excited and then divided up into individual slices. 3-D imaging also allows for the secondary spatial reconstruction of specific anatomic structures on a different, arbitrarily selected plane at a later time (see Fig. 7-3).

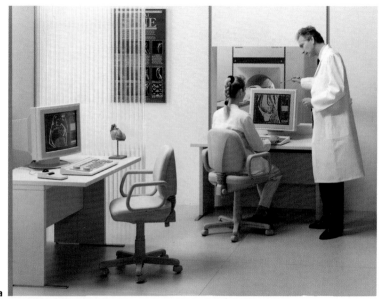

a

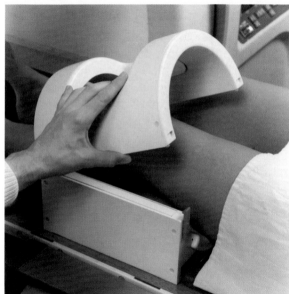

b

Fig. 7-1a, b. 1.5 Tesla Magnetom imager (Siemens, Er-langen, W. Germany) (**a**), The patient's knee is placed within a special knee coil (**b**)

7.2
Menisci

The anterior and posterior horns of the menisci are best visualized on sagittal sections, and the central portion is best seen on coronal views (Fig. 7-2). Radial reconstructions can be made when the 3-D imaging technique is used. This permits a complete anatomic reconstruction in which all segments of the meniscus

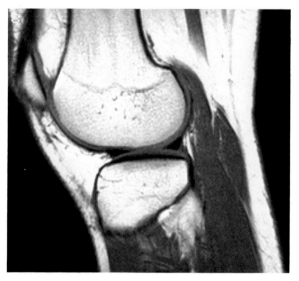

Fig. 7-2. Intact anterior and posterior horns of the lateral meniscus

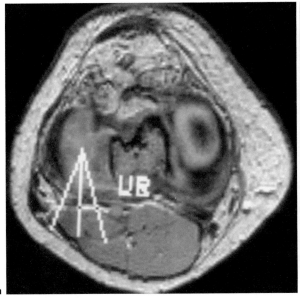
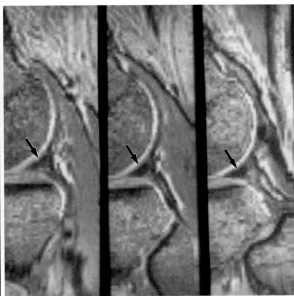

a b

Fig. 7-3a, b. Reconstruction of the medial meniscus in 3-D technique. Selected planes of section *(white lines)* **(a).** Following reconstruction, the characteristic trian-gular shape of the medial meniscus is portrayed on each of the selected planes **(b)**

Table 7-1. Classification of meniscal lesions. (After Reicher [593a])

Grade	MR appearance	Pathology	Tearing
0	Low, homoge-neous signal in-tensity	None	None
I	Punctate area of increased signal intensity on one section, does not communicate with the meniscal sur-face	Mucoid degen-eration	Unlikely
IIa	Multiple punctate sites of increased signal intensity	Extensive mu-coid degenera-tion	Likely
IIb	Linear hyperin-tensity that does not communicate with the meniscal surface		
III	Longitudinal or irregular area of increased signal intensity, defor-mation, displace-ment of fragments	Tear communi-cating with the meniscal sur-face	Definite tear

are portrayed in their characteristic wedge-shaped cross section (Fig. 7-3).

The classification of Reicher has proven use-ful for categorizing the appearance of meniscal lesions on MR images (Table 7-1, Fig. 7-4).

Meniscus lesions of grade I or grade II severity cannot be detected by arthroscopy, be-cause they consist of structural changes within the substance of the meniscus. It is likely that these changes will eventually progress to a frank tear, and indeed the precursor lesions may themselves produce clinical symptoms re-sembling a chronic meniscal lesion, although locking does not occur. Differentiation is re-quired from the physiologic areas of increased signal intensity that may be seen in meniscal tissue. These areas are regularly shaped and may be found in many parts of the meniscus (see Fig. 7-4).

Grade III meniscal lesions can be visualized by arthroscopy. They appear as fissures or tears of variable depth.

MRI has been found to have a high specific-ity, sensitivity, and accuracy in the diagnosis of

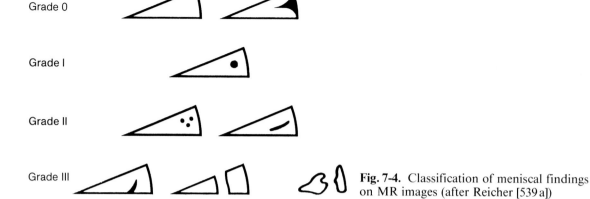

Grade 0

Grade I

Grade II

Grade III

Fig. 7-4. Classification of meniscal findings on MR images (after Reicher [539a])

meniscal lesions (Table 7-2). The reported rate of false-positive results is between 5% [459] and 20% [600], that of false-negative results between 3% and 33% [600].

Thus, MRI is a powerful technique for the diagnosis of meniscal pathology (Fig. 7-5). While it is true that a meniscal lesion can be correctly diagnosed by clinical examination in 60%–90% of cases, it is not uncommon for symptoms of a lateral meniscal tear or retropatellar lesions to be projected medially [627], creating the erroneous impression of a medial meniscal tear. MRI is most rewarding in cases where the clinical examination cannot definitely exclude a meniscal lesion, and typical meniscal symptoms are present.

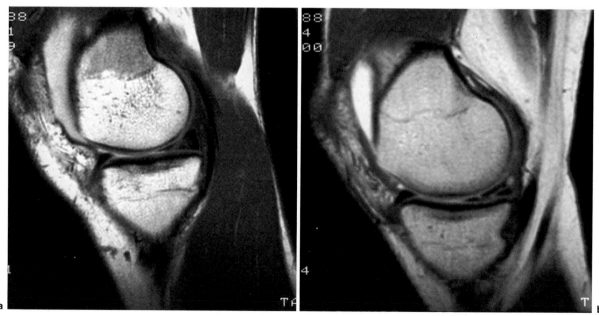

a

b

Fig. 7-5 a, b. Lesion of the posterior horn of the medial meniscus (**a**). In some cases contrast can be enhanced by the intraarticular injection of gadolinium-

DTPA (**b**). Inferior longitudinal tear with an associated horizontal tear

Table 7-2. Sensitivity, specificity, and accuracy of MRI in the diagnosis of meniscal lesions (MM = medial meniscus, LM = lateral meniscus)

Author	Year		Specificity	Sensitivity	Accuracy
Mandelbaum	1986	MM	82%	96%	100%
		LM	95%	75%	91%
Jung	1988		83%	88%	94%
Minkoff	1988	MM	94%		89%
		LM	95%		83%
Polly	1988	MM	100%	96%	98%
		LM	95%	67%	90%
Silva	1988				49%
Jackson	1988	MM	89%	98%	93%
		LM	99%	85%	97%
Glashow	1989		84%	83%	

7.3
Cruciate Ligaments

7.3.1
Anterior Cruciate Ligament

The entire course of the ACL can be visualized on sagittal scans when the leg is positioned in slight external rotation (10°–20°). A similar evaluation can be made on paraxial views (Fig. 7-6). In examinations were 3-D imaging is used, the course of the ligament can be visualized by reconstruction.

The ACL has a higher MR signal intensity than the PCL. Accordingly, it does not appear as a homogeneously dark (low-signal) band like the PCL, but more as a nonhomogeneous dark structure permeated by brighter zones of higher signal intensity. This nonhomogeneous signal pattern is attributed to the interposition of fat between the divergent collagen fibers, especially in the distal portions of the ligament (Fig. 7-7).

Tears of the ACL can be detected clinically by the Lachman test (see Fig. 3-19), but their exact location (proximal, central, distal) cannot be ascertained. Nor is it possible to exclude an acute partial tear of the ACL in patients with hemarthrosis and a positive Lachman test with a firm end point. Lesions of the ACL are of variable prominence on MR im-

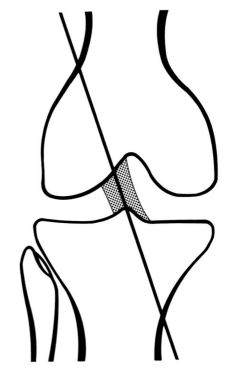

Fig. 7-6. Paraxial scan planes for demonstrating the ACL

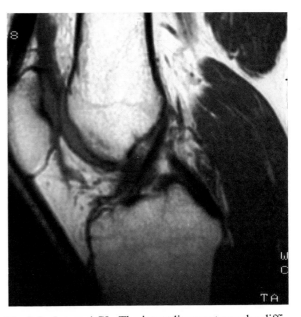

Fig. 7-7. Intact ACL. The intact ligament may be difficult to distinguish from surrounding soft tissues

ages and can be classified using the system of Reiser [545 a] (Fig. 7-8).

MRI can not only confirm the diagnosis of an ACL tear with very high accuracy (Table 7-3) but can also pinpoint the location of the tear.

The study can also disclose coexisting lesions of the cartilage or menisci. The site of the ligament tear has an important bearing on treatment planning. A proximal or distal tear can be managed by reattachment of the ligament, combined with an augmentation procedure. A midsubstance tear, on the other hand, is usually managed by primary reconstruction of the ligament e. g. with an homologous substitute.

MRI has a strong role in the evaluation of postoperative problems following ACL reconstructions. The patient who develops or retains an extension deficit following ACL reconstruction is an excellent candidate for MRI, which can clearly demonstrate the reconstructed ligament, its sites of tibial and femoral attachment, and the surrounding tissue (Fig. 7-9). It may be found, for example, that the extension loss results from placing the tibial insertion site too far anteriorly, or from hypertrophic changes in the transplant or surrounding tissue (see Fig. 2-25 b).

Table 7-3. Specificity, sensitivity, and accuracy of MRI in the diagnosis of ACL lesions

Author	Year	Speci-ficity	Sensi-tivity	Accuracy
Mandelbaum	1986	100%	100%	100%
Jung	1988	82%	100%	95%
Haller	1988	100%		100%
Glashow	1988	82%	61%	
Minkoff	1988	87%		80%
Jackson	1988	96%	100%	97%
Polly	1988	100%	97%	97%

A slowly progressive extension loss after ACL reconstruction also can be investigated by MRI. Osteophytes, only faintly visible on radiographs, are frequently causative. Osteophytes that do not contain bone marrow are poorly demonstrated by MRI.

Following autologous cruciate reconstructions, MRI is of some value in assessing the intraligamentous condition of the transplant and classifying its structure [241, 543]. Initial studies indicate that clinical and MRI findings do not always concur. In some clinically stable knees that underwent ACL reconstruction, for example, MRI demonstrated only fibrous tissue instead of a uniform ligamentous structure [241].

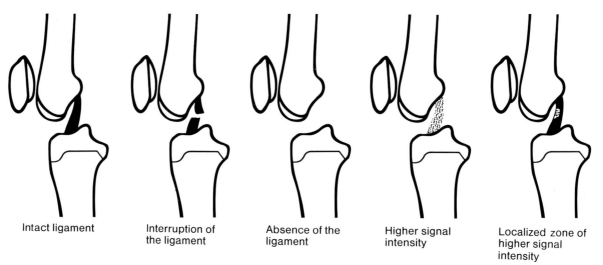

Intact ligament   Interruption of   Absence of the   Higher signal   Localized zone of
                       the ligament   ligament   intensity   higher signal
                                                                                         intensity

Fig. 7-8. Classification of MRI findings in ACL lesions (after Reiser [545 a])

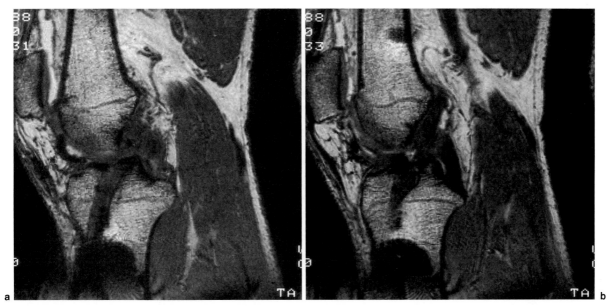

Fig. 7-9 a, b. MRI examination following ACL reconstruction with an alloplastic substitute. The course of the drill channel in the proximal tibia appears normal (**a**). The ligament passes over the lateral femoral condyle in the over-the-top position (**b**)

7.3.2
Posterior Cruciate Ligament

The PCL appears on MR images as a curved, posteriorly convex structure of uniformly low signal intensity. MRI is useful for evaluating the course and continuity of the ligament (Fig. 7-10).

The clinical diagnosis of a PCL lesion is quite difficult compared with the diagnosis of an ACL tear. It is not unusual to find a negative posterior sag and negative posterior drawer test in patients with an acutely torn PCL [299]. Thus, MRI can assist in the diagnosis of a suspected PCL injury in cases where clinical findings are equivocal (Fig. 7-11).

In chronic cases, imaging should be performed with contiguous thin (< 4 mm) sagittal slices to ensure that a possible absence of the PCL is not overlooked (Fig. 7-12).

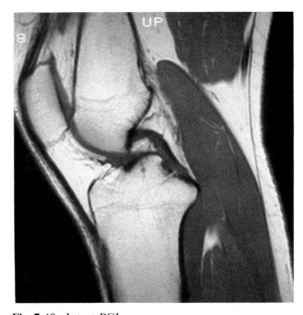

Fig. 7-10. Intact PCL

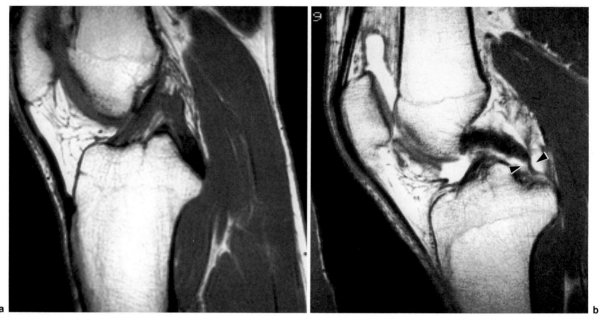

Fig. 7-11a, b. Proximal rupture (**a**) and distal attenuation *(arrows)* (**b**) of the PCL

7.4
Cartilage

The cartilage can be demonstrated on axial, coronal, and sagittal planes. Axial views are best for visualizing the retropatellar cartilage.

Clinical signs are of limited value for assessing the condition of the cartilage. Pain, recurrent effusion, and palpable crepitus are non-specific signs that are features of many other disorders. On plain radiographs, secondary changes such as joint-space narrowing and osteophytosis provide the only visible evidence of degenerative cartilage disease. Even arthrography and articular CT can demonstrate only superficial cartilage changes.

Similarly, arthroscopy can demonstrate all superficial cartilage lesions but tells us little about the structural integrity of the cartilage or

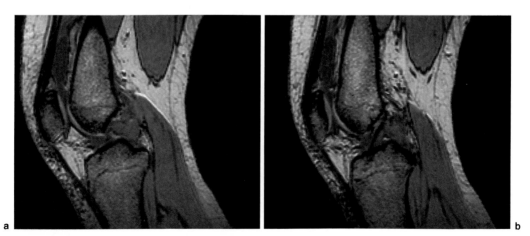

Fig. 7-12a, b. "Absent" PCL (**a, b**). The ligament is sought on multiple contiguous slices. The ACL appears as a structure of higher signal intensity (**b**)

its thickness. MRI provides a noninvasive technique for acquiring this kind of information.

Recent investigations, including our own studies, indicate that MR gradient-echo sequences with intermediate FLIP angles (FISP 30° and 40°, FLASH 30° or 40°) are ideally suited for cartilage examinations. This was demonstrated experimentally by imaging the retropatellar cartilage in a human patella autopsy specimen. Longitudinal defects 1 mm deep, 2 mm deep, and extending to the subchondral bone were created in the cartilage, and the specimen was imaged using various spin- and gradient-echo sequences (Fig. 7-13).

The proper imaging sequences can demonstrate pathologic changes in both the femoral and the retropatellar cartilage. A comparision of arthroscopic and MR findings in patients with retropatellar chondromalacia showed that MRI had a sensitivity of 95%, a specificity of 66%, an accuracy of 88%, a positive predictive value of 90%, and a negative predictive value of 20%, with a prevalence of 76% [545]. Grade I chondromalacia of the retropatellar cartilage is manifested by a nonhomogeneous signal pattern on MR images. Structurally, however, the cartilage is still intact and shows no evidence of surface irregularities. The presence of surface irregularities implies grade II chondromalacia, while full-thickness changes extending to the subchondral bone signify grade III disease (Fig. 7-14).

If osseous involvement is present in addition to cartilage changes, as in osteochondritis dissecans (Fig. 7-15) or osteonecrosis (Fig. 7-16), MRI is helpful in forming an impression of the extent of the pathology. In the case of osteochondritis dissecans, the absence of a fluid rim around the osteochondral fragment is noted when the cartilage surface is intact.

MRI is also useful for tracking the postoperative course of the knee following a subchondral abrasion chondroplasty or Pridie drilling procedure. Filling of the cartilage defect by fibrous tissue can be confirmed, and the optimum timing for a follow-up arthroscopic examination can be determined.

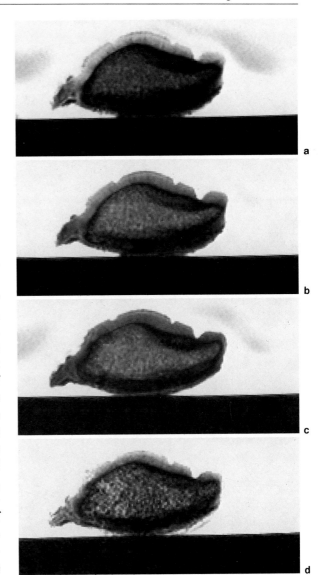

Fig. 7-13a-d. Determination of optimum imaging sequences for the diagnosis of cartilage lesions. Artificially produced lesions of the retropatellar cartilage were imaged using various gradient-echo sequences: FISP 10 (**a**), FISP 30 (**b**), FISP 50 (**c**), and FISP 90 (**d**). The lesions are demonstrated best by the FISP 30 sequence (**b**)

In patients who developed new complaints following osteochondral grafting, König [372] used MRI to identify the cause (e.g., medullary edema, exudative synovitis, cartilage edema, degenerative cartilage changes with fibrocartilage formation, circumscribed cartilage defects). Again, gradient-echo sequences were found to be advantageous for portraying the

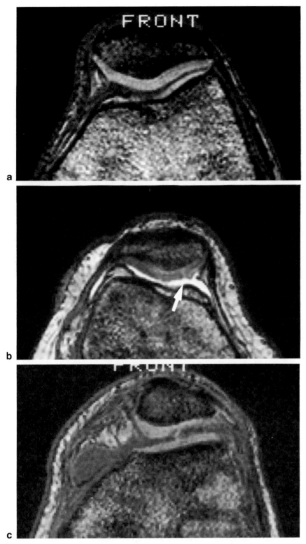

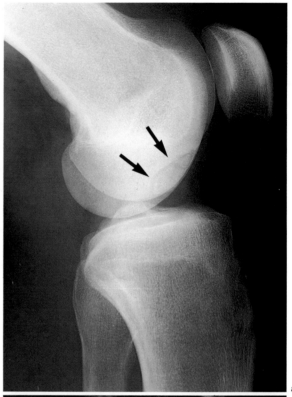

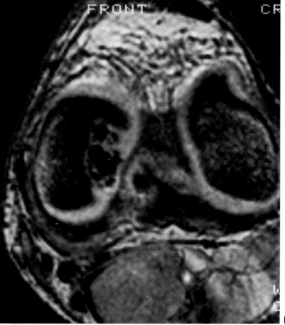

Fig. 7-14a-c. Intact retropatellar cartilage (**a**). Structural irregularities and small fissures in grade II chondromalacia (**b**). Deep fissuring and full-thickness cartilage defects in grade III chondromalacia (**c**)

cartilage changes. Spin-echo sequences proved better for evaluating the osseous portion of the graft.

Fig. 7-15a, b. Osteochondritis dissecans of the medial femoral condyle. Radiographic findings (**a**). MRI defines the total extent of the lesion (**b**)

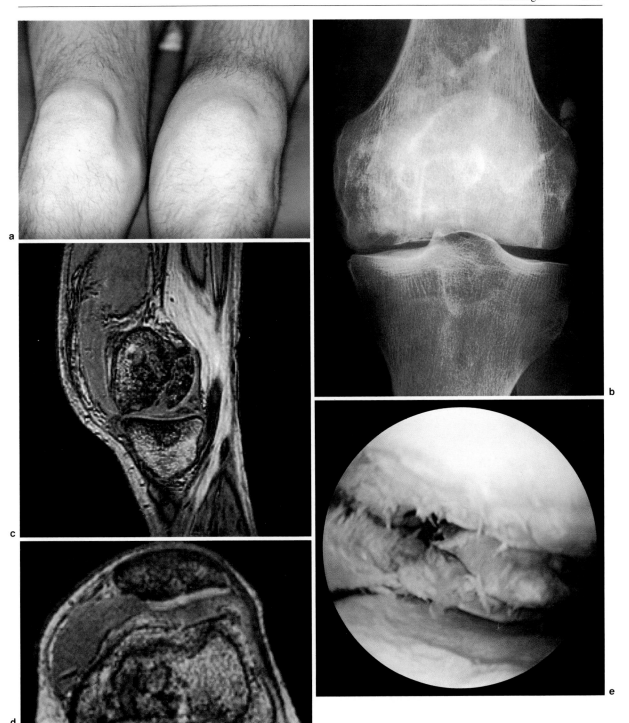

Fig. 7-16a–e. Pronounced knee joint effusion three days after a rotational injury in a 36-year-old dialysis patient (**a**). Radiographs show massive osteonecrosis (cortisone therapy), a positive Rauber's sign on the medial tibial plateau, and multiple intraarticular loose bodies (**b**). The sagittal MR image (**c**) defines the true extent of the cartilage damage on the medial femoral condyle and reveals a peripheral meniscal tear. The transverse image shows a cartilage defect involving the entire medial patellar facet (**d**). MR findings were confirmed by arthroscopy, which revealed multiple loose bodies, osteochondral fragments, and a degenerative, fibrillated medial meniscus (**e**)

7.5
Periarticular Soft Tissues

MRI can demonstrate periarticular mass lesions such as tumors, meniscal cysts, Baker cysts (Fig. 7-17), as well as thickenings of the patellar ligament like those encountered in jumper's knee.

7.6
Synovial Membrane

In rheumatoid patients it is not unusual to find enormous thickenings and deposits on the normal synovial membrane. Frequently these are accompanied by cartilaginous changes. Both can be detected by MRI (Fig. 7-18).

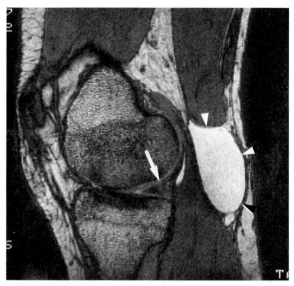

Fig. 7-17. Baker's cyst *(arrowheads)* and lesion of the posterior horn of the medial meniscus *(arrow)*

7.7
MR Arthrography

The intraarticular injection of a contrast-enhancing material (gadolinium-DTPA) is currently undergoing clinical trials in Münster, West Germany, and in Vienna, Austria. Initial results indicate that contrast enhancement with Gd-DTPA increases the sensitivity of MRI in the detection of cartilage lesions [233]. Our own clinical experience shows that the information content of the examination can be significantly increased in selected cases.

The ACL is more easily distinguished from surrounding structures on contrast-enhanced MR images, in some cases permitting the more reliable identification of incomplete tears. Contrast enhancement with Gd-DTPA can also aid in the diagnosis of meniscal lesions (see Figs. 7-5b, 7-11b, 7-17). Of course, contrast injection sacrifices a major advantage of MRI, its noninvasiveness, and many more clinical studies are needed to substantiate the diagnostic value of MR arthrography in the knee.

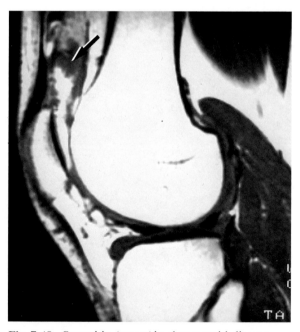

Fig. 7-18. Synovitis *(arrow)* in rheumatoid disease

7.8
Concluding Remarks

MRI can be applied to the diagnosis of a great many diseases and articular disorders. Realistically, however, its role should be limited to cases in which MR images can supply pertinent information not furnished by the clinical examination. For certain indications, we regard MRI as an important adjunct to the diagnostic spectrum (Table 7-4).

Not infrequently, MRI performed after major arthroscopic procedures reveals multiple intraarticular metallic artifacts which degrade the image quality. These artifacts are produced by fine metal debris that has been abraded from the surface of the operating instruments.

Table 7-4. Indications for MRI of the knee joint

1. Extension deficit following ACL reconstruction or refixation
2. Detection of cartilage lesions
3. Follow-up of cartilage operations
4. Follow-up of osteochondral graft procedures
5. Localization of tear site in ruptures of the ACL
6. Evaluation of the PCL
7. Tumors
8. Indeterminate mass lesion
9. Unexplained meniscal symptoms in patients with negative clinical meniscal tests
10. Preoperative detection of coexisting lesions
11. Unexplained joint complaints in cases where surgery is contraindicated

These particles cause the patient no discomfort, and they cannot be detected clinically or radiographically. They can, however, cause some deterioration of the MR image.

8
Sonography

Sonography is a very widely used diagnostic technique offering numerous advantages (Table 8-1) that have long been appreciated in the clinical imaging of abdominal, retroperitoneal, vascular, and gynecologic disorders. In orthopedics, ultrasound has been used for many years in the early detection of congenital hip dysplasias. But sonography is also playing an increasingly important role in the diagnosis of lesions of other joints (shoulder, knee), tendons, and muscles. A great variety of injuries and diseases of the knee joint can be diagnosed with ultrasound (Table 8-2) [145, 187, 205, 206, 258, 269, 456, 556].

8.1
Instrumentation

We use the Toshiba model SSA 100-A real-time ultrasound imager with a 5-MHz and 7.5-MHz sector transducer (Fig. 8-1). The 5-MHz transducer is preferred for soft-tissue examinations, especially in obese patients. We operate the scanner in the normal video mode in which echogenic areas appear bright and hypoechoic areas appear dark. The inverse format (black on white) like that used in sonography of the infant hip is not recommended for scanning of the soft tissues and knee joint.

We use a video printer, video cassette recorder, and multiformat camera to make records of the sonographic examination.

Table 8-1. Advantages of sonography

1. Causes no known side effects.
2. Limits need for invasive diagnostic procedures.
3. Can be freely used even in infants and small children.
4. Easy to use.
5. Requires little time.
6. Economical.
7. Can be performed as bedside or outpatient procedure.
8. Permits differentiated soft-tissue diagnosis.
9. Can demonstrate muscles, tendons, and joints.

Table 8-2. Structures and lesions about the knee joint that can be demonstrated with ultrasound

1. Baker's cyst
2. Meniscal lesions (tear, cyst)
3. Hematoma
4. Abscess
5. Effusion
6. Disorders of the patellar ligament (e.g., jumper's knee)
7. Osteochondritis dissecans
8. ACL and PCL
   - Acute complete tears
   - Old tears with associated effusion
   - Traumatic or inflammatory swelling
9. Medial collateral ligament
10. Synovitis
11. Bursitis
12. Soft-tissue tumors
13. Periarticular osteochondromas
14. Bone fragments (including bipartite patella)
15. Loose bodies
16. Epiphyseal plate fracture and separation
17. Vascular abnormalities: thrombosis, aneurysm, or occlusion of the popliteal artery
18. Soft-tissue infiltration by bone tumor
19. Patellar tracking disorders
20. Cartilage thickness

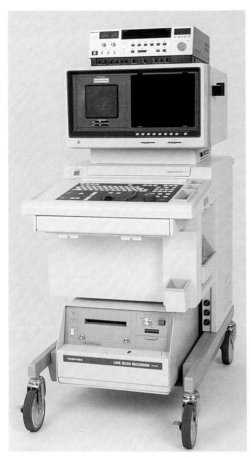

Fig. 8-1. Ultrasound scanner (Toshiba SSA 100-A)

Table 8-3. Recommended procedure for ultrasound scanning of the knee, after Röhr [556]. The structures that can be visualized are shown in parentheses

1. Suprapatellar longitudinal and transverse scans.
2. Suprapatellar transverse scan in the flexed knee (femoropatellar articular surfaces).
3. Infrapatellar transverse scan in the extended knee (femoropatellar articular surfaces).
4. Infrapatellar longitudinal scan (patellar ligament, infrapatellar bursitis? lesion of tibial tuberosity?).
5. Medial longitudinal scan (medial collateral ligament, meniscal cyst?).
6. Medial longitudinal scan in 90° flexion with maximum external rotation of the tibia (medial collateral ligament, central portion of medial meniscus).
7. Infrapatellar longitudinal scan in maximum flexion with slight external rotation (about 15°) of the transducer (ACL, infrapatellar fat pad).

The patient is moved to the prone position for scanning the posterior joint regions.

8. Posteromedial longitudinal scan in slight flexion (posterior horn of medial meniscus) and in 60°–80° flexion with neutral, internal, and external rotation of the tibia (lesions of posterior meniscus horn).
9. Posterior intercondylar longitudinal scan (PCL, posterior capsule).
10. Posterolateral longitudinal scan in extension (posterior horn of lateral meniscus, popliteus region) and in flexion with neutral, internal, and external rotation of the tibia (posterior horn of lateral meniscus).
11. Posterior transverse scan (without rotation) at various levels (ACL, PCL, fibrous posterior capsule).
12. Posterior transverse scan with the tibia internally rotated (ACL).

8.2
Examination Procedure

Ultrasound scanning is performed over several compartments of the knee joint, making this examination considerably more time-consuming than sonography of the hip (approx. 20–30 min). In every case the healthy knee should also be examined to furnish a baseline.

Like arthroscopy, the sonographic examination should follow a systematic routine to ensure that no pathology is overlooked. We base our procedure on that recommended by Röhr [556] (Table 8-3).

Every ultrasound examination should include scans of the blood vessels in the popliteal fossa, because vascular diseases in this region (aneurysms, occlusions, thrombosis) can be a source of knee complaints [556].

8.3
Menisci

Sonography is being used with increasing success for the diagnosis of meniscal pathology [205, 206, 556]. The posterior horns of the medial and lateral menisci, the most common locations for injury, are the areas most accessible to ultrasound (Figs. 8-2 through 8-6). The anterior horn of the medial meniscus is frequently difficult to visualize [556].

When performed by an experienced examiner, sonography is approximately 70-90% accurate in the diagnosis of meniscal lesions [205, 206]. Sometimes scans will show intrameniscal structural changes, similar to those seen on MR images, which do not have the typical appearance of a meniscal tear. These may represent changes within the substance of the meniscus that have not yet led to a tear but will probably culminate in a tear with passage of time.

When scanning the meniscal posterior horn, the examiner should also examine the posterior compartment of the knee joint for evidence of disease (Fig. 8-7).

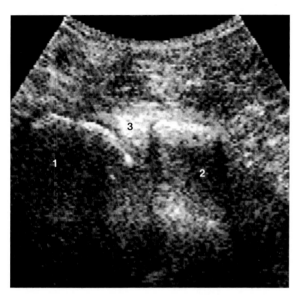

Fig. 8-2. Intact posterior horn of the medial meniscus. Medial femoral condyle *(1)*, medial tibial plateau *(2)*, posterior horn of medial meniscus *(3)*

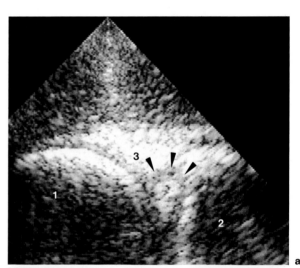

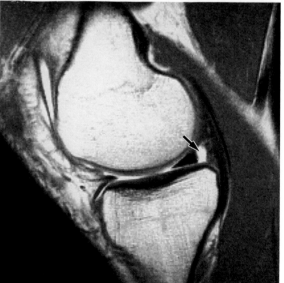

Fig. 8-4a, b. Posterior longitudinal tear of the medial meniscus *(arrow)* (**a**). A thin peripheral rim of meniscus is preserved *(3)*. Medial femoral condyle *(1)*, medial tibial plateau *(2)*. The meniscal tear is also demonstrated by MRI *(arrow)* (**b**)

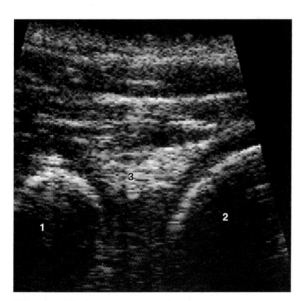

Fig. 8-3. Meniscal remnant six months after partial meniscectomy. Medial femoral condyle *(1)*, medial tibial plateau *(2)*, remnant of medial meniscus *(3)*

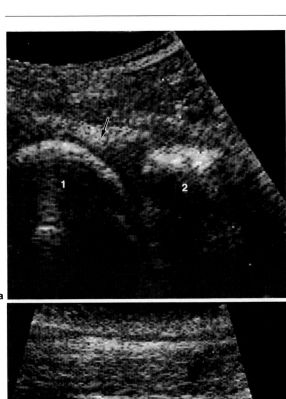

a

b

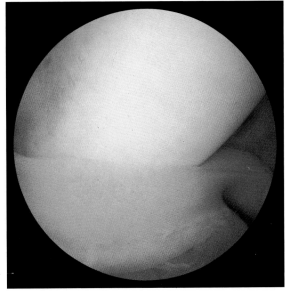

d

Fig. 8-5a-d. Bucket-handle tear of the medial meniscus with a small peripheral remnant *(arrow)* (**a**). Elsewhere on the peripheral remnant there is a break in the meniscal contour consistent with a second tear *(arrow)* (**b**). Contralateral side with intact meniscus *(arrow)* (**c**). Arthroscopy revealed a bucket-handle tear whose principal fragment had displaced into the intercondylar fossa and a posterior longitudinal tear (**d**). Medial femoral condyle *(1)*, medial tibial plateau *(2)*

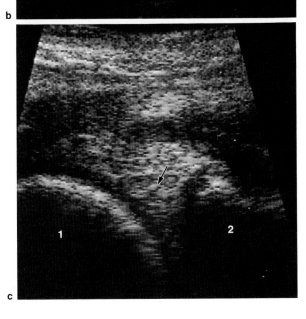

c

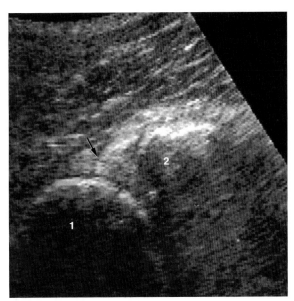

Fig. 8-6. Posterior longitudinal tear of the medial meniscus *(arrow)*. Medial femoral condyle *(1)*, medial tibial plateau *(2)*

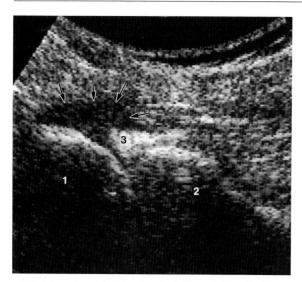

Fig. 8-7. Enlargement of the posteromedial recess *(arrows)* in a woman with rheumatoid arthritis. The patient experienced continual posteromedial knee complaints since undergoing open synovectomy two years earlier. At arthroscopy, the posteromedial recess was found to be filled with hypertrophied synovium. Medial femoral condyle *(1)*, medial tibial plateau *(2)*, posterior horn of medial meniscus *(3)*

8.4
Cruciate Ligaments

While tears of the ACL can be readily diagnosed clinically by means of the Lachman test (see Sect. 3.3.3), the exact location of the tear cannot be established by clinical methods. This accounts for the value of sonography in cruciate ligament injuries. An experienced sonographer can examine even the proximal part of the ACL, including its area of origin. This is easier in cases where the patella rides fairly high when the knee is completely flexed. Old ACL tears are difficult to evaluate with ultrasound unless effusion is present [556].

Sonographic documentation of the Lachman test provides an indirect means of evaluating anterior displacement following rupture of the ACL [577]. In this technique the transducer is mounted on a positioning device that is secured to the knee. Scans are taken to determine the deflection angle (slope of the tibial plateau relative to the plane of the ultrasound

beam) in the resting position and during application of a maximum anterior drawer stress in the slightly flexed knee (Lachman test). If the ACL is torn, the difference in the deflection angles will differ significantly from that in healthy controls [577]. This technique also can reproducibly evaluate knee laxity following a ligament reconstruction procedure. In contrast to machine laxity testing (see Sect. 9.3), the results of the ultrasound examination are not adversely affected by the soft tissues, even in obese patients, because the measurement is performed entirely on bony structures.

Because injuries of the PCL cannot always be reliably excluded by clinical examination [299], there is interest in noninvasive techniques that can evaluate this structure without the use of ionizing radiation.

The distal and central portions of the PCL can be delineated with ultrasound (Fig. 8-8). Lesions of the ligament produce a widening of the ligament echo [258, 556]. In acute injuries, however, sonography cannot reliably distinguish between ligamentous tissue and hemorrhage, although this is easily accomplished by MRI. The proximal part and origin of the PCL usually cannot be visualized due to scattering of the obliquely incident sound beam on the walls of the intercondylar notch [258]. Nonetheless, sonography is a useful examination for suspected PCL injury, especially when one considers its relatively low technical and monetary costs compared with other modalities.

8.5
Collateral Ligaments

Röhr [556] presents the following classification of medial collateral ligament injuries based on their sonographic features:

Grade I   *(stretch injury):* Hypoechoic thickening of the medial collateral ligament. The ligament itself appears homogeneous but contains few internal echoes.

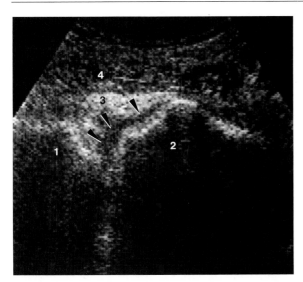

Fig. 8-8. Intact PCL *(arrows)*. Roof of the intercondylar notch *(1)*, posterior intercondylar portion of the tibial plateau *(2)*, posterior capsule *(3)*, gastrocnemius muscle *(4)*

Grade II *(partial rupture):* Hypoechoic thickening of the ligament, which contains a number of scattered internal echoes.

Grade III *(complete rupture):* Massive thickening with a combination of hypoechoic and hyperechoic areas.

Just as the Lachman test for anterior laxity can be documented sonographically (see above), the valgus test for medial laxity also can be quantified on ultrasound scans [53].

8.6
Femoropatellar Joint

Disorders of the femoropatellar joint, especially instability or uncentering of the patella, are difficult to detect by clinical examination alone. Sonography may be used to evaluate for tilting and lateralization of the patella and to determine the width of the femoropatellar joint space [145]. So far, however, relatively little research has been done on this application.

8.7
Cartilage

The thickness of the articular cartilage on the weight-bearing portion of the femoral condyles can be determined sonographically [6, 269]. As the knee must be scanned in complete flexion, this examination is not possible if the patient cannot adequately flex the knee. Neither can the examination be performed if there is an intraarticular effusion which separates the cartilage from the overlying soft tissues that normally appose to the front of the femoral condyles during flexion. The cartilage thickness can be determined with ultrasound only if the soft tissues are in contact with the cartilage. Accordingly, the articular cartilage is well delineated only when it is contrasted against the different acoustic impedances of the adjacent soft tissues and subchondral bone [269]. At present we have no personal experience with the sonographic determination of cartilage thickness.

8.8
Patellar Ligament

After rupture, insertional tendinopathy at the inferior pole of the patella, known also as "jumper's knee," is the most common disorder affecting the patellar ligament. While rupture of the ligament is easily diagnosed, the morphologic status of the proximal insertion of the patellar ligament cannot be adequately assessed by clinical examination alone.

The sonographic features of jumper's knee are characteristic [187]:

1. *Thickening or swelling* of the patellar tendon.
2. A *heterogenous tendon structure.* Hyperechoic areas may indicate scar tissue, circumscribed zones of fibrosis, or intratendinous calcifications. These calcifications and scars represent the final stage of a chronic inflammation. Hypoechoic areas represent inflammatory or edematous zones, fresh hematoma, or intraligamentous microruptures.

3. *Irregularities of the tendinous envelope,* which may appear thickened or poorly defined.

Fritschy [187] classified the morphologic tendon changes into three stages based on sonographic findings:

1. *Inflammatory stage* (initial stage). Characterized by edema of the tendon fibers. The tendon is swollen but still presents a homogeneous appearance.
2. *Irreversible anatomic lesions.* The tendon presents a heterogeneous structure (hypoechoic and hyperechoic areas).
3. *Final stage.* The tendinous envelope is irregular and thickened, and the tendon fibers appear heterogeneous, but swelling has subsided.

Sonography is also useful for following the progression of jumper's knee and confirming therapeutic response. It thus provides a sensitive diagnostic technique for evaluating the disorder and monitoring treatment [187, 265].

Since the patellar ligament is the preferred donor structure for autologous reconstructions of the ACL, sonography offers an excellent modality for the follow-up of these operations. While it might be assumed that the patellar ligament remains thin for a long period of time, and thus forms a site of weakness, the opposite is true. Dupont [139] showed that when the central 50% to 60% of the tendon is removed to replace the ACL, the remaining tendon quickly hypertrophies. Follow-up sonograms showed that the hypertrophy persisted for about one year after operation and then tended to regress [139].

8.9
Problems in Sonography

Sonography cannot be performed under optimum conditions in every patient. The following factors can complicate the sonographic evaluation of the knee [556]:

1. *Limitation of knee motion* (e.g., by an entrapped meniscus or loose body). Structures such as the ACL, which can examined only in complete flexion, or the central portion of the medial meniscus, which is best viewed in 90° flexion with the tibia in maximum external rotation, cannot be evaluated.
2. *Patella baja.* A low-riding patella hampers evaluation of the ACL on the longitudinal infrapatellar scan with the knee in complete flexion.
3. *Extreme obesity.* If the knee cicumference exceeds 50 cm, even the 5-MHz transducer will not have sufficient penetration to give a satisfactory view of the intercondylar notch.
4. *Presence of large osteophytes* in severe degenerative arthritis. The underlying soft tissues cannot be adequately evaluated.

8.10
Outlook

Sonography of the knee joint has not yet become widely established as a procedure for the diagnostic evaluation of knee disorders. But as experience with the modality grows and its advantages, limitations, and capabilities are more clearly appreciated, there is no question that the role of sonography will expand. The almost ubiquitous presence of ultrasound instruments in office and clinical settings can only accelerate this trend.

9
Machine Evaluation of Laxity

The problems of objectifying and quantifying clinical findings in laxity testing, along with the risks of radiation exposure to the patient and examiner, especially in stress radiography, have spurred the development of "nonradiographic" techniques of machine examination designed to provide a more objective and quantitative evaluation of knee joint laxity.

Various articular structures and functions can be examined with these techniques, owing largely to advances in microprocessor technology. "Nonradiographic" machine laxity testing is still in its early stages, however, even though many types of test apparatus have already been designed and implemented.

Of the imaging techniques that do not utilize ionizing radiation, the most promising are sonography, owing to its widespread availability, and MRI, which is reserved for special types of investigation (see Chap. 7 and 8).

The standard clinical examination can establish whether or not excessive knee laxity is present as a manifestation of ligamentous injury. Also, a gross assessment can be made as to whether the abnormal laxity is mild or severe. A truly quantitative evaluation cannot be made, however. When laxity is determined by stress radiography, numerous X-ray films are needed to supply the quality of information needed in modern knee diagnostics. If findings are inconclusive, it would be irresponsible to repeat the examination several days later as this would compound the radiation exposure. Nonradiographic techniques, on the other hand, may be repeated as often as desired.

One problem in machine testing is that the measuring apparatus or sensor must be applied to the soft-tissue envelope surrounding the knee joint. Shifting of the soft tissues can result in inaccurate readings unless the measurements are computer-corrected or proper allowance is made for the soft-tissue displacements.

9.1
Requirements

The apparatus for nonradiographic laxity testing must meet the same stringent standards as the positioning devices used in stress radiography (see Table 6-8).

As in the clinical examination, the patient undergoing machine laxity testing should be comfortably positioned so that there is little or no reflex muscle tension in the limb being examined. In some of the more complex devices, the leg is literally locked into position by the test apparatus. Each time before a subluxating force is applied to the knee, the patient is told to relax his muscles completely. Tensing of the quadriceps muscles can decrease laxity values by as much as 75% [442].

The length of the examination is another important factor, especially in anxious or acutely injured patients. With some devices, such as the Genucom (see Fig. 9-5) and KSS system (see Fig. 9-6), even an experienced examiner will require approximately 30 min to complete the procedure. An examination of this length can easily overtax the tolerance of both the patient and examiner.

Various types of apparatus have been developed for machine laxity testing:

1. Devices for evaluating varus-valgus laxity (medial and lateral opening of the joint space)
2. Devices for evaluating rotatory laxity

3. Devices for evaluating anterior and/or posterior displacement (drawer tests)
4. Goniometers
5. Complex testing apparatus

The force applied to the knee joint may be imposed at a constant level for a variable period of time (static test) or may be applied cyclically at varying intervals (dynamic test). The great majority of machine evaluations currently in use are of the static type.

9.2 Evaluation of Varus-Valgus Laxity

To date, numerous static and dynamic machine techniques have been described for the determination of varus-valgus laxity (Table 9-1).

In static tests a single force is applied to the medial or lateral aspect of the knee to provoke lateral or medial opening [25, 337, 363, 407, 618, 619]. For dynamic testing the tibia is loaded in varus and valgus by imposing a sinusoidal displacement at a designated torque and frequency [104, 530, 531, 702].

Klein [363] developed the first nonradiographic apparatus for the measurement of knee laxity. His "knee ligament testing instrument" consists of two sleeves, interconnected by a pivot, that fit over the thigh and lower leg and register motion on a mechanical dial indicator. Sprague [618, 619] projects a grid with angular degree lines onto the lower leg, applies a varus or valgus stress, and then takes measurements on photographs of the extremity. Kalenak and Morehouse [337] use a potentiometer to measure lateral and medial joint opening. Balkfors [25] reads varus-valgus displacement on a scale in angular degrees. Some dynamic instruments display their results as a continuous trace on an X-Y plotter, in which case the examiner must interpret the neutral point on transition from medial to lateral opening [103, 407, 530]. Pope [530] uses a linear potentiometer to determine the magnitude of valgus-varus deflection.

Table 9-1. Machine techniques for evaluating varus-valgus laxity

	Year	Pos	Ext	10°	20°	30°	Fl	Rot
Klein	1962	Si/Su	x					n.d.
Sprague	1965	Sit	x	S				n.d.
Kalenak	1975	Sit	x	S				n.d.
Crowninshield	1976	Sup					15°	DF
Pope	1976	Sup	D			D		DF
Lowe	1977	Sup	D	D				n.d.
Narechania	1977	Lat	D			D		n.d.
Markolf	1978	Sup	D		D			NR
Pope	1979	Sup			x			ER
Balkfors	1982	Sup	D		D			n.d.
Genucom	1983	Sup					D	D
Acufex	1987	Si/Su					D	D

Legend for Tables 9-1 through 9-5:
Position of subject (Pos); tibial rotation (Rot); sitting (Sit); defined neutral rotation (NR); lateral decubitus (Lat); defined external rotation (ER); supine (Sup); defined internal, neutral, and external rotation (INER); sitting and supine positions (Si/Su); tibial rotation defined by foot plate (F); neutral rotation defined by foot plate (FNR); external rotation defined by foot plate (FER); knee joint extended (Ext); knee joint flexed (Fl); flexion angle defined by flexing knee over support (S); apparent position, not defined (x); force stated in kg, N or Nm; defined position (D); manual force of undefined magnitude (Man); position or force level not defined (n.d.)

Besides these individual techniques, varus-valgus testing may be but one function of a more complex apparatus that is able to test additional components of pathologic knee joint motion [3, 154, 422].

So far, none of the techniques described for the exclusive testing of varus-valgus laxity have found significant routine clinical application. This is understandable when one considers that varus-valgus testing is not sufficient in itself to adequately evaluate a capsuloligamentous lesions of the knee.

9.3
Evaluation of Rotatory Laxity

Various machine tests have been devised for the active and passive determination of rotational laxity (Table 9-2). There is considerable disagreement among the results of many of these studies (Table 9-3).

Shoemaker [596] measured 41° of pure tibial rotation with the knee flexed 20°, and 47° of rotation with the knee flexed 90°. The range of foot rotation is twice as great as that of pure tibial rotation. Besides differences in equipment, the lack of agreement among different authors probably relates to variations in test conditions. Thus, while hip flexion and the applied force influence the rotatory laxity of the knee [596], some test procedures do not take these factors into account.

Little would be gained by the routine clinical use of these machine tests due to the relative unimportance of the isolated determination of rotatory knee laxity.

Table 9-2. Machine techniques for evaluating rotatory laxity. (Legend see Table 9-1)

Author	Year	Pos	15°	20°	30°	45°	60°	90°
Crowninshield	1976	Sup						D
Markolf	1978	Si/Su		D				D
Bargar	1983	Sit						D
Ross	1932	Sit				x		x
Ruepp	1977	Sit						D
Khasigian	1978	Sit						D
Osternig	1978	Sit				D		D
Zarins	1983	Lat	D		D		D	D

Table 9-3. Measured ranges of rotation

Author	Year	Flexion angle					
		20°	45°	60°	90°	120°	135°
Meyer	1853			52°	42°	33°	
Fick	1911				50°		
Ross	1932		34°		31°		34°
Hallen	1965				26°		
Ruetsch	1977				36°		
Khasigian	1978				68°		
Shoemaker	1982	82°			91°		
Zarins	1983		72°	73°	74°		

9.4
Evaluation of Anterior-Posterior Laxity

9.4.1
Problem of the Neutral Position

The standardization and reliability of machine test procedures are a major concern, regardless of the technical complexity of the apparatus. They are significantly influenced by the problem of the neutral position, i.e., the difficulty of determining the neutral or starting position of the tibia when there are coexisting lesions of the ACL and PCL. This problem has not yet been satisfactorily resolved.

In theory the neutral position should first be determined in the normal knee and then transferred to the injured knee, the rationale being that each side will tend to have equal laxities when placed in identical examination positions. One problem that remains, however, is the tendency for the tibia to sag posteriorly under its own weight and the weight of the apparatus fastened to the lower leg while the patient lies supine, for example, with the knee flexed.

This problem can be avoided by determining the total anteroposterior displacement of the tibia. This can be done by first pulling the upper end of the tibia anteriorly (starting point of the measurement) and then pushing it posteriorly (end point of the measurement). However, the individual drawer components cannot be accurately determined from the total extent of anteroposterior displacement. Since adequate means are not available for defining the neutral position for differentiating the anterior and posterior components of the total displacement, the initial or resting position of the knee is generally considered to be the "neutral" position.

Daniel [117] uses the "quadriceps neutral angle test" to identify the neutral position for drawer testing (see Fig. 3-53). He starts by finding the neutral position for the normal leg, i.e., the angle of knee flexion in which contraction of the quadriceps muscle does not produce anterior or posterior displacement of the tibia. Once the neutral angle has been found, the injured knee is positioned at the same angle, and testing is commenced.

9.4.2
Apparatus

Many types of apparatus and techniques have been developed for the measurement of anterior and posterior displacement (Tables 9-4 and 9-5).

Sylvin, using the apparatus of Lindahl, performed the first quantitative, nonradiographic measurements of anteroposterior knee laxity [642]. The individual components of the laxity also can be evaluated with this instrument, as Balkfors demonstrated [25].

Rodriguez was only able to measure a separate anterior or posterior component of tibiofemoral displacement [555]. Dandy's instrument [109] can determine the extent of the spontaneous posterior sag of the proximal tibia.

The manual application of an unknown or imprecisely defined force by the examiner [109, 332, 642, 659] is being abandoned in favor of machine techniques that can standardize the magnitude of the subluxating force, its site of application, and its direction. Cumbersome constraint systems that employ weights and pulleys, as described by Narechania [507] and Rodriguez [555], are being replaced by force sensors that can measure and indicate the tensile and/or compressive loads that are applied.

In the test instrument developed by Daniel et al., the KT-1000 arthrometer (Fig. 9-1), an audible tone signals when the designated force for measuring tibiofemoral displacement has been applied. This device permits standardized, quantitative laxity testing under a reproducible force with knee flexion and tibial rotation controlled by a knee support and foot rest [112, 113, 114]. This apparatus is currently the most widely used technique for the determination of anterior tibial translation [39, 397, 515]. The "compliance index," defined as the difference in the amount of translation at forces of 67 N and 89 N, is 3 times greater when the ACL is ruptured than when the ligament is intact (1 mm) [113]. Significant degrees of translation cannot always be achieved at the recommended stress levels of 67 N and 89 N. The maximal drawer test, which uses an applied force of 30–40 kg, elicits substantially greater anterior displacement comparable to that seen in manual examinations. As in the devices of Sylvin [642], Rodriguez [555], Dandy [109], and

Table 9-4. Machine techniques for evaluating anterior drawer. (Legend see Table 9-1)

Author	Year	Pos	Ext	20°	90°	Fl	Rot
Narechania	1977	Sup			D		INER
Markolf	1978	Si/Su	D	D	D		INER
Pope	1979	Sup				x	F
Sylvin	1975	Sup			x		n.d.
Rodriguez	1981	Sup		x	x		NR
Daniel	1982	Sup			S		FER
Jonsson	1982	Sit		D	D		n.d.
Edixhoven	1983	n.d.			x	25°	FNR
Genucom	1983	Sup				D	INER
Johnson	1984	Sup		x	x		n.d.
Shino	1984	Si/Su					?
Sodem-Calt	1984	Si/Su		D	D	x	F/n.d.
Stryker	1984	Sup		D	x		n.d.
Tittel	1984	Sup			x		n.d.
Acufex	1987	Si/Su				D	INER
Crawford	1987	Sup		D			n.d.
Harding	1987	n.d.	D	D	D		n.d.
Markolf	1987	Sup		D			F
Turner	1987					x	?
Calville	1988	Sup			S		NR

Table 9-5. Machine techniques for evaluating posterior drawer. (Legend see Table 9-1)

Author	Year	Pos	Ext	20°	90°	Fl	Rot
Markolf	1978	Si/Su	D	D	D		INER
Sylvin	1975	Sup			x		n.d.
Rodriguez	1981	Sup		x	x		n.d.
Daniel	1982	Sup			S		FER
Dandy	1982	Sup			x		n.d.
Edixhoven	1983	n.d.			x	25°	FNR
Genucom	1983	Sup				D	INER
Johnson	1984	Sup		x	x		n.d.
Shino	1984	Si/Su			x		?
Sodem-Calt	1984	Si/Su		D	D	x	F/n.d.
Stryker	1984	Sup		D	x		n.d.
Tittel	1984	Sup			x		n.d.
Acufex	1987	Si/Su				D	INER
Harding	1987	n.d.	D	D	D		n.d.
Turner	1987				x		

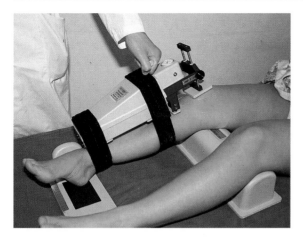

Fig. 9-1. KT-1000 arthrometer

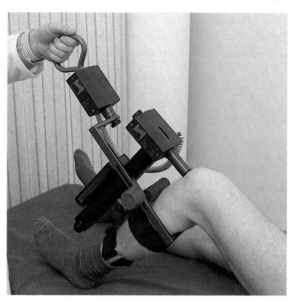

Fig. 9-2. CALT testing apparatus

Tittel [659], the measurements must be read from a scale.

Manual examinations can be assisted by computerized systems which electronically measure force and displacement and display laxity values in graphic form on a monitor screen or on a printout [144, 250, 593]. A microprocessor in the Computerized Accurate Ligament Tester (CALT, Sodemsystems) guides the examiner through a programmed sequence of steps, calculates the applied force and the extent of anterior and posterior displacement, and indicates the total anteroposterior displacement (Fig. 9-2). An accessory device can be used to hold the limb in defined positions of flexion and tibial rotation [611]. Fixation of the CALT apparatus to the lower leg can present problems, however. Because the apparatus is heavy and stands away from the lower leg, it has a tendency to tilt during use.

A small instrument that mounts easily to the lower leg is the Stryker Knee Laxity Tester (Fig. 9-3) [57]. This apparatus is so lightweight that tilting is not a problem. The extent of anterior tibial displacement is read from a scale. Generally it takes less than 5 min to complete the examination.

We have modified our positioning device for stress radiography [623] by adding an optoelectronic sensor which mounts anterior to the tibial tuberosity and measures anterior displacement of the tibia relative to the stationary femur. We have used this apparatus to determine anterior tibial displacement under specified stresses (3, 6, 9, and 12 kg) in 13 different joint positions that systematically cover the motion spectrum of the knee (Fig. 9-4; see also Fig. 3-2). The measurements are computer-processed and plotted graphically in the form of a three-dimensional "landscape" of displacement (see Sect. 9.6). However, routine clinical use of this system will require further refinement and simplification of the holding device and sensing process.

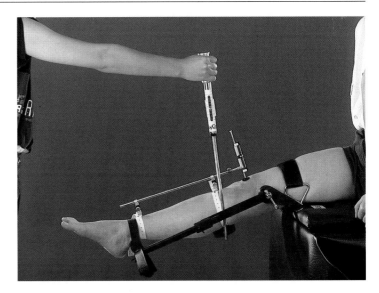

Fig. 9-3. Stryker Knee Laxity Tester, used here in performing the Lachman test. Knee flexion is controlled by a leg-holding fixture which also functions as a seat plate

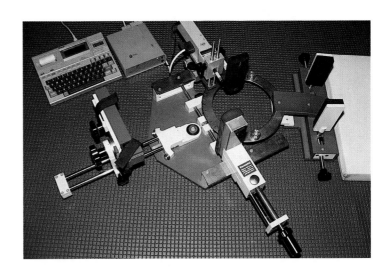

Fig. 9-4. Test setup in 30° flexion and neutral tibial rotation (Lachman test)

9.5
Goniometers and Complex Testing Apparatus

Complex test machines were developed in response to the clinical need to measure more than one laxity test with the same apparatus. Technically sophisticated goniometers have been described by Townsend [663] and Hang [247]. Like the CARS-UBC goniometer [330], these devices have been used chiefly for gait analysis and for determining the ranges of flexion and rotation.

Using an apparatus based on a modified dental chair, Markolf and his group have contributed much to the nonradiographic, quantitative machine laxity testing of the knee joint. They were able to measure varus-valgus and anteroposterior laxities while taking into account the rotational components of the elicited motions [27, 28, 422, 424, 596].

The most comprehensive diagnostic system to date is the Genucom Knee Analysis System, a complex unit consisting of an examination chair with a force-sensing system integrated into the seat and an electrogoniometer with six degrees of freedom that attaches to the lower leg. Data from the examination are individually processed by special software on a desktop computer, and the results are stored and can be graphically displaced on the monitor screen (Fig. 9-5) [154]. Varus-valgus and drawer laxity can be tested in arbitrary positions of flexion and tibial rotation on the Genucom, and this is the first system that can evaluate the femoropatellar joint, providing a graphic record of patellar tracking at various flexion angles while calculating the medial and lateral patellar pressures and the Q angle. It takes several minutes to calibrate the system before testing is begun, however, and a lengthy training period is needed before the examiner becomes proficient with the system (20 h according to Highgenboten and Jackson [284]).

The Knee Signature System (KSS) [3], a goniometer capable of measuring anteroposterior tibiofemoral displacement in response to a force applied by a separate force input device, can supplement the clinical examination by furnishing data on functional parameters, e. g., in the walking patient (Fig. 9-6) [3]. To date, however, there have been no detailed clinical studies on the diagnostic value of this system, nor has the system been compared with other, clinically proven devices (KT-1000 arthrometer, Stryker Laxity Tester).

Like the Genucom, the KSS requires time-consuming calibration before testing is begun, and secure fixation of the pole-like instrument may present difficulties.

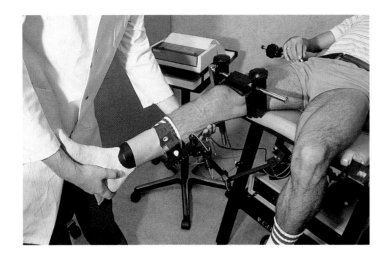

Fig. 9-5. Lachman test performed on the Genucom system

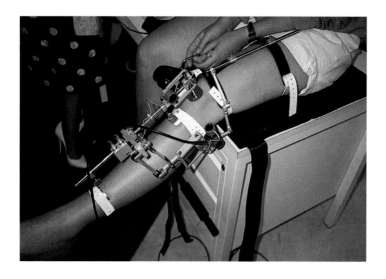

Fig. 9-6. KSS (Knee Signature System)

9.6
Graphic Representation
of Laxity Values

Machine laxity measurements necessarily involve the evaluation of one or more large bodies of collected data. In systems where the knee is tested in only one position, so that only the maximum laxity value is measured, there is no problem in determining and documenting the measured value.

When anterior displacement is measured in three different joint positions for both the lateral and medial tibial condyles, a minimum of six measurements are obtained, or 12 if both knees are examined. If posterior drawer is additionally tested, 24 values must be registered and processed. Simply tabulating these numbers would be of little practical benefit. It would be far more useful to represent the data in an easy-to-comprehend graphic form that would give the examiner a clearer appreciation of laxity responses.

While it is true that the measured values can be processed by manual computation, there is a high risk of error in the manual transferring of data. Manual methods are also very time-consuming. On the other hand, more complex mathematical procedures can be implemented at reasonable costs of time and personnel only if there is appropriate software available that can be run on a high-performance desktop computer.

9.6.1
Two-Dimensional Representation of Laxity

Most graphic representations of laxity values are two-dimensional. The aspect of greatest interest to the examiner is the deflection or length change that is elicited by a given force in relation to a specified initial or neutral position. Thus, force-displacement curves are the most common mode for the graphic representation of test data. Other factors such as tibial rotation and knee flexion angle must be kept constant. The two-dimensional graph, then, portrays laxity only as it exists at a given point in time in a designated limb position.

A widely used method for the graphic representation of anterior and posterior laxity was developed by Markolf, Mensch, and Amstutz [421]. The test results are plotted in the form of a curve with the applied forces recorded on the ordinate (anteriorly directed forces on the positive side, posteriorly directed forces on the negative side) and tibial displacement recorded on the abscissa (anterior displacement on the positive side, posterior displacement on the negative side). Before testing is begun, the system is calibrated to establish the zero or neutral point (where the ordinate and absissa intersect). Then an anterior stress is applied. Passive recovery of the tibia to its initial position is additionally recorded (broken line in Fig. 9-7). When the abscissa is reached, the posteriorly directed stress is applied, and passive tibial recovery is again recorded. These curves can be used to determine anterior "stiffness" (defined as the steepness of the curve upslope under an anterior stress of 50 N), anterior laxity (defined as the anterior tibial displacement at 200 N), and total laxity (defined as the total tibial displacement between an anterior and posterior stress of 200 N) (Fig. 9-7).

Ligamentous lesions have the effect of decreasing the slope of the force-displacement curve or shifting the position of the curve on the y axis. To record this curve, the measurement must be performed at the same time the force is applied. The Genucom (see Fig. 9-5) and KSS instruments (see Fig. 9-6) register the test results in the form of loading curves, with one curve generated for each joint position. Thus, if the healthy and injured knees are examined, say, in five different joint positions, a total of ten (!) curves are recorded. Interpretation is manageable if one patient is tested, but if several patients are being tested as part of a larger study, several hundred graphic records must be analyzed and interpreted.

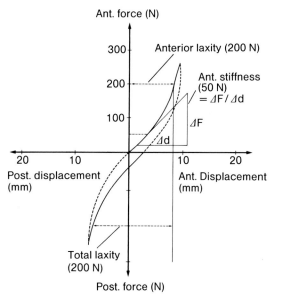

Fig. 9-7. Anterior and posterior loading curves of Markolf

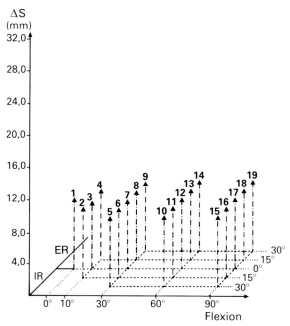

Fig. 9-8. Three-dimensional coordinate system with test grid covering 19 different joint positions. Anterior-posterior displacement is plotted in mm on the y axis, flexion on the x axis, and rotation on the z axis. *ER* external rotation, *IR* internal rotation (after [625])

9.6.2
Three-Dimensional Representation of Laxity

If the results of a laxity test are to be represented in a way that takes into account knee flexion and tibial rotation as independent variables, a two-dimensional plot like the force-displacement curve does not provide a sufficient graphic representation. To solve this problem, we worked with Prof. Werner (†) and Dr. H. Stenzel (Institute of Applied Mathematics, Rheinische Wilhelms University, Bonn) to develop a coordinate system for plotting knee laxity responses in three dimensions.

Flexion, tibial rotation, and the measured drawer displacement (in mm) form the three axes of the coordinate system. Over the area bounded by the x and z axes, representing the motion spectrum of the knee joint (see Fig. 3-2), the measured displacement values are plotted on perpendicular lines at the points where the measurements were performed (Fig. 9-8).

In experimental studies involving the planned sectioning of ligaments, we obtained standard stress radiographs in 19 different joint positions (see Fig. 3-58–3-62). In nonradio-

graphic studies performed in patients and normal subjects (see Fig. 9-4), we determined anterior and posterior laxity responses in 13 different joint positions (Figs. 9-9 and 9-10).

Measurements in any biologic system are naturally subject to variations and disturbances, which ordinarily are corrected by taking averages or mean values in cases where the parameters of the measured quantity do not change. More complicated, nonlinear values like those measured in laxity tests can be plotted in the form of fitted curves constructed by a technique known as the least squares method. Our experience with mathematical calculations and computer-generated plots of "landscapes" has shown that the test data are fitted best by a third-degree polynomial curve.

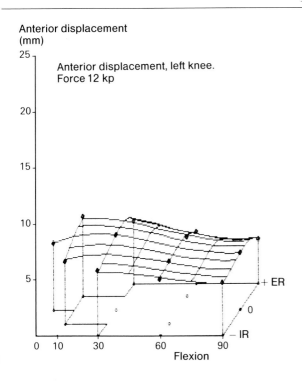

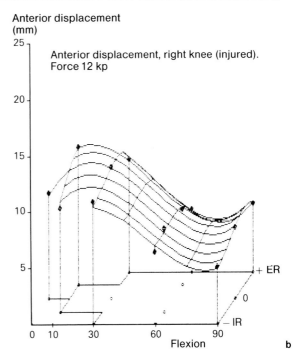

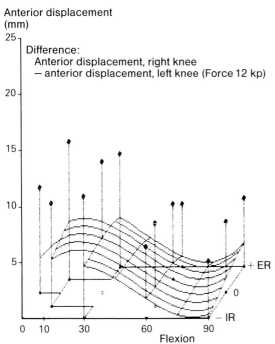

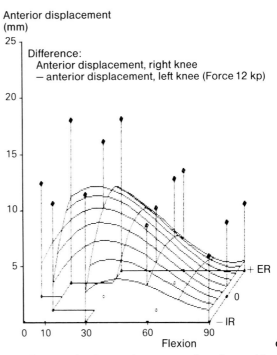

Fig. 9-9 a-d. Nonradiographic assessment of anterior displacement, recorded as a three-dimensional "landscape" of the left intact knee (**a**) and right injured knee (**b**). The computer-generated "difference landscape" shows up to 7 mm of anterior displacement at a small flexion angle, consistent with a tear of the ACL (**c**).

The difference landscape in a second patient with more pronounced clinical instability signs (positive pivot shift test) shows significant anterior displacement at a small flexion angle (**d**). *IR* internal rotation, *ER* external rotation (anterior force 120 N)

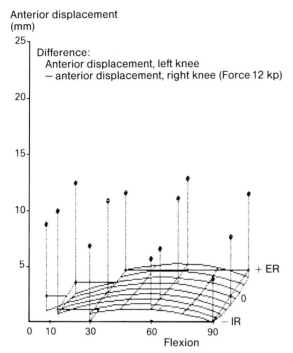

Anterior displacement
(mm)

Difference:
Anterior displacement, left knee
− anterior displacement, right knee (Force 12 kp)

Fig. 9-10. The "landscape" of a subject reporting no history of knee injury moves about the initial plane (anterior force 120 N)

9.7
Conclusion

Since more than 90% of ligamentous injuries of the knee joint can be diagnosed by a careful history and thorough clinical examination [235], the role of machine laxity testing must lie elsewhere. Obviously there is no rationale for performing machine testing on every "new" patient who presents with a suspected ligamentous injury.

The primary evaluation of the capsule and ligaments is accomplished by the clinical examination. If increased laxity is noted and it is difficult to determine clinically the amount of anterior or posterior tibial displacement in millimeters that is elicited by the applied stress, machine laxity testing is indicated. Especially in the functionally important positions of slight flexion, it can be difficult to determine the exact amount of tibial displacement by clinical means.

As stated earlier, the indication for machine

testing lies in the documentation and quantification of laxity. Machine testing is also used as a follow-up procedure to evaluate the success of operative or conservative treatment so that comparable results can be obtained.

So many types of test apparatus are available that it can be difficult to select a particular model. Simple devices such as the KT-1000 arthrometer, CALT, and Stryker Knee Laxity Tester are easy to operate and maintain, but their diagnostic capabilities are limited. On the other hand, more complicated systems like the Genucom and KSS require a long and intense learning period (up to 20 h) [284]. Calibration alone may take more time than would be needed to test several patients on simpler devices; the total examination time for one patient usually exceeds 30 min. Moreover, the complex devices can be extremely difficult to use in an operating room setting, despite the fact that quantitative laxity tests are most rewarding when performed under general anesthesia, when muscular relaxation is complete.

Because the quantification of tibial displacement at small flexion angles is a prime indication for machine laxity testing, other types of test (anterior drawer test in 90° flexion, posterior drawer test in 90° flexion, varus-valgus test) that can be performed with the more complex devices are of relatively minor importance. Sommerlath and Gillquist [612] compared a simple instrument (the Stryker Knee Laxity Tester) with a more complex device (the Genucom) and with manual clinical examination. In the Lachman test, the results of the Stryker instrument agreed with manual test results in 72% of cases, while those of the Genucom agreed in only 58%. Similar results were noted in tests of total anteroposterior laxity [612].

To date there have been few studies comparing the sensitivities, specificities, and accuracies of different test machines in patients with specific injuries and in normal controls. This particularly applies to the more complex devices, with very little research being done on the Genucom and none at all on the KSS. Studies in which, say, 20 healthy subjects are tested as a control population must be viewed critically in terms of their validity [284]. Other problems relate to the computer-assisted graphic processing of laxity values. While this may seem an attractive feature in some systems, further refinements are needed to make the graphic software more user-friendly. It would be desirable to have one graphic display that would enable the experienced examiner to determine the nature and extent of the ligamentous injury or identify the type of laxity that has developed.

We must ask, then, whether the substantial investment of time and equipment associated with the use of complex testing apparatus is in reasonable proportion to the diagnostic gain. These devices may well be useful for scientific and experimental investigations. Simple devices like the KT-1000 arthrometer and Stryker instrument are preferred for routine clinical applications owing to their speed and simplicity of use. It should be considered, however, that these devices provide only one measurement that is read from a scale. Unlike the radiographic Lachman test, the procedure does not furnish an objective record of, say, anterior tibial translation. Another advantage of the radiographic Lachman test is that it permits the separate evaluation of medial and lateral compartmental translation (see Fig. 6-47 e, f). The radiation exposure from two lateral radiographs is acceptable, even in repeat studies.

10
Rare Diagnostic Procedures

10.1
Radionuclide Scanning

For many years radionuclide scanning (scintigraphy) has demonstrated its value as a sensitive screening procedure for the diagnosis of inflammatory disease. Various scanning agents have been used, ranging from Tc-99 m-labeled phosphonates for 3-phase bone scanning to Tc-99-labeled nanocolloids and Ga-67 citrate for the nonspecific diagnosis of inflammation. More recent techniques involving the in vitro labeling of separated granulocytes with In-111 or Tc-99 m HMPAO or with Tc-99 m or I-123 antigranulocyte antibodies have displayed specific advantages (lower radiation exposure, higher sensitivity and specificity, sensitive to earlier changes, better availability, better image quality).

The combined application of bone scanning and leukocyte scanning can improve the specificity of nuclear medicine imaging procedures. Superior morphologic definition is achieved by tomographic imaging with a rotating gamma camera (SPECT = single photon emission computed tomography).

Leukocyte scanning is a sensitive technique for the diagnosis of granulocytic inflammatory processes. Often it can even distinguish a frank infection from a transient postoperative state that does not require treatment [589]. Bone scanning provides a sensitivity of 70%–100% depending on the timing of the examination, the scanning technique, and the site of the infection [587]. The imaging of meniscus tears with Tc-99 m pyrophosphate has shown a sensitivity of 56% (lateral meniscus tears) to 95% (medial meniscus tears, tears of both menisci) and a specificity of 93% [431].

It is still too early to assess definitively the value of leukocyte scanning in the diagnostic evaluation of knee disorders due to a lack of controlled studies in larger populations.

Numerous indications exist for radionuclide imaging of the knee (Table 10-1). The combination of bone and leukocyte scanning has proven particularly effective for the detection and localization of inflammatory processes (Figs. 10-1 and 10-2).

Bone scanning, with its high sensitivity and low specificity, can contribute to the early detection and follow-up of knee disorders. Leukocyte scanning is indicated when there is clinical suspicion of an inflammatory knee disorder or an osteomyelitic processes close to the knee joint. Image quality is not significantly degraded by the presence of an endoprosthesis or other metallic implant.

Table 10-1. Indications for radionuclide scanning of the knee

1. Localization of inflammatory foci
2. Aseptic necrosis of bone (osteochondritis dissecans of the femoral condyles or patella)
3. Sympathetic reflex dystrophy
4. Rheumatoid diseases
5. Paget's disease
6. Systemic bone diseases (osteoporosis)
7. Stress fractures
8. Metastases
9. Tumors
10. Degenerative joint diseases
11. Pain of unknown origin
12. Chronic pain

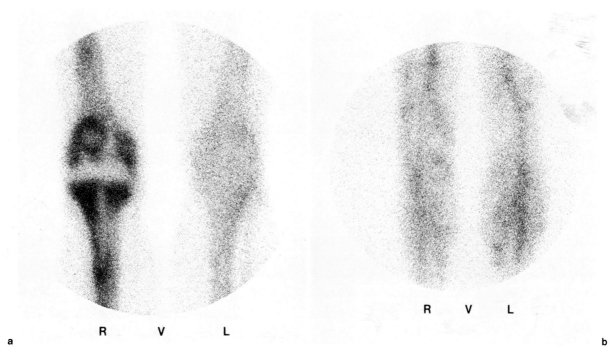

Fig. 10-1a, b. Suspicion of infection in a 60-year-old man with a total knee replacement. Bone scanning with Tc-99 m MDP shows a postoperative elevation of bone metabolism (**a**). WBC scanning with In-111-labeled leukocytes does not demonstrate a focus of infection (**b**)

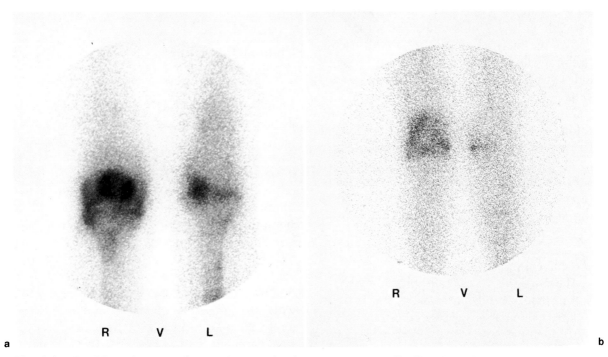

Fig. 10-2a, b. Man 32 years of age who sustained open injuries of both knees; the right knee was operatively explored. Bone scanning with Tc-99 m MDP shows an elevation of bone metabolism in all areas of the right knee and in the medial compartment of the left knee (**a**). Leukocyte scanning with I-123-labeled monoclonal antibodies shows increased uptake in all portions of the right knee and in the medial compartment of the left knee. This implies an infection involving the right knee joint and a local inflammatory process in the medial compartment of the left knee (**b**)

10.2
Thermography

Noncontact infrared thermography is a technique for recording infrared radiation emitted from tissues without touching the patient.

Since thermographic procedures are very sensitive to external conditions, the European Society for Thermology and the American Academy of Thermology have defined standard conditions for the examination room (18° room temperature), patient preparation, examination technique, and type of equipment needed. The patient must not ingest any vasoactive substances prior to the examination. Activities that raise tissue temperatures, such as sauna bathing or therapeutic exercise, should also be avoided in the hours preceding the examination.

In one study, thermography demonstrated an 85% accuracy rate in the diagnosis of meniscal lesions [598]. Thermograms in patients with femoropatellar pain syndrome showed a typical patellar "hot spot" in 96% of cases (n = 56) with a temperature rise of 1°–3°C above the normal level [599]. Arthroscopic findings were positive in only 49% of these patients (with grade 1 or grade 2 chondromalacia).

A temperature rise of up to 2°C is also seen during 4–6 weeks following the rigid internal fixation of a fracture. The temperature returns to normal when fracture healing is complete. This contrasts with the persistent hyperthermia (up to 2°C) that is associated with the loosening of an implant (e.g., a total knee prosthesis). Temperature elevations as high as 4°C have been recorded thermographically in the presence of infection [380].

Thermography is a costly procedure that is still in the experimental stage as far as its use in knee examinations is concerned. Its only indication at present is for the documentation of "hot spots" in knee joints affected by sympathetic reflex dystrophy (Fig. 10-3).

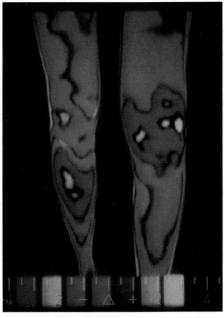

Fig. 10-3. Thermography of both knee joints in a patient with sympathetic reflex dystrophy of the left knee. The thermogram of the left knee shows marked hyperthermia of the entire joint and especially of the patella, which normally appears as a "cold spot" (blue area in the right knee)

10.3
Phonoarthrography

Many joints, including the knee, emit sounds during motion of the articular surfaces. Abnormalities in the knee joint such as meniscal tears, loose bodies, and retropatellar chondromalacia can amplify the sounds to the point that they becomes audible even to bystanders. The patient becomes aware of a snapping, crackling, or grating in the knee. The auscultation of joint sounds with a stethoscope has been practiced for many years [45, 376, 613, 724]. The intensity of the sounds is strongly influenced by the content of the knee joint, with effusion producing an essentially "silent" joint and pannus-like thickenings of the capsule leading to muffled sounds. Sound intensity is also affected by the load on the joint during motion (e.g., squatting) and by the quickness of the movement. According to Sonnenschein [613], the character of the sound depends mainly on the change in the tissue that is generating the sound (cartilage, fibrotic capsule, cartilage deposits).

Special microphones can be used to record the "patellar click" and crepitations in the femoropatellar joint. Background noises, most conspicuous in rapid movements, distort the sound recording [437], so some examiners use an accelerometer in place of an acoustic microphone [438].

Pässler [518] has developed a new phonoarthrographic technique in which intraarticular sounds are recorded with a special high-sensitivity microphone applied over the patella. The flexion angle at which the sounds are elicited gives important information on the location of cartilage pathology. The knee flexion angle is measured during the examination with a goniometer attached to the side of the leg (Fig. 10-4). Joint sounds are provoked by having the patient move the knee through its range of motion, the frequency or rate of the flexions being controlled by a ball pendulum (green ball in Fig. 10-4). The sounds picked up by the microphone and the flexion angles measured by the goniometer are relayed to an analog-to-digital converter via an amplifier and are processed on a personal computer, which creates a graphic readout (Figs. 10-5 and 10-6).

The healthy knee joint often emits a sound in maximum flexion. When degenerative disease is present, sounds can be recorded over the entire range of flexion. But with retropatellar cartilage damage, according to Pässler [518], sounds are elicited over a more limited range, especially between 20° and 60° of flexion (Figs. 10-5 and 10-6).

If the initial encouraging results are confirmed, phonoarthrography will provide a noninvasive technique for testing the retropatellar cartilage under functional conditions, i.e., under loading. Through this technique, we may be able to detect retropatellar cartilage damage in patients with ACL insufficiency or femoropatellar pain syndrome. In patients undergoing ACL or PCL reconstruction, phonoarthrography may provide a noninvasive means for determining the operative procedure that would cause the least damage to the femoropatellar cartilage. However, further studies are still needed on the diagnostic capabilities of this phonoarthrographic technique.

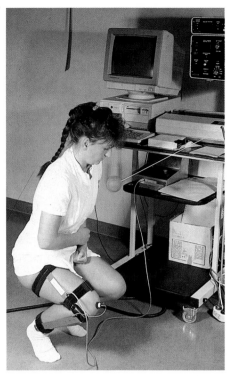

Fig. 10-4. Phonoarthrographic examination technique (after Pässler [518])

10.4 Vibration Arthrography

The vibrations emitted by moving joints are detected and recorded by small accelerometers, whose readings are not significantly affected by skin friction or background noise.

In subjects with healthy knees, three signal types have been recorded with varying frequency: a physiologic patellofemoral crepitus, recorded over the patella in 99% of subjects; a patellar click; and a "lateral band phenomenon," present in 22% of subjects on the lateral side of the joint [436]. In symptomatic knees, pathologic signals were recorded from approximately 85% of patients with meniscal injuries, plica syndrome, or degenerative cartilage changes [436, 438]. Especially in patients with patellofemoral cartilage disease, vibration arthrography was positive before radiographic changes became apparent. Meniscal surgery had the effect of reducing the intensity of the

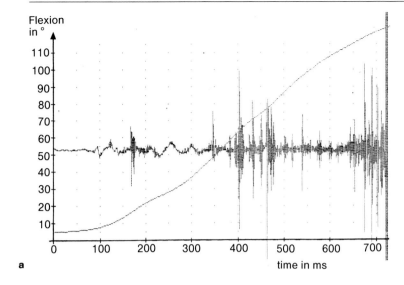

a

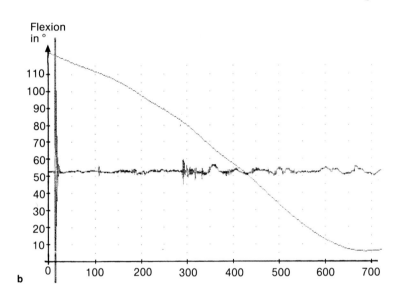

b

Fig. 10-5a, b. Phonoarthrographic findings. Pathologic joint sounds between 20° and 90° flexion as evidence of retropatellar cartilage damage in a chronically ACL deficient knee (**a**). Pathologic sounds are not recorded in the intact contralateral knee (**b**). Sounds at high flexion angles represent a physiologic phenomenon

pathologic meniscal signal by a factor of 10. McCoy [436] states that vibration arthrography is also useful for determining the efficacy of arthroscopic meniscectomy.

With further technical refinements and the miniaturization of sensors, phonoarthrography or vibration arthrography may well become an important noninvasive screening procedure for knee disorders.

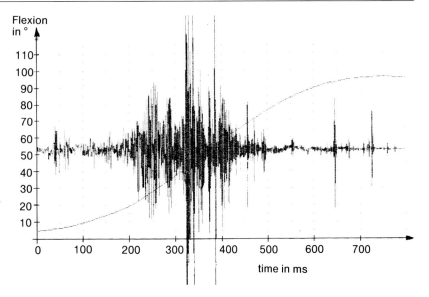

Fig. 10-6. Phonoarthrographic findings in a 60-year-old woman with severe retropatellar cartilage disease. The sound intensity is maximal between 20° and 70° of flexion. Extensive grade III and IV retropatellar chondromalacia was noted at arthroscopy

11
Arthroscopy

Arthroscopy of the knee joint is an effective, widely practiced procedure for the diagnosis and treatment of virtually all forms of intraarticular pathology. As a result, there is a tendency to utilize arthroscopy very liberally and perhaps hastily, even in cases where diagnosis could have been satisfactorily accomplished by a thorough clinical examination. Arthroscopy, whether diagnostic or operative and whether performed in an inpatient or outpatient setting, should stand at the end of the "diagnostic chain." The main danger of arthroscopy lies in its too-frequent, uncritical application.

In this section we shall limit our attention to diagnostic arthroscopy, which forms the basis for operative arthroscopic procedures. Details on operative arthroscopy may be found in the textbooks and atlases by Johnson [325], O'Connor [499], Glinz [212], Henche and Holder [273], Löhnert and Raunest [400], and Chassaing and Parier [91].

11.1
Historical Background

In the early 1800s, physicians began using optical instruments to inspect human body cavities. The earliest publications described procedures and methods for examining the bladder, vagina, rectum, and pharynx. Takagi, in 1918, was the first author to write on the endoscopic examination of the human knee joint. His initial attempts to examine cadaveric knees with a cystoscope were not very successful, so in 1920 he designed a simple arthroscope – still without a lens system – for the examination of tuberculous knees [643, 644]. In 1921, the Swiss physician Eugen Bircher [44] reported his initial experience with arthroscopic examinations in cadaveric knees and also in 18 patients (Fig. 11-1). He praised arthroscopy as being superior to all other methods of examination, but at that time he was unable to stimulate much interest in the procedure among his colleagues.

Besides being the first to successfully use arthroscopy clinically, Bircher gave an accurate prediction of its future development:

"The method of arthroendoscopy permits us to visualize the interior of the joint and evaluate pathologic changes, and thus to confirm the diagnosis by visual observation. In this respect it is superior to all other methods of examination and, like endoscopy of the bladder, can identify patients who require operative treatment. Also like cystoscopy, it will meet with resistance but undoubtedly will gain ground and progress until it becomes as indispensable as cystoscopy itself" (Bircher 1922).

Between 1930 and 1960, a great many scientists developed an interest in arthroscopy [75, 76, 432, 676, 704]. In the 1930's, Harry Mayer and Leo Finkelstein of the Hospital for Joint Diseases in New York developed an arthroscope 8 mm in diameter for performing biopsies. In 1931, Michael S. Burman, now regarded as the pioneer of arthroscopy in the United States, worked with the instrument manufacturer Wappler to design an arthroscope that embodied important basic features of present-day instruments. Burman, in collaboration with Finkelstein and Mayer, performed numerous cadaveric studies which laid the groundwork for the clinical application of the instrument. Following the insertion of a 4-mm-diameter trocar, the joint was irrigated and distended with Ringer's solution and then inspected with a 3-mm direct-view arthro-

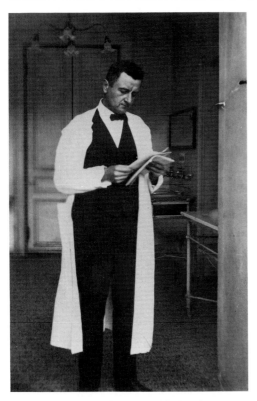

Fig. 11-1. Eugen Bircher (1882–1956)

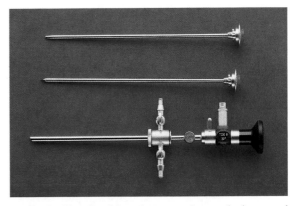

Fig. 11-2. Sheath with arthroscope inserted, sharp and blunt trocars. The plane of the spigots is rotatable (Storz)

11.2 Equipment

Diagnostic arthroscopy is a costly and technically demanding procedure. The basic equipment consists of the arthroscope, sheath (trocar sleeve), sharp and blunt trocars (Fig. 11-2), and a light source and connecting cable to the arthroscope.

11.2.1 Arthroscopes

Three types of arthroscope are most commonly used: the 0° direct-view arthroscope and the 30° and 70° oblique arthroscopes (Fig. 11-3).

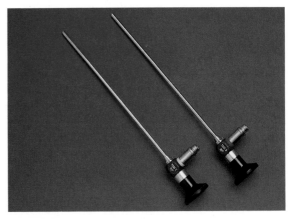

Fig. 11-3. Arthroscopes (30° and 70° wide-angle scopes, Storz)

scope. Burman described various approaches to the knee joint and researched the potential applications of arthroscopy in the hip, ankle, shoulder, and elbow. However, technical deficiencies aroused the skepticism of many colleagues, and unfortunately the *Arthroscopic Atlas* compiled by Burman remained unpublished.

The great resurgence of interest in arthroscopy since 1960 can be credited largely to the development of the No. 21 arthroscope by Watanabe, a pupil of Takagi [691–693]. In subsequent years O'Connor [499] developed the first operating arthroscope and may be listed with Gillquist [207, 208] of Sweden, Dandy [108] of Great Britain, Johnson [325] of the United States, and Henche [272, 273] of Germany as a pioneer of modern arthroscopic technique.

Today, diagnostic and operative arthroscopy hold a significant place in the day-to-day clinical practice of every orthopedic department and trauma unit.

The mainstay of diagnostic knee arthroscopy is the 30° oblique scope, which can be rotated to visualize almost the whole interior of the joint.

Older arthroscopes transmitted their images through a series of small, thin lenses separated by air spaces. The English physicist Hopkins greatly improved upon this system by his discovery of rod-lens optics. This system provides better image quality, a wider viewing angle, and increased image brightness, which is particularly advantageous in arthroscopes with an optical system of small diameter. Wide-angle arthroscopes contain fewer air-glass interfaces than conventional scopes, which significantly reduces the scattering of reflected light at the interfaces.

A basic distinction is drawn between the viewing angle of an arthroscope and its visual field. In an 30° arthroscope, the viewing angle is directed 30° obliquely relative to the long axis of the scope. The viewing angle is always directed opposite to the side of the scope that carries the light cable. Thus, if the scope is held with the light cable at the top, the viewing angle will be directed 30° downward in a 30° oblique scope. The visual field of a wide-angle arthroscope is approximately 90° in a gas medium. The visual field in a fluid medium is decreased by about 25%–30% due to the higher refractive index of water.

The arthroscope (4 mm diameter) is positioned within the sheath (5 mm diameter), which is equipped with two spigots for the inflow and outflow of irrigating fluid. The space between the sheath and arthroscope forms the channel through which the fluid is delivered and removed.

Sheaths 5.5 mm or 6 mm in diameter are also available. The larger space between the arthroscope and sheath allows for more rapid filling of the joint space and eliminates the need for a separate large-gauge inflow cannula, especially in minor arthroscopic operations.

The arthroscope is connected to the light source (cold light or xenon light) by a cable. When the eyepiece of the scope is coupled to a sensitive video camera, a light intensity of 250 W will be sufficient to visualize all com-

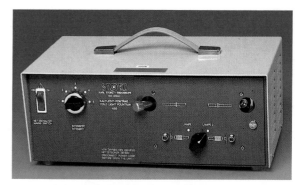

Fig. 11-4. Cold-light source (250 W, Storz)

partments in the knee, even those that are difficult to illuminate (e. g., the suprapatellar pouch) (Fig. 11-4).

11.2.2
Video System

The examiner can inspect the joint directly through the eyepiece of the arthroscope. However, this requires that he proceed very carefully to avoid contamination, for the hand that guides the arthroscope is considered to be unsterile. Also, he may find it difficult to demonstrate arthroscopic findings to an assistant, for even the slightest change in the position of the scope will shift the visual field away from the area of interest and hamper communication between operator and assistant. This can be especially troublesome in operative arthroscopy.

For these reasons it is advantageous to use a video system consisting of a video camera, a monitor, and possibly a videotape recorder. The monitor image is visible to all persons in the operating room and can be correspondingly discussed and interpreted (Fig. 11-5). This not only provides a teaching and learning tool for the operating staff but also enables the conscious patient (under peridural anesthesia) to witness the "live transmission" from his knee joint. This can help many patients, especially those with severe degenerative changes, to better understand the cause of their complaints and why it may not be possible to restore the joint to complete health.

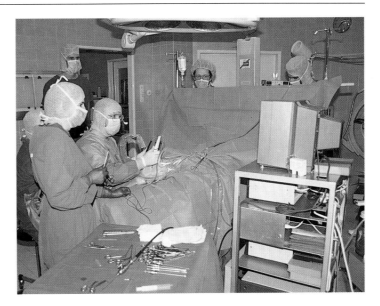

Fig. 11-5. Video arthroscopy. The monitor is placed where it can be viewed by the operator, assistant, scrub nurse, and other OR personnel. Arthroscopic operations can be performed under sterile conditions. The video camera is encased in a sterile, transparent plastic sleeve

Modern microprocessor technology has made it possible to develop color video cameras of very small size. Besides the traditional tube cameras (Fig. 11-6), tubeless solid-state cameras (Fig. 11-7) have become available. The tube cameras offer excellent color reproduction and image quality and have sensitivities as high as 5 lux, permitting the use of a lower-wattage light source. The latest generation of solid-state cameras offer enhanced sensitivities with automatic brightness and contrast control and a high line resolution picture (Fig. 11-7).

Both tube cameras and solid-state cameras can be sterilized by soaking in disinfectant solution. However, due to the potential corrosive action of the solution on the camera body and seals, we prefer to enclose the camera preoperatively in a sterile, transparent plastic sleeve that fastens to the arthroscope (Fig. 11-5). This also avoids the danger of the disinfectant causing a reactive synovitis in the joint [252]. The plastic makes it difficult to exchange arthroscopes (e. g., replace the 30° scope with a 70° scope), because the camera has to be rewrapped.

If a change of arthroscopes is planned, a special adapter should be used which attaches to the eyepiece of the scope [370].

11.2.3 Probe

All pathologic conditions in the knee joint cannot be diagnosed by inspection alone. Some lesions can be identified only by palpation of the involved structure. This is accomplished with a probing hook passed into the joint through a separate instrument portal (Fig. 11-8).

The probe should bear length markings at

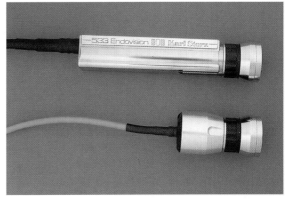

Fig. 11-6. Tube camera (Endovision 533), sensitivity 5 lux (top), and small solid-state camera (TV Endopocket 536, bottom), which plugs into any standard TV monitor, sensitivity 5 lux (Storz)

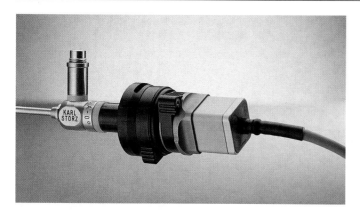

Fig. 11-7. High-resolution solid-state camera (Endovision 538) with the new signal system CMOS-Process 55 (noise factor 55 dB), S-VHS technique, automatic color adjustment, resolution 320 000 pixel for 380 horizontal lines, light sensitivity 5 lux, weight 30 g, size 22 × 36 mm. An available light amplifier which permits signal amplification of 100 % is integrated in the camera. Dark areas of the joint, e. g., the superior recess, can be evaluated more satisfactorily. A high-speed diaphragm is also available which reduces over-exposures and light reflections by as much as a factor of 10. With the four control buttons on the camera body all functions together with color correction can be used by the examiner on demand. The available light amplifier and the high-speed diaphragm are automatically reset to the starting value when normal degrees of brightness are reached (Storz).

5-mm intervals to help the examiner estimate the size or extent of pathologic findings (loose bodies, meniscal tears). Without these markings, the less experienced examiner may find it difficult to judge sizes due to the approximately 10:1 to 30:1 magnification factor in a fluid medium.

The probe can be used to check the tension and integrity of the ACL and to elevate the meniscus and inspect and palpate its undersurface and submeniscal cartilage areas. When pressure is applied to the meniscus, old meniscal scars will feel hard beneath the probe while inferior, incomplete tears and degenerative areas will feel soft.

11.2.4
Documentation

The documentation of intraarticular findings is necessary both for the patient's information and to aid communication among health professionals (teaching, science). Arthroscopic images may be documented with a video recorder or by still photography.

If extremely high image quality is desired, a good solution is to use the semiprofessional U-Matic video recording system, which employs three-quarter inch tapes. Even copying and editing can be done with minimal loss of image quality. However, a standard one-half inch VHS cassette recorder is more economical and usually provides a record of acceptable quality. Also, the VHS system is so widely used that the patient can be given a copy of the video cassette to take home if he so desires.

Very high-quality slides can be taken with a reflex camera by attaching a special lens to the camera and holding the lens up to the eyepiece of the arthroscope. However, this method of documentation is very time-consuming and leads to sterility problems. Additionally, it requires a light source that has built-in through-the-lens synchronization. After taking the pictures, moreover, the operator must rescrub and change gowns before proceeding with the examination.

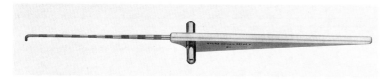

Fig. 11-8. Arthroscopic probe with length markings (Storz)

Documents of acceptable quality can be made simply and cheaply by taking still photographs of the monitor image, assuming the video camera and monitor produce an image of acceptable quality. We use a single-lens reflex camera (e. g., Minolta Dynax 7000i) with auto-aperture set to a shutter speed of 1/4 or 1/8 second. A tripod should always be used for exposures in this range. We take the pictures on normal daylight film with a speed of 100 ASA/21 DIN or 200 ASA/24 DIN (Fujichrome, Ektachrome).

A simple but reliable documentation system is a video printer, which can be used to record the most important findings.

11.3
Preparation

Arthroscopy requires the same aseptic technique used in other operative procedures on the knee such as internal fixations and ligament reconstructions. It may be performed under general, peridural, or spinal anesthesia. Local anesthesia is possible, but we rarely use it.

It is best, for practical and organizational reasons, to follow a standard "house procedure" when preparing and positioning the patient, draping the field, setting up the irrigation system, and laying out the instruments.

11.3.1
Positioning

The patient is examined in the supine position. Either of two methods may be used for positioning the leg:

1. The leg is extended on the surface of the table (Fig. 11-9). A padded lateral post is attached to the side of the table at the level of the distal third of the thigh. The leg can be placed against this post for the application of valgus stress during examination of the medial compartment.
2. The leg is flexed over the edge of the table (Figs. 11-10 and 11-11). This requires the use of a special leg holding device (leg holder) that attaches to the middle third of the thigh. Our device differs from other leg holders in that it has no bulky side clamps (Fig. 11-10). It fits so flat against the thigh that it does not interfere with procedures such as drilling a femoral channel in ACL or PCL reconstructions or reattaching the posterior horn of the lateral meniscus. In addition, the leg holder can be opened or removed without violating asepsis. This is advantageous, for example, when the arthroscopy must be followed by an open reconstruction of the posteromedial or posterolateral corner.

To obtain a bloodless field for arthroscopy, we exsanguinate the limb by wrapping it with a

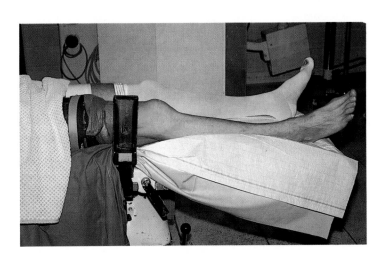

Fig. 11-9. With the leg extended, a padded lateral post mounted about a handswidth proximal to the patella can be used as a fulcrum for applying valgus stress

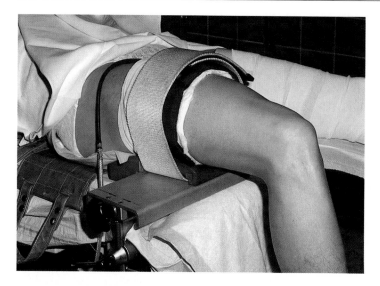

Fig. 11-10. Leg holder (Aesculap)

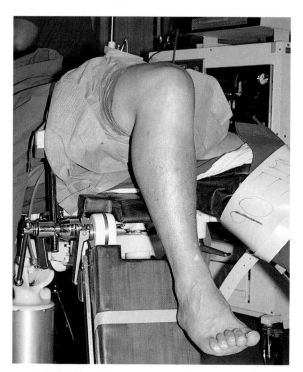

Fig. 11-11. The leg is flexed over the edge of the table while the leg holder secures the thigh

rubber Esmarch bandage and then inflate the tourniquet on the thigh. The tourniquet should never remain inflated for more than 120 min.

11.3.2
Draping the Leg

Disposable, waterproof drapes are applied whenever irrigating fluid is used. After the skin has been degreased and prepared circumferentially with iodine, the entire operating area is draped with waterproof material (Fig. 11-12).

The draping procedure will be very time-consuming and inefficient if all the draping materials are individually packaged. It is better to use a special arthroscopic drape set (e. g., Klinidrape 100, Mölnlycke) that contains all materials needed to drape the patient for arthroscopy, including a waterproof gown for the operator.

We do not use an incision drape for diagnostic or operative arthroscopy. However, we do use an incision drape in cases where the arthroscopy is be followed by a major open knee operation.

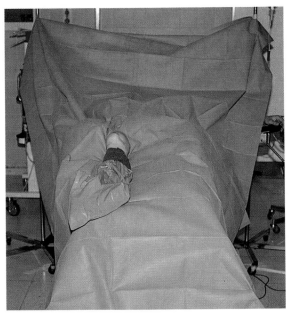

Fig. 11-12. The extended leg and surrounding area are draped with waterproof material (Klinidrape 100, Mölnlycke). The operator and assistant wear waterproof gowns

Table 11-1. Advantages of gas arthroscopy [362]

1. Better image quality
2. Better visualization in hemarthrosis
3. Easier to distinguish between old and recent tears of the ACL
4. Rapid distention of the joint space

Table 11-2. Disadvantages of gas arthroscopy

1. Gas leakage through the incision, causing loss of distention
2. Vision obscured by bubbles in residual intraarticular fluid
3. Soiling of optics by blood
4. Fogging of optics by condensation (especially when a high-energy light source is used)
5. Danger of cutaneous emphysema from gas entering the soft tissues
6. Need for gas insufflator
7. Danger of gas embolism

11.3.3 Irrigation System

The joint space is distended with gas, fluid, or a combination of both media (first gas, then fluid). Arthroscopy in gas offers several advantages (Table 11-1) but has numerous disadvantages as well (Table 11-2).

Foaming, a frequent complaint in gas arthroscopy, can be minimized by first washing out the joint with irrigating fluid.

Since two fatal cases of air embolism were described following arthroscopy in patients with bony injuries (avulsed intercondylar eminence, tibial plateau fracture) [231], gas arthroscopy is considered to be contraindicated in patients with hemarthrosis or a fresh bony injury that exposes the cancellous spaces.

By contrast, arthroscopy in a fluid medium displays numerous advantages (Table 11-3), especially in cases where arthroscopic surgery is proposed [362].

Minor disadvantages of fluid arthroscopy, such as the obstruction of vision by "waving" synovial fronds or the need to use waterproof drapes, must be tolerated. Also, the examiner must adjust to the "aquarium effect" of the fluid medium [273], which affords a view markedly different from the appearance of the arthrotomized joint (Fig. 11-13).

Irrigation may be performed with Ringer's solution, physiologic saline, or an electrolyte-free solution (e. g., Purisole SM, Fresenius). An electrolyte-free solution should be used if the diagnostic arthroscopy is to be followed by intraarticular electrosurgery (electroresection). For all arthroscopies – whether diagnostic or, as in more than 95% of cases, operative – we suspend two bags, each containing 3000 or 5000 ml of *Purisole SM,* from a ceiling fixture (Fig. 11-14) or from a tall i. v. pole. The pressure of the irrigating fluid is controlled by adjusting the level.

If a roller pump is available, the desired fluid pressure can be set directly on the instrument. Gas and fluid arthroscopy can be combined to exploit the advantages of each medium. In this case the joint is flushed several times with irrigating fluid and then distended with gas for the examination. If surgery is to follow, the gas is released and the joint is distended with fluid.

Table 11-3. Advantages of arthroscopy in fluid media

1. Economical

2. Fluid stream clears the joint of
   - cellular debris (may be therapeutic, relieving pain in degenerative joint disease)
   - small and minute loose bodies
   - hemarthrosis
   - fibrin deposits

3. In operative arthroscopy, permits use of
   - electrosurgical instruments
   - suction punches
   - motorized instruments (shavers, cutters, etc.)

It is convenient to place all the equipment for video arthroscopy (monitor, U-Matic recorder, light source, etc.) on a wheeled cart where all components are easily seen and accessible. To eliminate tangled cords, the cart is equipped with a central power strip that supplies current to all instruments. The cart itself has one power cord that plugs into an electrical outlet in the operating suite. The cart is easily wheeled from one side of the table to the other for multiple examinations in the course of a day, without the need for time-consuming rearranging of equipment.

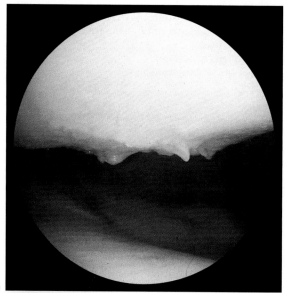

a

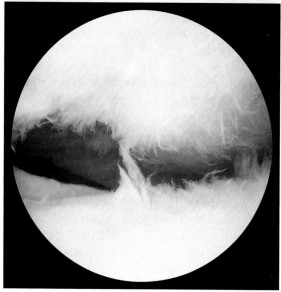

b

Fig. 11-13a, b. Comparison of gas and fluid arthroscopy. At first sight, these appear to be views of two completely different cases. Distention of the knee joint with gas (**a**) presses down small fronds of cartilage and synovium, and surface has a glistening appearance. When the joint is distended with fluid (**b**), the synovial and cartilage fronds "float" in the medium. When interpreting the findings, the examiner must keep in mind the essential difference between a gas and fluid distending medium

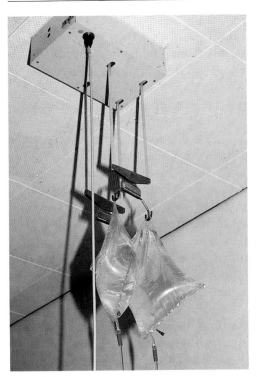

Fig. 11-14. Ceiling suspension with bags of irrigating fluid (Purisole SM, Fresenius)

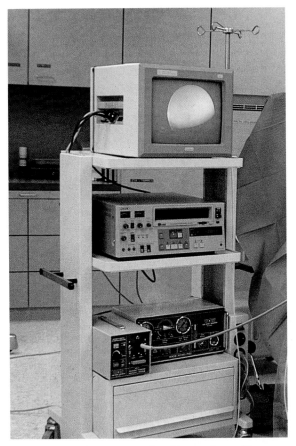

Fig. 11-15. Arthroscopy unit with monitor, video cassette recorder, light source, and roller pump

11.4
Portals

Selecting the correct sites of insertion for the arthroscope and other instruments is essential for the smooth conduct of the examination. If the portal for the arthroscope is unfavorably placed, only a portion of the joint interior can be inspected [519, 520]. Significant iatrogenic cartilage damage can result from attempting to "force" the arthroscope or instrument to the desired location [91, 129, 637].

11.4.1
Arthroscopic Portal

Of the many existing approaches (Fig. 11-16), we prefer a *high anterolateral* portal for insertion of the arthroscope. This has become our standard approach, and we use a low antero-

lateral portal only if arthroscopic lateral release is planned. The high anterolateral portal is located by palpating the patellar apex and lateral border of the patellar ligament with the thumb while the knee is flexed to approximately 70° (Fig. 11-17). A skin incision about 0.5 cm long is then made at the level of the patellar apex. A sharp-pointed knife (No. 11 blade) is used, carrying the incision through the subcutaneous tissue and fibrous capsule.

In the classic insertion technique, described in many textbooks, the sheath and sharp trocar are first inserted through the skin incision. Then, once the fibrous capsule has been penetrated, as evidenced by a decrease in resistance, the sharp trocar is changed for a blunt trocar or obturator.

However, many arthroscopists no longer consider it necessary to use a sharp trocar, es-

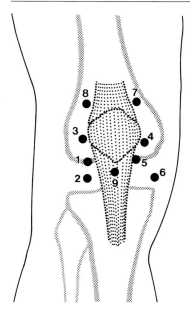

Fig. 11-16. Arthroscopic approaches: High anterolateral approach (level with the patellar apex, lateral to the patellar ligament) *(1)*; low anterolateral approach *(2)*; midpatellar lateral approach *(3)*; midpatellar medial approach *(4)*; high medial approach (gives instrument access to lateral meniscus and posterior horn of medial meniscus) *(5)*; suprameniscal medial approach (gives more anterior or medial instrument access, depending on the lesion and the degree of valgus laxity) *(6)*; suprapatellar medial *(7)* and lateral *(8)* approach; transligamentous (Gillquist's) approach *(9)*

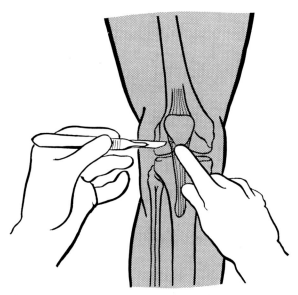

Fig. 11-17. Location of the high anterolateral arthroscopic portal. The patellar apex and lateral border of the patellar ligament are palpated, and a stab incision is made at the level of the apex. (From [637]

pecially since the sheath with blunt trocar presents a uniform tip that can pass through the subcutaneous tissue and fibrous capsule. Eliminating the sharp trocar not only eliminates the changing of trocars but also provides a significant safety reserve for the cartilage. Deep iatrogenic cartilage lesions are unlikely to occur even if the tip suddenly enters the joint space and comes into contact with the cartilage (see Fig. 11-66). Thus, after the skin incision is made and the knee is flexed to approximately 70°, the sheath with blunt trocar is carefully advanced in the direction of the ACL with a twisting motion. The right index finger (in a right-handed operator) is held against the sheath about 2–3 cm back from the tip to act as an "emergency brake" to prevent plunging.

Another important safety factor is the careful insertion of the sheath with a slight rotatory screwing motion. This reduces tissue resistance and makes the insertion easier to control. When the tip is directed toward the ACL, plunging of the sheath may damage the synovial investment of the cruciate ligament but will not harm the cartilage on the medial and lateral femoral condyles. A decrease in resistance signifies that the sheath and trocar have entered the intraarticular space. At that point the knee is carefully extended while the sheath is simultaneously advanced toward the medial suprapatellar recess, the thrust of the instrument being contained within the broad suprapatellar pouch. Then the blunt trocar is changed for the arthroscope (30° wide-angle scope), which is coupled to the sterily wrapped video camera.

If inserted too far laterally and superiorly, the sheath may enter the space between the capsule and synovium. If the inflow of irrigating fluid is started at that time, the synovial membrane will balloon into the joint space and hamper further inspection once the interior of the joint has been reached.

If the sheath is inserted too horizontally (toward the medial joint line) while the knee is still flexed, it may enter the infrapatellar fat pad. The irrigating fluid will then distended the fat pad, making the rest of the examination more difficult.

For these reasons, fluid inflow and suction through the sheath should be started, and the joint space distended, only after it has been confirmed that the tip of the sheath is within the joint space.

If hemarthrosis is present, the joint should be thoroughly irrigated before the arthroscope is inserted. For this the blunt trocar is removed, the open end of the sheath is manually occluded, and the joint is alternately irrigated and suctioned until the efflux is clear. Only then is the arthroscope with attached camera inserted and the joint space redistended. Alternatively, a separate instrument portal can be established, and large organized clots can be extracted with a grasping forceps or removed with a motorized shaver device.

11.4.2
Instrument Portal

The location of the instrument portal is determined on the basis of arthroscopic findings. Optimum placement of this portal will facilitate probing and any subsequent arthroscopic surgical measures. It will also decrease the risk of iatrogenic cartilage damage caused by the forced probing of poorly accessible sites.

Pathologic findings and ligamentous laxity vary greatly in degree from one patient to the next. In some cases the joint space is large and accessible, while in others the space can hardly be opened even by a strong valgus stress. Some tears may be found in the lateral meniscus while others are located in the posterior horn area of the medial meniscus. Consequently, there is no standard instrument portal that can give optimum access to all intraarticular structures.

The instrument portal is formed using the *cannula method* under arthroscopic visual control (Fig. 11-18 and 11-19).

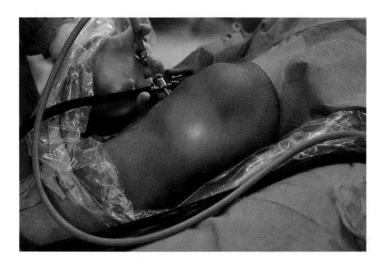

Fig. 11-18. Transillumination

11.4.2.1
Creation of the Instrument Portal

The approximate location of the instrument portal is determined by transilluminating the skin with the arthroscopic light (Fig. 11-18). The examiner then palpates the joint in that area while watching the monitor for the bulge in the joint capsule made by the palpating finger. At that site he inserts a cannula percutaneously into the joint under visual control (Fig. 11-19a). If the puncture is correctly placed, the cannula should be able to reach the target structure (e. g., the posterior horn of the medial meniscus) (Fig. 11-19b). If the structure cannot be reached with the cannula, it will be even more difficult to reach with the larger probing hook. And if arthroscopic surgery is required, the instruments will either be unable to reach the area or reach it with an exorbitant risk of iatrogenic cartilage injury.

In this situation it is prudent to remove the cannula and reinsert it at a slightly different site. Multiple punctures are less damaging than an incorrectly or unfavorably positioned portal that complicates all subsequent maneuvers. Once the optimum location for the instrument portal has been found, a sharp-pointed knife (No. 11 blade) is introduced to make a longitudinal incision in the fibrous capsule and synovium (Fig. 11-19c). The blade should point upward so that if it slips, it will not damage the meniscus. Care is taken that incisions of equal length are made through the skin, subcutaneous tissue, and fibrous capsule. Thus, a small skin incision over a large capsular incision will permit a large amount of irrigating fluid to leak from the joint and collect in the subcutaneous tissue, while a large skin incision over a small capsular incision will make it very difficult to introduce the probe and operating instruments. After the instrument portal has been created, the probe is introduced (Fig. 11-19d). The operator should be aware that any change in the position of the knee joint, such as a change in flexion angle, will cause a relative shifting of tissue layers that may hamper or prevent the reinsertion of instruments.

11.4.2.2
Location of the Instrument Portal

The site of the instrument portal is particularly crucial to the success of arthroscopic operations. Although arthroscopy continues to be important diagnostically, the main focus of interest is on arthroscopic surgery. Using this method, the surgeon can operate on pathologically altered structures with small instruments passed into the joint through the instrument portal, known also as the working portal. Thus, the portal must not only permit atraumatic probing but above all must meet the very rigorous requirements of arthroscopic surgery. Unnecessary contact between instruments and cartilage must be avoided.

The medial suprameniscal instrument portal is most commonly required (Fig. 11-20). Sited just proximal to the base of the meniscus, this portal gives access to the entire medial meniscus, provided there is sufficient medial joint laxity (Fig. 11-21). If the ligaments are tight and greatly restrict opening of the medial joint space, the location of the instrument portal assumes particular significance. The narrower the joint space, the farther medially the instrument portal should be placed. Thus, in a tight joint with minimum valgus laxity, the portal should be placed immediately in front of the anterior border of the medial collateral ligament (Fig. 11-21b). If the joint has ample valgus laxity, on the other hand, any suprameniscal portal will give access to the medial meniscus (Fig. 11-21c).

The posterior horn of the medial meniscus also can be reached directly through a high medial approach. Entry is made just medial to the patellar ligament at the level of the patellar apex (cf. high anterolateral arthroscopic portal). After the leg is placed in the "figure-four" position (with the lower leg crossed over the contralateral thigh, see Fig. 11-57), this portal will also give instrument access to all portions of the lateral meniscus. However, we recommend making this portal for probing of the lateral compartment only after the leg has been moved to the figure-four position.

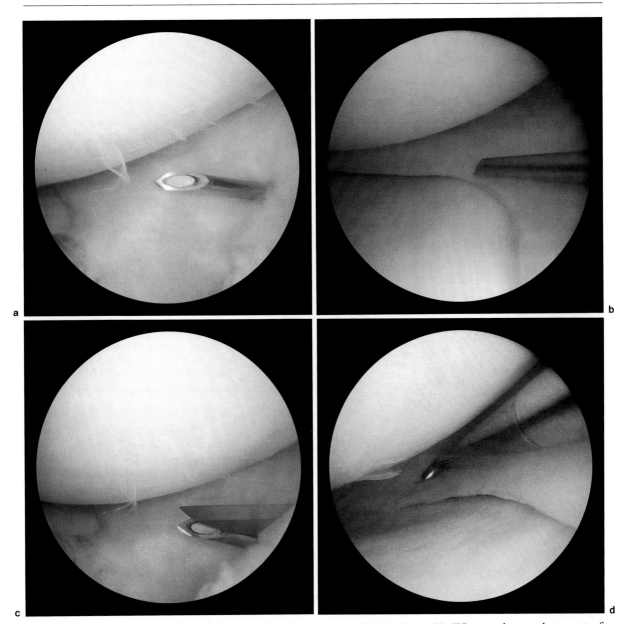

Fig. 11-19 a–d. Creation of a medial suprameniscal instrument portal under arthroscopic control. A cannula is inserted under visual control immediately above the medial meniscus (**a**), and it is determined whether the cannula can reach the suspicious posterior portion of the medial meniscus (**b**). When optimum placement of the puncture site is confirmed, the fibrous capsule and synovium are incised with a scalpel (blade points upward to protect the meniscus) (**c**). Finally the probing hook is inserted for palpation of the meniscus (**d**)

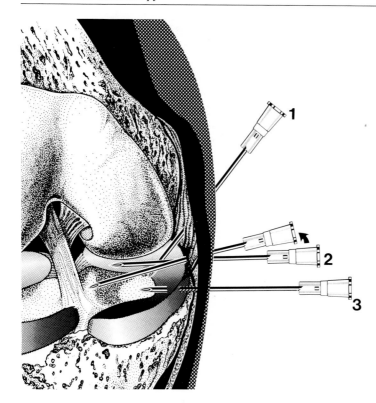

Fig. 11-20. Medial suprameniscal instrument portal made with the cannula technique. If the puncture is made too far superiorly, access is obstructed by the femoral condyle *(1)*, and probing of the meniscus will be difficult. Puncture just above the meniscus gives adequate freedom of movement while giving access to the ACL and posterior meniscal areas *(2)*. Placing the portal too far distally jeopardizes the meniscus *(3)* [from Strobel et al. (1989) Arthroskopische Untersuchung des Kniegelenkes. Deutscher Ärzteverlag, Cologne]

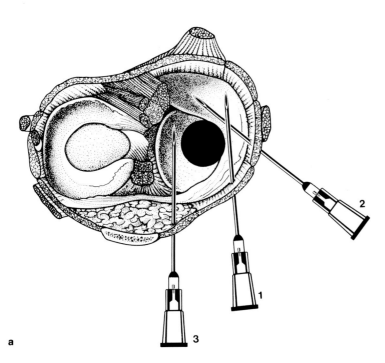

a

Fig. 11-21a–c. Location of the suprameniscal portal as a function of valgus laxity. **a** Normal valgus laxity: Only part of the medial femoral condyle lies on the suprameniscal entry plane *(black area)*. The posterior parts of the meniscus cannot be reached with a cannula inserted too far anterior to the medial collateral liga-ment; access is blocked by the medial femoral condyle *(1)*. A cannula inserted slightly anterior to the medial collateral ligament will miss the femoral condyle and can reach the posterior portion of the meniscus *(2)*. The posterior horn is directly accessible through a high medial approach *(3)*.

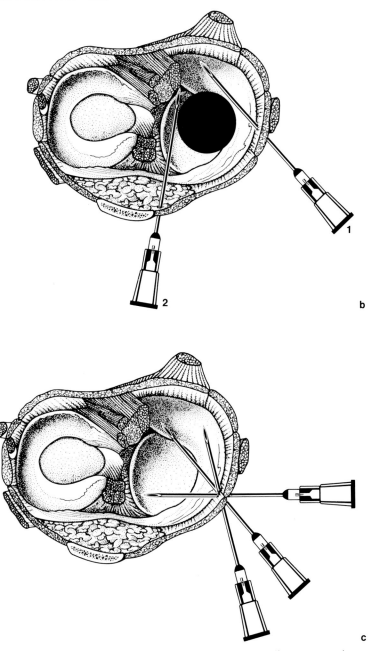

Fig. 11-21.b, c. b Minimal valgus laxity (tight knee): The medial femoral condyle obstructs access on the suprameniscal plane *(black area).* The cannula is inserted just anterior to the medial collateral ligament *(1).* If the cannula were inserted more anteriorly, the intervening femoral condyle would deflect it away from the posterior meniscus. The posterior horn of the medial meniscus can be reached directly through an approach just medial to the patellar ligament at the level of the high anterolateral arthroscopic portal *(2).* **c** Marked valgus laxity in a patient with hyperlaxity or torn medial ligaments: As the femoral condyle is not on the suprameniscal plane *(missing black area),* it does not obstruct access. Selection of the approach is simple. All portions of the meniscus are accessible from any suprameniscal portal (after [637])

11.4.3
Triangulation

The simultaneous manipulation of the probe and arthroscope can be especially difficult for the inexperienced examiner, because the probe is not always easy to bring into the optical field of the arthroscope. DeHaven [119] has described an improved technique for two-puncture diagnostic arthroscopy based on the principle of triangulation. In this technique the probe and arthroscope are held so that their tips form the apex of an imaginary triangle. If the operator keeps the triangulation principle in mind while guiding the arthroscope and probe – analogous to eating with a knife and fork – he should have no difficulty bringing the tips of the instruments together. Usually the probe can be visualized by slowly withdrawing the scope until the tip of the probe comes into view.

The probing hook is used to check the articular cartilage for projections, defects, and areas of softening. The menisci are probed for the presence of submeniscal or incomplete tears, and the ACL is probed to assess its tension and continuity.

11.5
Orientation and Systematic Joint Inspection

Like the clinical examination, the arthroscopic examination of the knee should be done in a systematic manner. While the sequence in which the structures and compartments are inspected may vary from one examiner to the next, the routine must guarantee that no intra-articular pathology is overlooked (Table 11-4).

Orientation during arthroscopy is often difficult for the novice, because the scope reveals only a fraction of the joint interior at one time. It is like trying to become oriented on a large map by looking at an area only 2×2 cm in size. A meaningful interpretation of findings is possible only if there are clearly identifiable

Table 11-4. Systematic routine for arthroscopic examination of the knee joint

1. Retropatellar cartilage
2. Suprapatellar pouch
   - Suprapatellar plica
3. Lateral recess
   - Popliteus tendon
   - Lateral aspect of lateral meniscus
4. Patellofemoral joint
5. Medial capsule
   - Mediopatellar plica
6. Medial compartment
   - Medial meniscus
   - Medial femorotibial articular surface
7. Intercondylar notch
   - Infrapatellar plica
   - ACL
   - Posterior horn of medial meniscus
   - Posteromedial recess
   - PCL
8. Lateral compartment (knee is moved to "figure-four" position)
   - Lateral meniscus
   - Popliteal hiatus
   - Lateral femorotibial articular surface

points or landmarks that can serve as a basis for orientation.

When the examiner looks directly through the arthroscope, the angle of vision in a 30° oblique scope is directed 30° downward when the light cable points upward (Fig. 11-22). Conversely, when the light cable points down, the angle of vision is directed upward.

The position of the light cable is an important aid to orientation.

When arthroscopy is performed without a video system, the examiner can easily become oriented by the position of the light cable. But when a video camera is used, the location of the intraarticular structure on the monitor does not always correspond to its true anatomic location (Fig. 11-23). It must be determined, then, which parts of the image are superior, inferior, medial, and lateral in the anatomic sense. Again, the position of the light cable provides a crucial aid to orientation once the arthroscopic system has been tentatively "calibrated" by an easily recognized feature. The calibration process is aided by external palpation, for the bulge made by the palpating finger is clearly visible on the monitor.

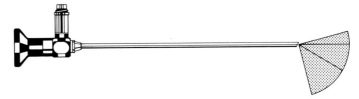

Fig. 11-22. In the 30° wide-angle arthroscope, the viewing angle is directed 30° downward when the scope is positioned with the light cable at the top. The visual field *(shaded area)* is approximately 90°

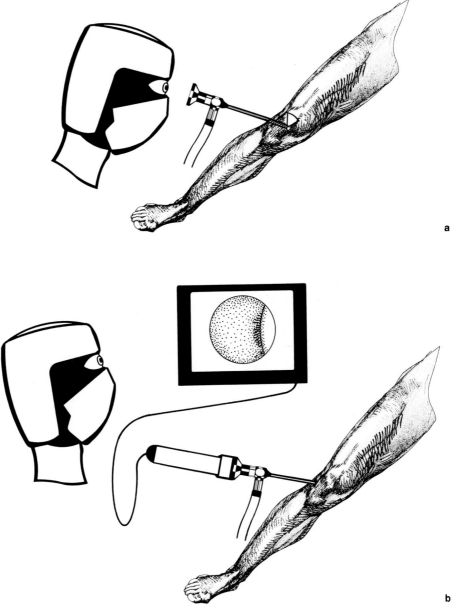

Fig. 11-23a–c. Direct inspection through a 30° wide-angle arthroscope with the light cable down demonstrates the anatomic structure in its true superior location (**a**). When a video camera is used, the structure (e. g. the patella) may not be displayed at the top of the monitor, as one would expect, but on the left or right side (**b**) or even at the bottom.

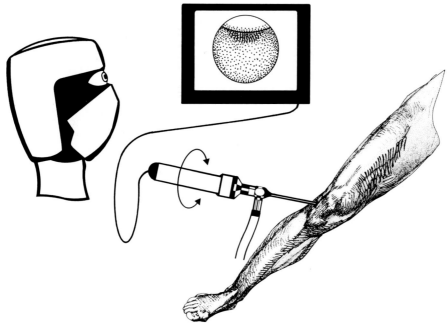

Fig. 11-23c. By carefully rotating the camera relative to the arthroscope, the monitor image can be corrected to portray the structure in its true anatomic position (**c**)

Orientation in video arthroscopy, like the examination itself, should follow a standard routine. The first step is to ensure that the anatomic structures which are uppermost in the extended knee joint (retropatellar cartilage, posterior surface of quadriceps tendon) are displayed at the top of the monitor screen. This is accomplished by carefully loosening the connection between the video camera and arthroscope and rotating the camera relative to the scope.

First the retropatellar cartilage is displayed at the top of the monitor.

Once this gross orientation has been established, right-left orientation is accomplished by positioning the video image as if the observer were looking into the knee joint from the anterior side. Thus, the medial meniscus of a right knee is displayed on the right side of the screen, the medial meniscus of a left knee on the left side. Besides transillumination of the skin with the arthroscopic light (Fig. 11-18), this orientation is aided by digital palpation over the joint line. The examiner can easily see the palpating finger over the medial capsule and determine whether the mediolateral orientation on the monitor is correct or requires further adjustment. The articular surfaces of the femorotibial joint and the meniscal plane should be horizontal on the monitor.

Numerous readjustments may be necessary during inspection of the various joint regions, and the novice may find that numerous "reorientations" are required. One should never attempt to examine the joint without proper orientation; this would pose an excessive risk of iatrogenic cartilage and ligament damage and would preclude a meaningful diagnostic assessment. If orientation is lost, the examiner should regain it by identifying one or more landmark features (retropatellar cartilage, medial meniscus, ACL) and correct the monitor image accordingly.

11.6
Arthroscopic Anatomy and Pathologic Findings

11.6.1
Retropatellar Space

The main problem after insertion of the arthroscope is to establish proper orientation; this is essential before the examination may proceed. First the arthroscope is rotated 180° so that the light cable points downward (Fig. 11-24). In a 30° oblique scope, this maneuver will direct the viewing angle 30° upward. Normally, in the extended knee, the retropatellar cartilage will appear as a glistening white area at the top, side, or bottom of the screen as the arthroscope is slowly pulled back from the suprapatellar pouch. The camera is rotated relative to the arthroscope until the retropatellar cartilage is displayed at the top of the screen. Manual pressure on the patella confirms that the feature shown is really the undersurface of the patella and not the opposing patellar surface of the femur.

11.6.1.1.
Cartilage

The intact hyaline articular cartilage appears arthroscopically as a smooth, white, pearly layer that feels firm and resilient when probed.

Cartilage changes are notoriously difficult to diagnose clinically and radiographically in their early stages, when X-rays generally show no abnormalities. In these cases arthroscopy can be helpful in assessing the extent and location of cartilage lesions, which can be graded using the classification of Ficat [166]:

Grade I: *Edematous change* (cartilage surface can be indented with the probe, Fig. 11-44).

Grade II: *Fibrillated* cartilage with fissures, chondral flaps, and ulcerations that do not reach the subchondral bone.

Grade III: *Deep fibrillation* with full-thickness chondral separations exposing the bone (Fig. 11-25).

Retropatellar cartilage changes chiefly affect the medial facet and the inferior portion of the patella (Fig. 11-26). Affected areas can be probed from a medial instrument portal so that the cartilage lesions can be positively identified as retropatellar and evaluated as to their depth and extent [81, 91]. Inspection of the lateral patellar facet is facilitated by manually tilting the patella medially while rotating the scope so that the light cable points medially.

Lesions of the retropatellar cartilage are among the most common arthroscopic findings. It is not unusual to find pronounced degenerative retropatellar changes even in patients who are clinically asymptomatic and have no femoropatellar complaints. Conversely, it is common to find grade I or grade II

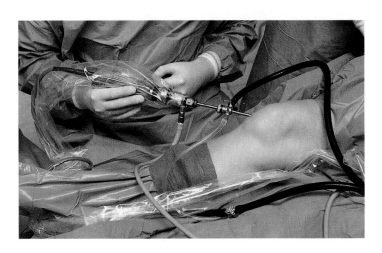

Fig. 11-24. Position of the arthroscope for examination of the retropatellar cartilage. The viewing angle is directed upward, as signified by the "down" position of the light cable

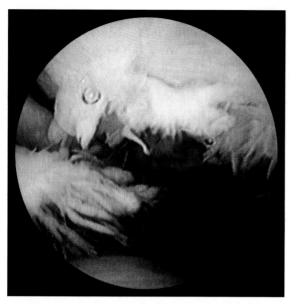

Fig. 11-25. Grade III chondromalacia of the retropatellar cartilage, characterized by deep fibrillation and fissuring with cartilage fragments floating in the joint

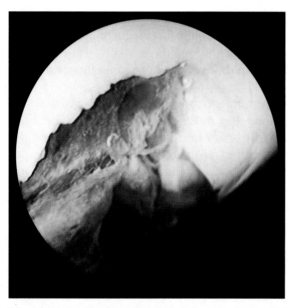

Fig. 11-26. Fresh osteochondral defect on the medial patellar facet following dislocation of the patella

chondromalacia in young patients who are experiencing severe knee pain. With otherwise normal clinical findings, it is tempting in these cases to refer the complaints to the chondromalacia. However, it is better diagnostic procedure to evaluate for functional disturbances of the femoropatellar joint in cases of this kind. The term chondromalacia merely describes a morphologic condition and does not necessarily have pathogenic significance or denote a pathologic entity. Accordingly, the morphologic retropatellar changes must always be interpreted within the context of the clinical presentation (see Sect. 5.1). Retropatellar cartilage changes of some degree are found in nearly 100% of patients over 50 years of age.

11.6.2
Suprapatellar Pouch

Having acquired orientation from the retropatellar cartilage, the examiner pushes the arthroscope up into the suprapatellar pouch. The arthroscope is rotated so that the light cable points medially, and the monitor image is reoriented to give a satisfactory view of the suprapatellar pouch.

The floor of the pouch (anterior surface of the femur) is viewed by rotating the arthroscope an additional 90° so that the light cable points upward.

11.6.2.1
Synovium

The healthy synovium is smooth and transparent and displays fine vascular markings. The floor of the compartment (anterior femoral surface) is studded with transparent synovial villi that contain a small central blood vessel. Interspersed among them are yellowish villi with a very high fat contant; these have no pathologic significance.

In mechanical synovitis, the villi lose their transparency and become completely or partially opaque (Fig. 11-27). This contrasts with their appearance in inflammatory synovitis, which is marked by a proliferation of clublike synovial fronds. The synovial membrane may be smooth, edematous, hyperemic, or sclerotic [91, 364]. Rarely, a synovial chondromatosis may be seen in which chondromas have detached to form multiple loose bodies (Fig. 11-28).

If findings are suspicious, it is recommended that a synovial biopsy be performed with a biopsy forceps passed through the instrument portal (Fig. 11-27).

11.6.2.2
Suprapatellar Plica

Besides the synovium and its villi, attention must be given to the various synovial duplications and plicae, which can exhibit their own forms of pathology [249, 270, 271, 560].

Inspection of the suprapatellar pouch will reveal a plica of variable prominence that usually appears as a crescent-shaped fold just superior to the patella. In some cases, however, this plica may completely separate the suprapatellar pouch from the rest of the joint space [91, 271, 560], preventing distention of the pouch with the irrigating fluid. This possibility should be considered if distention of the femoropatellar space is found to be inadequate with the knee extended.

11.6.3
Lateral Recess

The arthroscope is turned so that the light cable points up and the viewing angle is directed downward.

Loose bodies and small cartilage fragments floating in the joint may be found in the lateral recess or the lateral suprapatellar recess (Fig. 11-29).

To enter the lateral recess, the tip of the scope is moved downward and posteriorly over the lateral femoral condyle. The direct route is often obstructed by synovial folds of variable prominence (Fig. 11-30). In this case it is helpful to withdraw the arthroscope with a gentle twisting motion until the obstructing plica comes into view and then readvance the scope posteriorly to the level of the lateral joint line, the lateral aspect of the lateral meniscus, and the popliteus tendon (Fig. 11-31).

Following *dislocation of the patella,* arthroscopy may reveal osteochondral and/or chon-

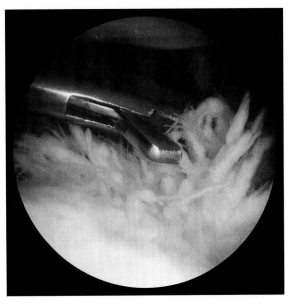

Fig. 11-27. Synovitis with marked hypertrophy of the synovial villi in the suprapatellar pouch in degenerative joint disease. Synovial biopsy was performed

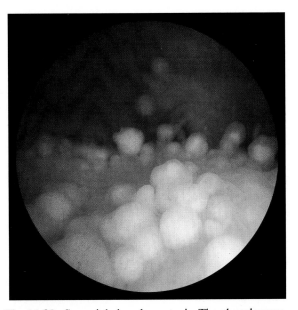

Fig. 11-28. Synovial chondromatosis. The chondromas are produced by the synovium and are released into the joint

dral fragments or cartilage contusion marks with associated hemorrhage on the lateral aspect of the lateral femoral condyle.

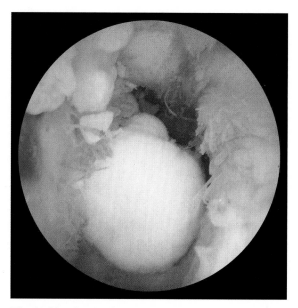

Fig. 11-29. Large loose body in the lateral recess. There is coexisting synovitis with fine and coarse villi

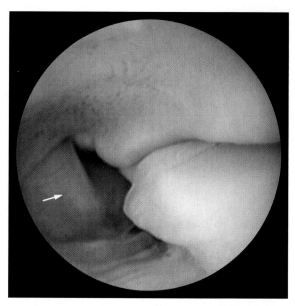

Fig. 11-31. View of the lateral recess showing the lateral aspect of the lateral meniscus, an osteophyte on the lateral femoral condyle, and the popliteus tendon *(arrow)* posteriorly

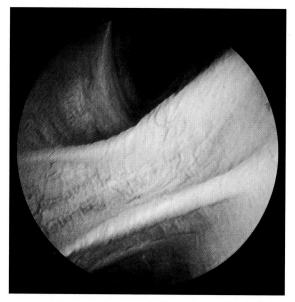

Fig. 11-30. Variable synovial plicae are encountered in the lateral recess. Note the fine vascular markings in the thin synovial membrane

11.6.4
Patellofemoral Joint

The patellofemoral contact area is evaluated by slowly flexing the extended knee joint while observing the retropatellar space through the arthroscope (Fig. 11-32). The scope is pushed in the direction of the medial capsule and turned so that the light cable points toward the tibia. Because cartilage lesions on the undersurface of the patella are frequently associated with cartilage changes on the patellar surface of the femur, this view should not be omitted.

Observation of patellar tracking will also show whether there is a tendency toward lateral patellar subluxation or excessive lateral patellofemoral pressure. Additionally, the examiner should watch for contusion marks, hemorrhages, and tears in the medial retinaculum that may signify a previous patellar dislocation (Fig. 11-33).

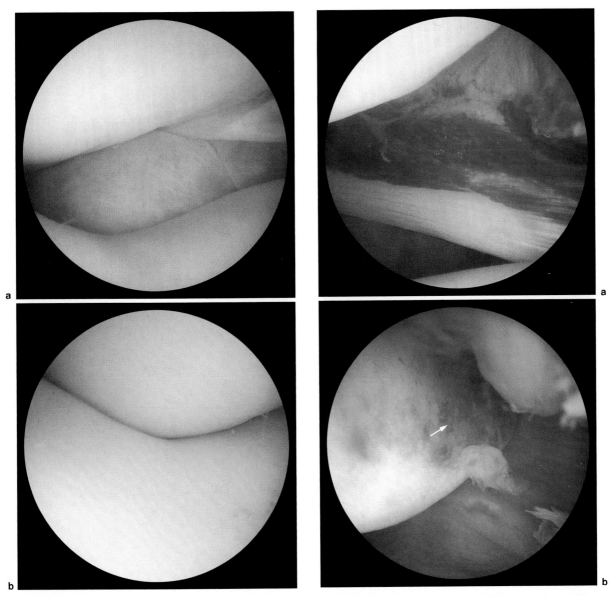

Fig. 11-32a, b. The femoropatellar joint space is widely open in extension (**a**) and narrows as the knee is flexed. As flexion increases further, the point where the patella contacts the femur can be identified (**b**), This view demonstrates a central area of patellofemoral contact

Fig. 11-33a, b. Tear and hemorrhage in the medial retinaculum (**a**) and contusion marks *(arrow)* on the medial patellar facet (**b**) secondary to dislocation of the patella

11.6.5
Medial Compartment

Following inspection of the retropatellar space, the tip of the scope is advanced toward the medial suprapatellar recess and then swept over the medial femoral condyle in the direction of the medial joint space (light cable points medially).

A synovial fold, the mediopatellar plica, may be encountered on the anteromedial capsule wall (Fig. 11-34).

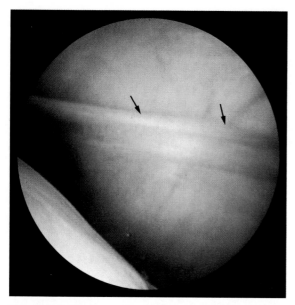

Fig. 11-34. Mediopatellar plica *(arrow)* on the antero-medial capsule

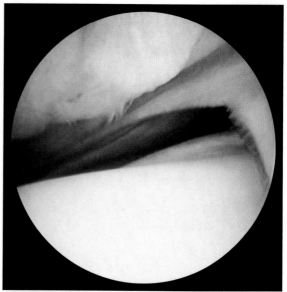

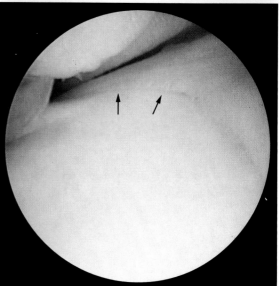

Fig. 11-35 a, b. Hypertrophied mediopatellar plica (**a**). As flexion increases, the distance between the femoral condyle and plica dwindles until impingement occurs *(arrows)* (**b**)

11.6.5.1
Mediopatellar Plica

The mediopatellar plica (medial shelf) is a roughly vertical fold of synovium located on the medial wall of the joint cavity. It has the greatest clinical relevance of all the synovial folds [271, 365]. If the plica is fibrotic or enlarged, it assumes an almost "meniscus-like" appearance and may impinge against the medial femoral condyle during flexion of the knee (Fig. 11-35). Cartilage damage occurring in that area can cause pain in the medial part of the joint or slightly above the joint line. The mediopatellar plica reportedly exists in 20%–50% of the population [396, 581]. According to Hempfling [271], the plica should be considered pathologic only if it has produced cartilage lesions on the medial femoral condyle or the undersurface of the patella (medial shelf syndrome, plica syndrome).

A large, hypertrophic mediopatellar plica not associated with cartilage changes is considered to be a normal anatomic variant.

11.6.5.2
Medial Meniscus

The arthroscope is turned so that the light cable points medially (Fig. 11-36). From that position the medial structures (meniscus, tibial lateau, femoral condyle) are inspected. For easier orientation, the medial meniscus in the left knee is displayed on the left side of the

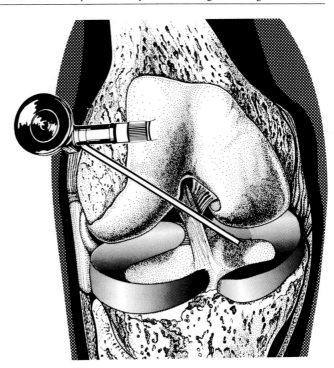

Fig. 11-36. Visualization of the medial compartment (light cable points medially). A valgus pressure is applied in slight flexion (10°) to open up the medial joint space (from [637])

monitor, while the medial meniscus in the right knee is displayed on the right side. The application of a valgus stress to the slightly flexed knee will make the medial compartment easier to inspect. The entire posterior horn of the medial meniscus cannot be visualized unless medial instability or hyperlaxity is present.

In very tight joints it can be difficult to demonstrate any of the posterior portion of the meniscus, and the posterior horn cannot be visualized. In this case the tip of the scope is moved toward the central portion of the meniscus, the tibia is externally rotated, and the medial joint space is opened by a valgus stress with the knee in slight flexion (5°–10°). Usually this maneuver will demonstrate most of the posterior segment of the meniscus. If the knee is flexed too far (e. g., to 30° or 40°), the meniscus will recede and its posterior portions cannot be inspected.

The intact medial meniscus displays a sharp, uniform free border. Almost the entire meniscus can be inspected when the medial joint space is stressed open (Figs. 11-37 and 11-38). Small undulations in the posterior portion of the meniscus usually have no pathologic sig-

nificance, but palpation is indicated to exclude tears in those areas (Fig. 11-39). Conspicuous lesions such as radial tears, longitudinal tears, meniscal flaps, bucket-handle tears, and complex degenerative changes can usually be detected by inspection alone (Figs. 8-6d, 11-40 to

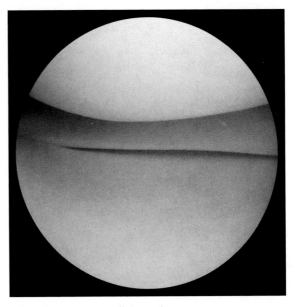

Fig. 11-37. Intact medial meniscus

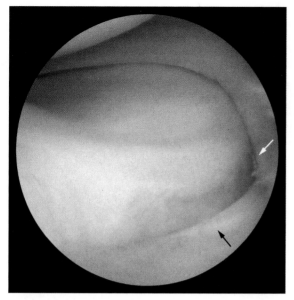

Fig. 11-38. Medial meniscus intact in its central portion. The anterior segment *(arrow)* leaves the medial tibial plateau. Probing should be done to exclude hypermobility of this segment

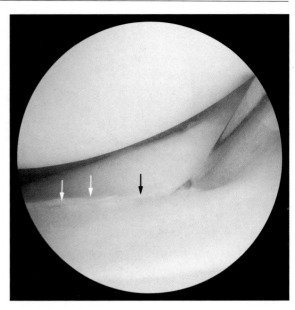

Fig. 11-40. Posterior longitudinal tear *(arrows)* delineated with the probe

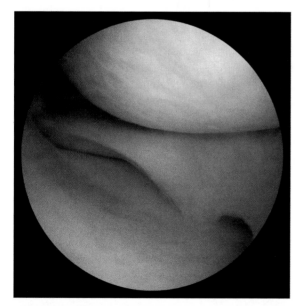

Fig. 11-39. Small undulation in the posterior portion of the meniscus in a joint with marked valgus laxity. Probing is necessary to exclude a posterior longitudinal tear of the meniscus

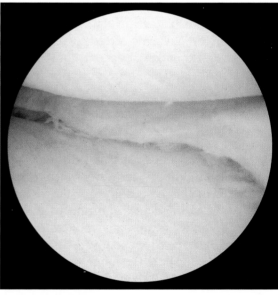

Fig. 11-41. Slight degenerative fraying of the free border of the meniscus

11-43). After a medial instrument portal is established, the firmness of the meniscosynovial junction is tested with the probe. The meniscus is elevated to uncover any submeniscal lesions such as horizontal tears or partial-thickness inferior longitudinal tears. The surface of the meniscus is probed under pressure to detect hidden lesions and evaluate the consistency of the meniscal tissue. Hard fibrous areas signify an old rupture or degenerative changes that have not yet progressed to a frank tear. With a partial-thickness inferior longitudinal tear, the free border of the meniscus will protrude under the pressure of the probe.

On finding a very small medial meniscus, the examiner may be tempted to diagnose an "intact but small medial meniscus." However, this type of finding may actually represent a bucket-handle tear of the meniscus. This can be resolved by pulling the scope back and examining the intercondylar notch for a displaced bucket-handle fragment that can be reduced or redisplaced with the probe (Fig. 11-42).

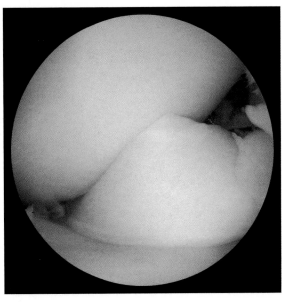

Fig. 11-42. Bucket handle tear displaced in the medial compartment

11.6.5.3
Medial Femorotibial Joint

Cartilage changes involving the femoral condyles and tibial plateau tend to occur posteriorly in the major load-bearing area, so the knee joint should be adequately flexed for inspection of that region (Fig. 11-44).

Degenerative changes with denuded bone areas and osteophytes are easy to demonstrate by arthroscopy (Fig. 11-45). Often they are associated with pathologic changes in the menisci and synovium.

11.6.6
Intercondylar Notch

The intercondylar notch with the ACL and infrapatellar plica is reached by withdrawing the tip of the scope (light cable points medially).

If the posterior horn of the medial meniscus was difficult to see from the medial compartment, it can be directly visualized by carefully pushing the arthroscope toward the posterior capsule, the tip of the scope passing medial to the ACL (Figs. 11-46 and 11-47). The posterior horn can be probed through a medial supra-meniscal portal placed close to the patellar ligament.

Loose bodies of variable size also may be detected in the intercondylar region (Fig. 11-48).

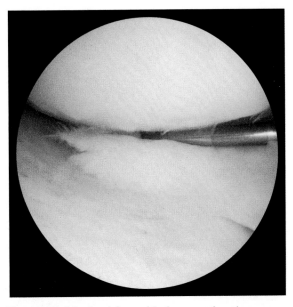

Fig. 11-43. Meniscal flap with degenerative changes

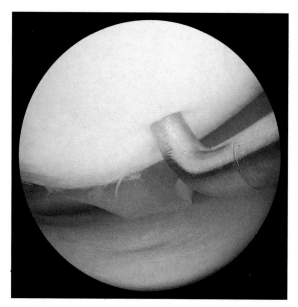

Fig. 11-44. Grade I chondromalacia on the medial femoral condyle. Note the persistence of the depression made in the medial tibial plateau by the probe

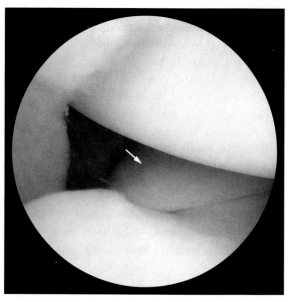

Fig. 11-46. Intact posterior horn of the medial meniscus *(arrow)*, visualized by traversing the intercondylar notch medial to the ACL

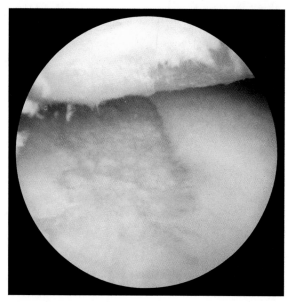

Fig. 11-45. Advanced degenerative changes with exposure of bone on the medial femoral condyle and tibial plateau in an osteoarthritic knee with varus deformity

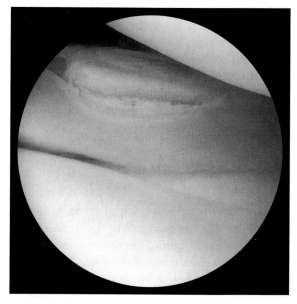

Fig. 11-47. Fleck of blood on the posterior horn of the medial meniscus, consistent with a longitudinal meniscal tear

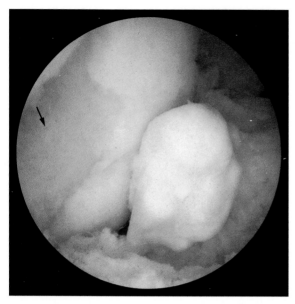

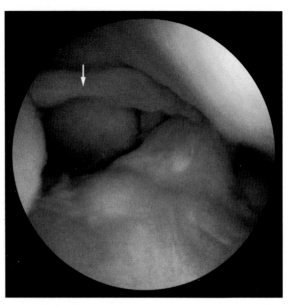

Fig. 11-48. Large loose body in the intercondylar area from old osteochondritis dissecans. The "crater" is located on the medial femoral condyle *(arrow)*

Fig. 11-49. The infrapatellar plica *(arrow)* runs separate from the ACL

11.6.6.1
Infrapatellar Plica

The infrapatellar plica (Fig. 11-49) is a fold of varying prominence extending from the roof of the intercondylar notch to the infrapatellar fat pad. If hypertrophied, the plica may obstruct the view of the ACL and may even be mistaken for the ACL by an inexperienced examiner (Fig. 11-50).

11.6.6.2
Anterior Cruciate Ligament

Arthroscopic evaluation of the ACL is difficult only if vision is obstructed by an enlarged infrapatellar plica. If this is the case, the tip of the scope can be withdrawn and pushed past the lateral side of the plica to view the ACL from a more lateral aspect.

Generally the ACL is easy to visualize, and it can be probed to evaluate its continuity and tension. Since proximal tears are the most common, the area about the origin of the ligament should be inspected first. For this the arthroscope is tilted slightly toward the tibia and turned so that the light cable points downward. This directs the arthroscopic view up into the intercondylar notch.

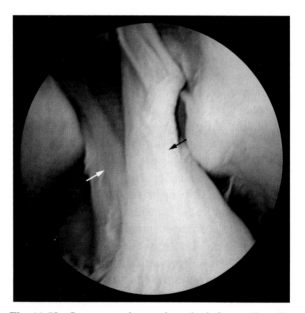

Fig. 11-50. On cursory inspection, the infrapatellar plica *(arrow)* may be mistaken for the ACL. The latter is located farther posteriorly *(white arrow)*

In acute injuries where the ACL appears grossly intact, it is common to find hemorrhagic areas beneath the synovium covering the ligament (Fig. 11-51). In acute tears, the probe is

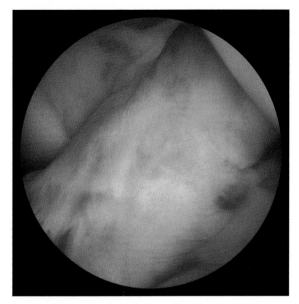

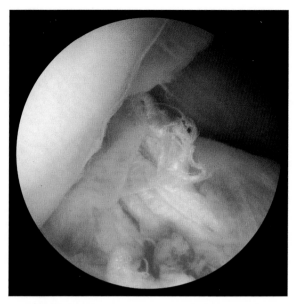

Fig. 11-51. Subsynovial hemorrhagic areas of the ACL following a hyperextension injury

Fig. 11-52. Inspection suggests an incomplete tear of the ACL. However, a complete tear can be excluded only by palpation with the probing hook

used to sort out the individual fibers. One may encounter both complete and partial tears with torn ligament fibers protruding in a fungus-like mass (Figs. 11-52 and 11-53). Sometimes inspection is hampered by an accompanying synovitis (Fig. 11-54) or by swelling of the infrapatellar fat pad.

Old partial and complete tears of the ACL are characterized by the clubbed appearance of the torn fibers (Fig. 11-55), which may become displaced into the medial or lateral joint compartment and produce signs mimicking those of an entrapped meniscus.

When an ACL tear occurs in the setting of a chronic capsuloligamentous instability, problems may be encountered during inspection of the joint compartments due to relative twisting of the tibia and femur as a result of the abnormal laxity.

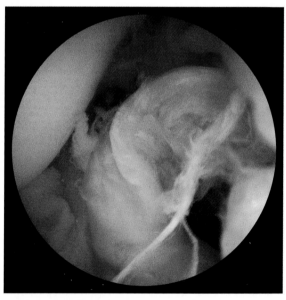

Fig. 11-53. Fresh, complete tear of the ACL

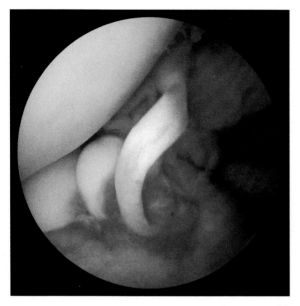

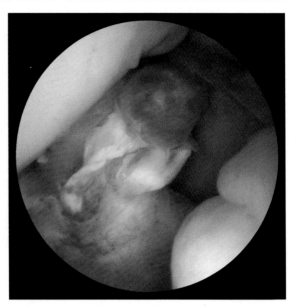

Fig. 11-54. ACL tear with accompanying synovitis (three weeks postinjury)

Fig. 11-55. Clublike distention of ACL fibers (five weeks postinjury)

11.6.7
Lateral Compartment

For inspection of the lateral compartment, the arthroscope is trained on the triangle formed by the lateral femoral condyle, lateral tibial plateau, and ACL (Fig. 11-56). While the scope is held in that position, the leg is moved to the "figure-four" position (Fig. 11-57) in which the knee is flexed and the lower leg is crossed over the contralateral thigh.

11.6.7.1
Lateral Meniscus

The leg having been moved to the figure-four position, the first structure seen in the lateral compartment is the posterior horn of the lateral meniscus (Fig. 11-58). The central and anterior portions of the meniscus, the free border of the meniscus (Fig. 11-59), the anterior horn region, and the popliteal hiatus with the popliteus tendon can also be inspected.

Like the medial meniscus, the lateral meniscus can exhibit a variety of pathologic conditions (Figs. 11-60 to 11-62). Though it is more mobile than the medial meniscus, the healthy

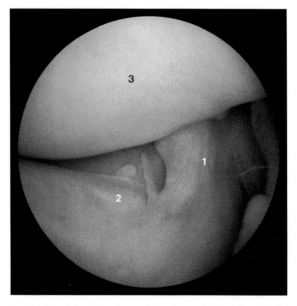

Fig. 11-56. Visualization of the lateral triangle. Medial: ACL *(1)*; inferior: anterior horn of lateral meniscus *(2)* and lateral tibial plateau; superolateral: lateral femoral condyle *(3)*

lateral meniscus cannot displace in front of the lateral femoral condyle.

The portals for the arthroscope and probe do not need to be changed for selective palpa-

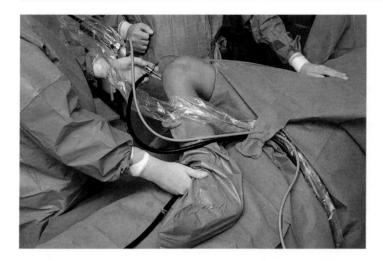

Fig. 11-57. Placement of the leg in the figure-four position (light cable points medially and is tangential to the joint line). Manual pressure on the medial side increases the varus stress and further opens up the lateral joint space

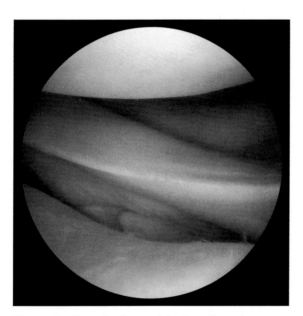

Fig. 11-58. Posterior horn of the lateral meniscus

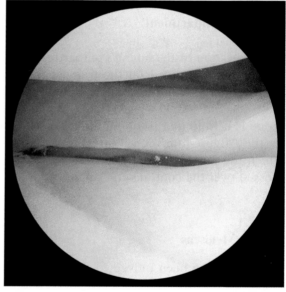

Fig. 11-59. Overview of an intact lateral meniscus

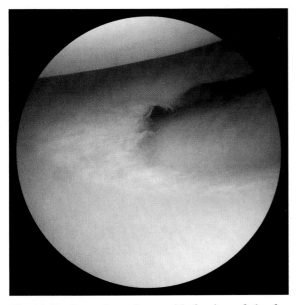

Fig. 11-60. Lateral meniscus with fraying of the free border

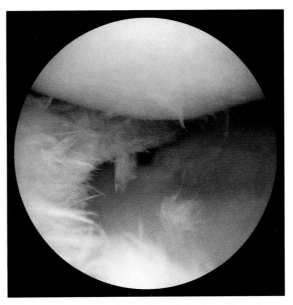

Fig. 11-61. Degenerative lesion of the lateral meniscus and exposure of bone at the lateral tibial plateau

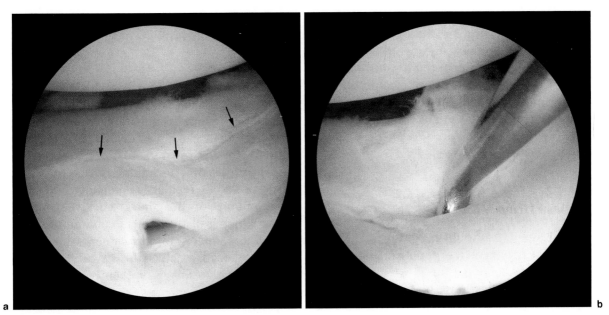

a   b

Fig. 11-62a, b. Longitudinal tear of the lateral meniscus *(arrows)* (**a**). The probe defines the extent of the tear (**b**)

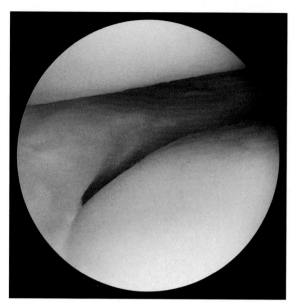

Fig. 11-63. Remnant of lateral meniscus 18 years after an open lateral meniscectomy

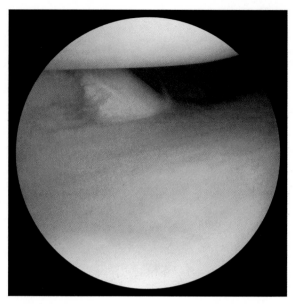

Fig. 11-64. Inspection of the popliteus tendon. The lateral tibial plateau is not visible. A complete discoid lateral meniscus is present

tion of the lateral meniscus. The medial instrument portal just needs to be placed proximal and close to the patellar ligament (high medial approach). Placing the portal too low, directly above the meniscal plane, would hinder smooth passage of the probe into the lateral compartment, for the intercondylar eminence might deflect the probe up toward the lateral femoral condyle.

11.6.7.2
Popliteal Hiatus

Special attention should be given to the posterolateral region of the popliteal hiatus with the popliteus tendon (Fig. 11-64). The hiatus sometimes contains loose bodies that may remain invisible until brought into view with the probe. An isolated injury of the popliteus tendon is possible but rare.

When the systematic inspection of all joint compartments has been completed, the leg is returned to the original position, and further measures are carried out after the appropriate instrument portals have been established.

11.7
Problem Situations

A variety of problems can arise during arthroscopy which make it difficult or impossible to conduct a smooth examination.

If the video camera is defective, it may be difficult for the operator to revert to conventional arthroscopic technique. These risks can be decreased by regular maintenance and careful handling of the shock-sensitive camera. Sharp kinking of the camera cable in the area where it connects to the camera should be avoided, because defects in the cable can degrade the video image or even result in complete image loss.

Besides regular maintenance, equipment-related problems can be minimized by following these rules:

1. Never force the tip of the arthroscope through bony passages.
2. Perform intraarticular instrumentation only when viewing conditions are optimal.

11.7.1
Yellow-Out, White-Out

The inexperienced arthroscopist is likely to experience a "yellow-out" or "white-out" in which everything on the monitor becomes whitish or yellowish and no anatomic features can be identified (Fig. 11-65). This situation is based on errors of technique. It is not the fault of the procedure itself.

A yellow-out or white-out can have various causes (Table 11-5). The most frequent cause, after faulty insertion of the arthroscope, is improper positioning of the arthroscope. It should always be kept in mind that when a 30° oblique arthroscope is used and is held with the light cable pointing up, the viewing angle is directed 30° downward. Often a yellow-out can be eliminated simply by rotating the arthroscope to move the lens away from the joint capsule or infrapatellar fat pad.

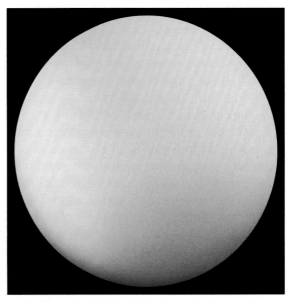

Fig. 11-65. Yellow-out

11.7.2
Red-Out

When hemarthrosis is present, bloody fluid will drain from the joint when the sheath is inserted and the obturator removed. Insertion of the arthroscope at that time would produce a uniformly reddish monitor image on which nothing can be identified. This is avoided by first irrigating the joint cavity until the outflow is completely clear of blood.

If a red-out occurs during the arthroscopic examination, the joint should be copiously irrigated as described until adequate visibility is restored. If necessary, one can attempt to fill and lavage the joint more rapidly and control the extravasation of blood by increasing the pressure of the irrigating fluid (i. e., turning up the pressure on the roller pump or suspending the bags at a higher level) or by passing a large-gauge inflow cannula into the suprapatellar pouch.

With an older hemorrhagic effusion, the joint will contain blood clots of varying size which often cannot be removed by simple aspiration – although this should be attempted initially with the arthroscope removed from

Table 11-5. Potential causes of yellow-out

1. Faulty insertion of arthroscope
2. Incorrect positioning of arthroscope
3. Failure to start inflow of irrigating fluid
4. Depletion of irrigating fluid supply
5. Adhesive bands
6. Hypertrophied synovial villi

the sheath. If a clot is lodged in front of a structure requiring inspection (e. g., the ACL), it can be mobilized and pushed aside with the probe or extracted with a small grasping forceps. This is the first step in converting diagnostic arthroscopy to operative arthroscopy ("removal of a loose body").

11.7.3
Extravasation of Fluid

If large incisions are made in the synovium and fibrous capsule while the skin incision is of minimal size, considerable fluid will escape into the subcutaneous tissue and make instrument insertion difficult. On completion of the arthroscopy, the knee will be found to be markedly distended in that area.

While extravasation is troublesome intraoperatively, it is rarely associated with postoperative complications, because most of the fluid is absorbed within a few hours. If extravasation seems excessive, the instrument portal or viewing portal may be left unsutured so that the dressing can help absorb the fluid [146].

Significant problems arise when marked extravasation of irrigating fluid occurs during the diagnostic arthroscopy, and an arthrotomic ligament reconstruction is planned for the same sitting. The tissue is edematous and distended, orientation is difficult, and the risk of infection is increased. If doubt exists, the ligament reconstruction should be postponed for a later sitting.

11.8
Complications

While the incidence of complications in arthroscopy is very low, the examiner should still know the potential complications that can arise (Table 11-6).

Though rare, the most feared complication of arthroscopy is intraarticular infection, which has a reported incidence of 0.01%–0.1% [91, 123, 129]. That is why a strict aseptic routine is mandatory in all diagnostic and operative arthroscopies. The interior of the joint must be protected from all unnecessary external influences.

Overvigorous intraarticular manipulations with the arthroscope, probe, or operating instrument can lead to cartilage damage. This danger calls for a meticulous operating technique with controlled instrument manipulations. This applies to the sheath itself, which can cause deep scoring or scraping of the articular cartilage at the time of insertion (Fig. 11-66). Iatrogenic cartilage lesions are disregarded in many studies. While it is granted that these lesions are difficult to detect, it is also true that iatrogenic cartilage damage is the most frequent complication of arthroscopy. Indeed, minimal cartilage lesions are caused by virtually every arthroscopy, even when per-

Table 11-6. Potential complications of knee arthroscopy

1. Infection
2. Iatrogenic lesions of:
   - cartilage
   - ligamentous structures
   - menisci
3. Introduction of particles from the incise drape
4. Nerve damage (infrapatellar branch of saphenous nerve)
5. Compartment syndrome
6. Effusion
7. Hemarthrosis
8. Tourniquet syndrome
9. Thromboembolism
10. Synovial fistula
11. Reflex sympathetic dystrophy
12. Intraarticular adhesions
13. Rare complications
    - Injury to popliteal artery
    - Fistula between prepatellar bursa and intraarticular space [237]
    - Osteomyelitis, meningococcal arthritis, bacteremia [93]
    - Rupture of semimembranosus bursa [74]
    - Pneumoscrotum [274]
    - Aneurysm of lateral inferior geniculate artery [419]
    - Herniation of infrapatellar fat pad [394]
    - Fatal air embolism [231]
    - Femoral fracture

formed by an experienced operator. It remains unclear, however, whether these lesions have true pathologic significance. Severe cases of iatrogenic arthroscopic cartilage damage are becoming more prevalent as arthroscopic operations are more widely practiced by less experienced operators.

Iatrogenic ligament injuries may be caused by the application of an excessive varus or valgus stress to the knee, even when the ligaments are initially intact. This is a particular danger in older patients. In other cases the applied stress may convert a partial ligament tear to a complete rupture. Iatrogenic meniscal injuries can occur when the instrument portal is placed too low. Incising the fibrous capsule with a pointed scalpel under conditions of poor visibility poses a particularly high and unnecessary risk of injury.

These rules should be followed to avoid iatrogenic injuries:

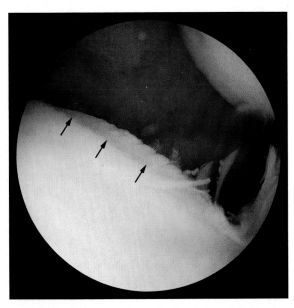

Fig. 11-66. Deep cartilage groove *(arrows)* gouged in the medial facet of the femoral trochlea by forced insertion of a sheath inadvertently armed with a sharp trocar (from [637])

1. Instrument maneuvers should always be carried out under arthroscopic visual control.
2. Instruments (arthroscope and probe) should never be moved forcibly within the joint space.
3. While an instrument is inside the joint, any change of knee position should be performed slowly and carefully.
4. If instrument access is found to be inadequate or unfavorable, it is better to establish a new accessory portal than inflict cartilage damage by attempting to work through an unsatisfactory portal.

Improper positioning of the leg can cause injury to the common peroneal nerve and lateral femoral cutaneous nerve. Very low instrument portals threaten the infrapatellar branch of the saphenous nerve.

Arthroscopy should be used with caution in patients with fresh, complex ligamentous injuries (dry joint), as a compartment syndrome can result from the dissection of irrigating fluid into the fascial compartments of the lower leg.

Mild mechanical irritation at the portals sometimes leads to local skin redness, which usually resolves spontaneously in one to two weeks.

To prevent effusion after extensive arthroscopic procedures, we conclude the arthroscopy by passing a No. 10 Redon suction drain into the joint through the arthroscopic sheath. The drain is removed on the first postoperative day or the second day at the latest to avoid a synovial fistula. Effusion prophylaxis is aided by wrapping the entire leg postoperatively with an elasticized compressive bandage.

While the incidence of complications in arthroscopy is low, the procedure is not complication-free. This is demonstrated by the study of Sherman et al. [591], who reviewed more than 2600 diagnostic and operative arthroscopies. Although they found a complication rate of 8.2% (!), that figure includes minor and very minor complications such as mild disturbances of wound healing and postoperative hematomas about the entry sites. Purely diagnostic arthroscopy showed the lowest complication rate by far, while the complication rate was highest in patients over 50 years of age and in cases where the tourniquet time exceeded 60 min, regardless of the nature of the operative procedure [591].

According to Dick et al. [129], iatrogenic cartilage lesions, with an incidence of 2%, are the most frequent complications of diagnostic arthroscopy. These authors observed no serious complications in any of the 3714 diagnostic arthroscopies reviewed.

Delee [123] reported on a multicentric study and evaluated 118,590 arthroscopies with a total of 930 complications (=0.78%). Small [608] reported the results of the largest study to date of the Committee on Complications of the Arthroscopy Association of North America covering 395,566 arthroscopies, of which 375,069 were arthroscopies of the knee. The total complication rate in this series was 0.56% (Table 11-7). The disadvantage of this huge study is that it involves a retrospective analysis of results. This makes it likely that the incidence of complications is understated while the number of arthroscopies is overstated [608]. In 1988, Small published the results of a prospective study involving 21 of the most experienced arthroscopists in the United States [609]. This series covered a total of 10,262 arthroscopies, of which 8741 were knee arthroscopies. A total of 173 complications (=1.68%) were reported (Table 11-8).

11.9
Indications for Diagnostic Arthroscopy

Purely diagnostic arthroscopy should be undertaken only after all clinical examination methods and tests have been exhausted. Besides furnishing a diagnosis (Table 11-9), arthroscopy aids in the detection of coexisting lesions and the planning of operative treatment (Table 11-10).

Because arthroscopy is a relatively nontraumatizing procedure and requires little time, we use it prior to ligament reconstructions to detect any coexisting injuries that might call for a different arthrotomy approach. It is not unusual to find clinically silent lateral meniscus lesions that can be managed arthroscopically by a partial meniscectomy or refixation.

When planning a corrective osteotomy, we first use arthroscopy to evaluate the condition of the articular cartilage that will be in the weight-bearing area after the bone is realigned. If inspection reveals significant cartilage pathology in that area, the chance for a successful operation is greatly reduced. The more extensive the cartilage damage, the greater the importance of early postoperative mobilization.

With a Baker's cyst, especially in older patients, arthroscopy often reveals severe intraarticular pathology causing increased synovial fluid production that perpetuates the cyst [535]. Thus, simple extirpation of the cyst is not curative as it merely eliminates the symptom of the underlying intraarticular disease.

When it comes to a choice between arthrography and arthroscopy, the latter should be chosen because it offers greater diagnostic certainty. As clinical experience grows, diagnostic arthrography is becoming largely obsolete, although it still can be rewarding in special types of investigation.

Table 11-7. Analysis of 2215 complications in 395,566 arthroscopies. (After Small [608])

Anesthesiologic complications	83
Instrument breakage	398
Ligamentous injuries	160
Femoral fractures	3
Nerve injuries	234
Vascular injuries	12
Infections	289
Thromboembolisms	752
Dystrophies	190
Other	94

Table 11-8. Analysis of 173 complications (100%) in 10,262 arthroscopic operations. (After [609])

Hemarthrosis, hematomas	60.1%
Infections	12.1%
Thromboembolisms	6.9%
Anesthesiologic complications	6.4%
Instrument breakage	2.9%
Reflex dystrophies	2.3%
Ligamentous injuries	1.2%
Fractures	0.6%
Nerve injuries	0.6%
Other	6.9%
	100.0%

Table 11-9. Indications for diagnostic arthroscopy

1. Hemarthrosis of unknown cause
2. Recurrent pain that is resistant to treatment
3. Recurrent effusions
4. Hemarthrosis in the chronically unstable knee
5. Recurrent locking of unknown cause

Table 11-10. Uses of arthroscopy in the detection of coexisting lesions and preoperative planning

1. Traumatic patellar dislocation (detection of cartilage damage)
2. Baker's cysts (determination of cause)
3. Medial instability with effusion (meniscal or cruciate ligament involvement?)
4. Before ligament reconstructions in chronically unstable knees (cartilage damage? lesion of meniscus?)
5. Before corrective osteotomies (to evaluate condition of cartilage)
6. Acute ligamentous injuries (involvement of meniscus? planning of arthrotomy approach)

11.9.1
Contraindications to Arthroscopy

Since arthroscopy is not a life-saving procedure, the patient undergoing arthroscopy should be in an optimum state of health. Appropriate medical and anesthesiologic preparation is advised in older patients, who are at increased risk for developing local as well as systemic complications [591].
Contraindications to arthroscopy are:

1. Unhealed cutaneous wounds on the leg or knee.
2. Infected skin eruptions about the knee.
3. Bony ankylosis.

Relative contraindications are:

1. Recent, extensive capsuloligamentous injury (danger of compartment syndrome).
2. Flu-like infections and other diseases that produce systemic effects.

If arthroscopy is elected for a fresh extensive capsuloligamentous injury, it should be performed by an experienced operator who can work quickly using the lowest possible fluid pressure.

11.10
Capabilities of Arthroscopic Surgery

Evolving beyond its role as a purely diagnostic method, arthroscopy has long been recognized primarily as an operative procedure that enables adequate treatment to be provided with very low morbidity [5, 91, 110, 147, 193, 208, 213, 219, 246, 325, 400, 440, 505, 582, 592].

Since Watanabe arthroscopically removed a small meniscal flap in May of 1962, operative arthroscopy has progressed at a staggering rate [499]. The development of small but stable operating instruments has led to the introduction of many new arthroscopic surgical techniques. Today there is scarcely a type of intraarticular pathology that cannot be treated arthroscopically. Large arthrotomies are avoided, and re-

habilitation is more rapid (Tables 11-11 and 11-12).

The disadvantages of operative arthroscopy include the duration of the procedure, which can be quite long even with an experienced operator; the demanding surgical technique; and the large and often costly instrumentarium.

The changes wrought by operative arthroscopy have been particularly marked in the area of meniscal surgery. Once it was common

Table 11-11. Advantages of arthroscopic surgery

1. Low morbidity
2. Short in-patient time or out-patient treatment
3. Early return to work
4. Low complication rate
5. No disturbance of proprioception
6. Very small scars
7. Allows concomitant treatment of associated injuries
8. Allows visually controlled surgery in hard-to-reach areas (e.g., the posterior horns of the menisci)

Table 11-12. Possible applications of arthroscopic knee surgery

1. Menisci
   - Partial meniscectomy
   - Subtotal meniscectomy
   - Total meniscectomy
   - Meniscus repair
2. Cruciate ligaments
   - Repair (incomplete tear)
   - Repair (complete tear)
   - Plastic reconstruction
3. Cartilage
   - Debridement
   - Subchondral abrasion chondroplasty
   - Drilling
4. Removal of loose bodies
5. Fixation of osteochondral fragments
6. Osteochondritis dissecans
7. Lateral release
8. Synovium
   - Biopsy
   - Partial synovectomy
   - Total synovectomy
9. Resection of mediopatellar plica
10. Removal of metal implants
11. Reefing of medial retinaculum for patellar dislocation
12. Arthrolysis
13. Tumor removal
14. Empyema
    - Placement of suction-irrigation tube
    - Synovectomy
    - Lavage
    - Debridement (removal of fibrin deposits)

practice to open the joint, examine the meniscus, and even proceed with total meniscectomy if the condition of the meniscus seemed questionable. Later a preference emerged in favor of a subtotal resection whenever possible. Today operative arthroscopy gives us the option of the "controlled partial meniscectomy." Only the pathologic portion of the meniscus is removed, the objective being to resect "as much of the meniscus as necessary but as little as possible" [213].

Because meniscal lesions are frequently associated with other injuries, arthroscopy is indicated before any meniscectomy is performed. This is done not only to pinpoint the location of the tear (clinical symptoms are sometimes manifested on the contralateral side) and ascertain its extent, but also to detect any coexisting lesions (e. g., cartilage damage). Accompanying injuries reduce the change of a successful operation and should be reported to the patient. For example, a coexisting ligamentous lesions or extensive cartilage damage will greatly reduce the prospects for a good or very good outcome following arthroscopic meniscectomy [5, 213, 400].

Terminology and Definitions

12
Terminology and Definitions

Mutual comprehension requires a consistent, generally valid, and unambiguous nomenclature for the description of tests, joint positions, and motions that occur in the healthy and injured knee.

Confusion has resulted from the use of different terms to denote the same condition, or from the use of terms that have diverse meanings. This has frequently led to situations in which clinical tests and their results are not uniquely defined, and knee injuries are diagnosed in terms of the outcomes of laxity tests. For example, "anterior drawer instability" and "valgus instability" are still given as diagnoses even though they do not identify the injured anatomic structures and give no information on the functional status of the knee. To be meaningful, the diagnosis of a ligamentous injury should always specify the anatomic structures that have been damaged [235, 495].

We owe a special debt to Noyes, Grood, and Torzilli [495] for addressing the problem of discrepancies in terms relating to the diagnostic evaluation of knee injuries. These authors began by analyzing the major articles on knee ligament injuries that have been published in the English language and cataloging the terms that were used. Then they compared the terms with one another and also with definitions taken from medical textbooks and from general and technical dictionaries. The results of this valuable research were reviewed by the International Knee Documentation Committee of the American Orthopedic Society for Sports Medicine (AOSSM) and the European Society of Knee Surgery and Arthroscpy (ESKA) and published in the 1989 article, "Definitions of Terms for Motion and Position of the Knee and Injuries of the Ligaments" [495]. The following definitions are taken largely from that publication.

12.1
Laxity

Laxity is defined in [495] as (1) slackness or lack of tension (a characteristic of a ligament) and (2) looseness, referring to a normal or abnormal range of motion of a joint.

Laxity as used in the orthopedic literature has two meanings, which can lead to confusion. When applied to a ligament, the term denotes a looseness or lack of tension in the ligament. Thus, many ligaments in the knee can be made tense or lax by changing the position of the joint (e. g., by rotating the tibia).

When the term is applied to a joint, a distinction should be drawn between abnormal (increased, pathologic) laxity and normal (physiologic) laxity. Increased laxity may be congenital (e. g., due to abnormal collagen synthesis, see Table 3-2) or acquired (e. g., due to injury).

Another problem is the lack of a clear dividing line between normal and abnormal laxity. We therefore use the term laxity when referring to or describing the degree of looseness of a ligament or a joint. The degree of laxity is defined in terms of laxity parameters (see Table 3-3).

The goal of laxity testing is to detect any increased mobility of the tibia relative to the femoral condyles in response to an applied force or stress and to determine the final or subluxated position [494]. Various tests can be performed to evaluate the laxity of a joint:

12.1.1
Passive Laxity Tests

In these tests the examiner applies a stress to the joint to produce a relative displacement of the tibia and femur. The patient must relax his muscles as completely as possible. The result of the test can be graded as

1+ = 0–5 mm or ° of pathologic motion
2+ = 6–10 mm or ° of pathologic motion
3+ = more than 11 mm or ° of pathologic motion

of the tibia relative to the femur. The resilience of the end point is also evaluated as being hard or soft (see Sect. 3.1.2.4). In the passive laxity tests, the magnitude of the applied stress depends on the individual examiner and consequently is not defined.

Examples of passive laxity tests:
- Valgus test
- Varus test
- Anterior drawer test
- Lachman test
- Posterior drawer test

12.1.2
Active Laxity Tests

In active laxity tests the patient himself moves the tibia relative to the femur by contracting individual muscles or muscle groups. During this time the examiner monitors the tibial displacement by visual observation or manual palpation. The end-point resilience cannot be evaluated. The main advantages of these tests are their painlessness and technical simplicity.

Examples of active laxity tests:
- Active quadriceps test in 30° flexion
- Active quadriceps test in 90° flexion
- Quadriceps neutral angle test

As in the passive laxity tests, the quantitative result relies on the subjective impression of the examiner. The grading of results as 1+, 2+, or 3+ is desirable but is often difficult. The force eliciting the tibial displacement is not defined.

12.1.3
Machine Laxity Tests

The degree of laxity can be objectively determined by means of a measuring apparatus (see Chap. 9) or by stress radiography (see Sect. 6.11).

The number of laxity parameters that can be tested or defined (see Table 3-3) depends on the type of positioning device that is used. Besides holding the knee in a designated position of flexion and tibial rotation, many devices are capable of measuring the force that is exerted on the knee.

It cannot be assumed that a patient with a pronounced, abnormally increased laxity is functionally disabled by that laxity. The degree of laxity, then, relates only indirectly to the functional status of the knee and the subjective well-being of the patient.

12.2
Instability

Instability is defined in [495] as a condition of a joint characterized by an abnormal increased range of motion (mobility) due to injury to the ligaments, capsule, menisci, cartilage, or bone.

The term instability is variously used in the literature to describe an event (symptom) or to characterize a condition. Thus, the term may refer to a complete loss of stability (complete giving-way), a partial or intermittent loss of stability (intermittent giving-way), or merely to a subjective feeling of instability that is described by the patient. None of these meanings takes into account the particular circumstances under which the episode occurs (e. g., during running, walking, jumping, or twisting).

We use the term instability only in the broad sense, e. g., to denote the subjective sensation described by the patient after a trauma ("It feels as if my lower leg is slipping forward or my knee wants to buckle") where there is simultaneous evidence of a pathologically increased laxity (positive laxity tests).

When one or more laxity tests are found to be positive, it cannot automatically be assumed that instability exists. This is illustrated by the fact that not all patients with a torn ACL complain of subjective instability even though a number of laxity tests are positive on clinical examination.

It is recommended that the term instability not be used to indicate episodes of giving-way, although this is still common practice. Neither should the word instability be used to describe the anatomic condition of a ligament. Unfortunately, the phrase "instability of the ACL" is still a common diagnosis [494].

12.3
Motion

Motion is defined as the process of changing position. The position change of an object can be quantified (1) by describing the distance the object travels during its motion or (2) by describing the displacement of the object between the starting point and end point of its path.

Two types of motion exist: rotation (motion about an axis) and translation (motion on a plane).

12.4
Displacement

This is defined as the net effect of a motion, the change in position of a body or particle between two points along its path without regard to the path followed [495].

Displacement, then, describes the extent or net effect of the change in position of a body. The motion of a rigid body, such as the tibia, consists of a change in position and a change in orientation. The change in position results from translation of the body, the change in orientation from rotation of the body. The unit of measure of translation is the meter, while rotation is measured in degrees. A displacing force must act upon the knee joint in order for displacement to occur. The amount of the displacement depends on the laxity parameters (see Table 3-3), on the magnitude of the force, its direction, and its point of application.

12.4.1 Rotation

Rotation is defined in [495] as a type of motion or displacement in which all points on a body move about an axis as a center, or a motion in which one point is fixed. The axis is commonly termed the axis of rotation.

During rotation, the points on a body move about an axis (the axis of rotation) and change their position at different speeds. The farther the points are located from the center of rotation, the greater their speed.

Rotation in the knee joint refers to motion about any of three axes: abduction-adduction (sagittal axis), flexion-extension (transverse axis), and internal-external rotation (vertical axis) (Figs. 12-1 and 12-2).

Rotation is measured in degrees.

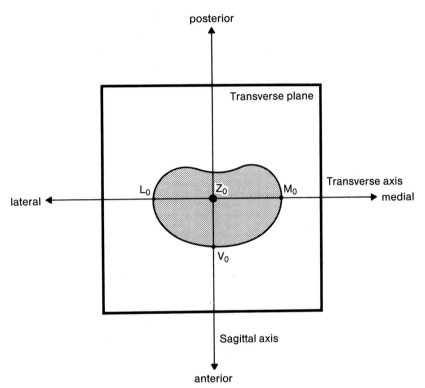

Fig. 12-1. Initial position (schematic model): Superior view of the transverse plane and tibial plateau. The center of the plateau *(point Zo),* where the axis of rotation is frequently located, lies at the intersection of the transverse, sagittal, and vertical axes. A lateral *(Lo)* and medial tibial point *(Mo)* lie on the transverse axis. The most anterior tibial point *(Vo)* lies on the sagittal axis. This initial position forms the starting point from which theoretically possible translations and rotations of the tibial plateau are described

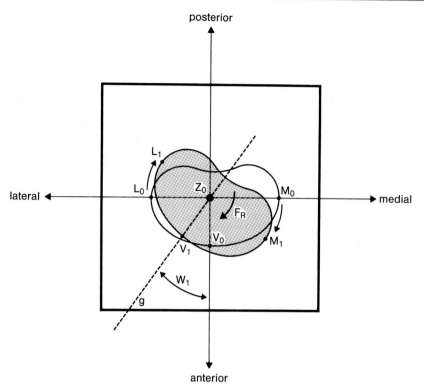

Fig. 12-2. External rotation produced by the force FR. Medial points *(Mo)* move anteriorly *(to M1)* while lateral points *(Lo)* move posteriorly *(to L1)*. The position of the tibial center *(Zo)* remains unchanged. In this case the axis of rotation passes through point Zo. The amount of rotation is determined by the angle W1 formed by the sagittal axis and the line g connecting V1 with Zo

12.4.2
Translation

Translation is defined in [495] as a type of motion or displacement of a rigid body in which all lines attached to it remain parallel to their original orientation.

Translation, then, describes a type of motion by which all points in a rigid body move parallel to a line on a plane (translational plane). All the points traveling an equal distance in the same direction and at the same speed.

In the knee, translation describes motion in which the medial and lateral condyles of the tibia, for example, move an equal distance forward (anterior translation) or backward (posterior translation) with respect to the femur (Figs. 12-3 and 12-4). Usually the reference point for determining the amount of translation is the center of the tibial plateau, i. e., the area of the intercondylar eminence (Figs. 12-3 and 12-4).

Motion of the medial or lateral compartment of the knee also can be described in terms of translation of the medial or lateral tibial plateau (see below).

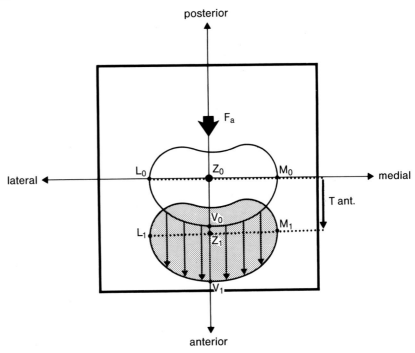

Fig. 12-3. Anterior translation. In response to the anterior force Fa, all points on the tibia *(Zo, Mo, Lo, Vo)* move the same distance *(arrows)* anteriorly *(Z1, M1,* *L1, V1).* The amount of anterior translation *(T ant)* is easily determined

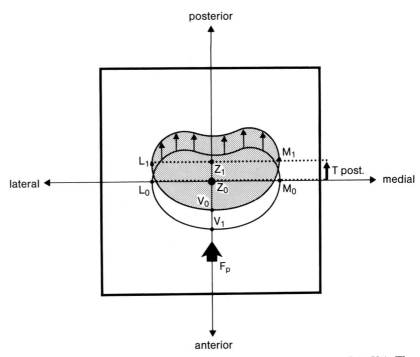

Fig. 12-4. Posterior translation. In response to the posteriorly directed force Fp, all points on the tibia *(Zo, Mo, Lo, Vo)* move the same distance *(arrows)* posteriorly on the transverse plane *(Z1, M1, L1, V1).* The amount of posterior translation *(T post)* is easily determined

12.5
Coupled Displacement and Motion

This is defined in [495] as a displacement or motion in one or more degrees of freedom that is caused by a load (force or moment) applied in another degree of freedom.

It is our view that coupled motions occur whenever a displacing force is applied to the knee, especially when a ligamentous injury is present.

An anteriorly directed force, like that applied to the knee in the anterior drawer test in 90° flexion or in the Lachman test, elicits an anterior displacement of the proximal end of the tibia. This anterior motion consists of several components (Figs. 12-5 and 12-6). Even when the knee ligaments are intact, an anteriorly directed force will produce some internal rotation of the tibia in addition to pure anterior translation. Moreover, it is likely that the rising tension of the ligamentous structures under the applied force will decrease the distance between the tibial plateau and femoral condyles, resulting in compression of the joint members (= proximal translation).

The amount of anterior translation produced by an anteriorly directed force and the amount of coupled displacement (e. g., medial translation, external rotation, lateral translation, or internal rotation) depend on the flexion angle of the knee, the position of tibial rotation at the start of the test, the amount of force applied, and the severity of the ligamentous lesion (Figs. 12-5 through 12-7).

If the force applied in the anterior drawer test elicits forward motion of the tibia, this motion is referred to as an anterior displacement or anterior drawer motion. The term anterior

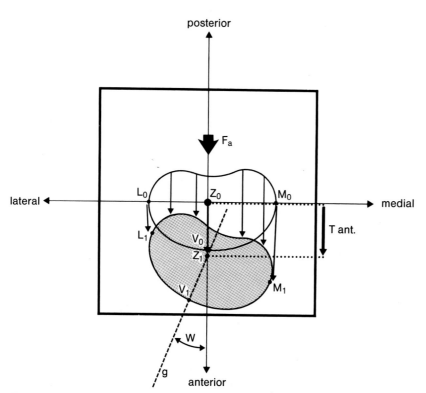

Fig. 12-5. Coupled motions produced by an anterior stress Fa. All points on the tibia *(Zo, Mo, Lo, Vo)* move varying distances forward *(Z1, M1, L1, V1)*. The amount of anterior translation *(T ant)* is determined by the anterior motion of the tibial center *(Zo)*. The angle between the sagittal axis and line g connecting Z1 and V1 determines the angle of rotation W. Anterior translation in this case is coupled with external rotation of the tibia

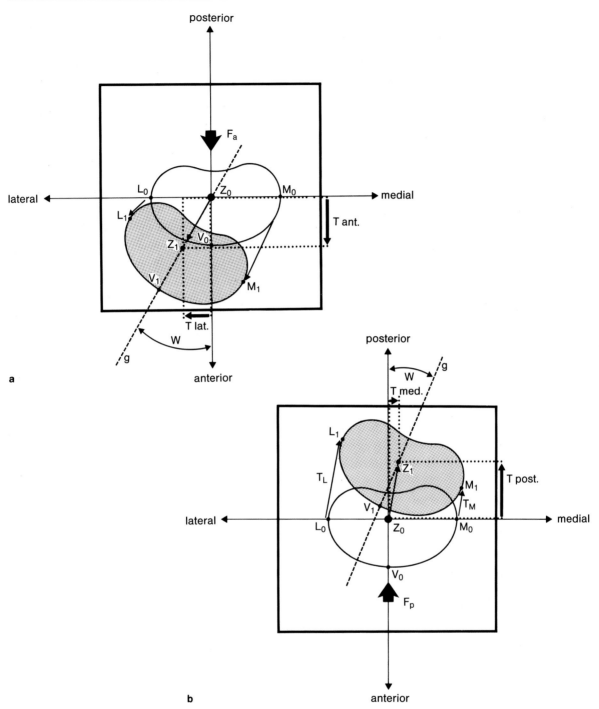

Fig. 12-6a, b. Examples of coupled motions produced by an anterior (**a**) and a posterior (**b**) stress. **a** All points on the tibia *(Zo, Mo, Lo, Vo)* move varying distances anteriorly and also laterally *(Z1, M1, L1, V1)*. The total displacement of the tibial center *(Z1)* represents the sum of an anterior translation *(T ant)* and a lateral translation *(T lat)*. The angle W between the sagittal axis and line g determines the amount of rotation. The medial and lateral tibial condyles undergo different amounts of displacement. Anterior translation in this case is coupled with motions of lateral translation and external rotation. **b** Opposite responses may be seen with a posteriorly directed force Fp, like that applied in a posterior drawer test. The force elicits a posterior translation plus coupled motions of medial translation and external rotation. The displacement of the tibial center from Zo to Z1 represents the sum of a posterior *(T post)* and medial *(T med)* translation (coupled displacement). The medial *(TM)* and lateral *(TL)* tibial points undergo different amounts of displacement

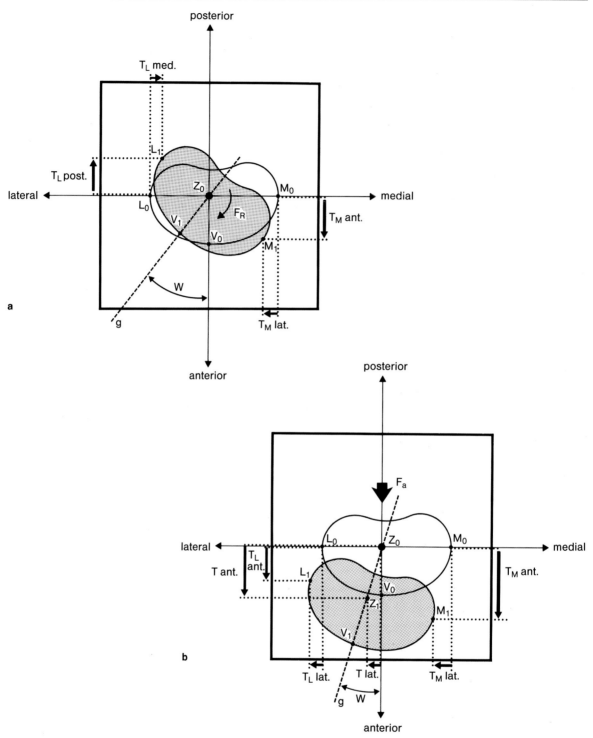

Fig. 12-7 a,b. Analysis of the translational components of rotation. **a** During external rotation, points on the medial side of the tibia (e. g. *Mo*) move anteriorly on the transverse plane *(M1)* while lateral points *(Lo)* move posteriorly *(L1)*. The rotational axis *(Zo)* remains unchanged. The motion of the medial point Mo to M1 during the rotation represents the sum of an anterior translation *(TM ant)* and a lateral translation *(TM lat)*. The same applies to the lateral point Lo. In this case the motion consists of a medial translation *(TL med)* and a posterior translation *(TL post)*. **b** In coupled displacements involving extensive translations and rotations in multiple degrees of freedom, the translations *(T ant and T lat)* can be stated not only for the tibial center *(Zo)* but also for the medial tibial points *(Mo, translation TM ant and TM lat)* and lateral tibial points *(Lo, translation TL ant and TL lat)*

translation also has become widely used for this type of motion. It is correct to speak of "anterior translation of the tibia" in describing a positive outcome of the anterior drawer test (see Fig. 12-3).

When translation is used as a synonym for displacement, it fails to take into account the coupled motions that may occur. That is why we have reservations about using the term translation in connection with clinical laxity testing. We prefer to use the term anterior or posterior displacement when describing the result of an anterior or posterior drawer test, and we use medial/lateral opening or medial/lateral displacement to describe the result of varus-valgus testing.

We believe that every stress exerted on the knee produces highly *complex displacements* of the tibia relative to the femur. Even with sophisticated measuring devices that register motion in all six degrees of freedom, the complex motions and displacements that occur during a laxity test can be analyzed only in approximate terms under laboratory conditions. In clinical laxity tests, the examiner must apply the displacement force to the tibia with his hands. In an anterior drawer test, for example, the examiner must direct the applied force precisely in the anterior direction. At the same time he attempts to register the resulting complex motion of the upper tibia. While the primary motion is relatively easy to assess (e.g., anterior displacement of the proximal tibia in

the anterior drawer test), it is extremely difficult to determine whether this motion fits the definition of a pure translation (see above) or whether it is associated with simultaneous internal or external rotation (motion about the vertical axis) or even with motions in other degrees of freedom, such as medial translation or axial compression. Nevertheless, the examiner should make an effort to recognize *coupled motions,* for example by trying to register the displacements of the medial and lateral joint compartments separately in the anterior drawer test. Feagin [159] has described a technique for this in which the examiner uses a special hand hold to fixate the tibia and femur (see Fig. 3-12). In this way the examiner can detect anterior translation as well as the rotational response of the tibia and can appreciate the separate translations of the medial and lateral tibial condyles (Fig. 12-7). The latter type of motion can also be described as anterior translation of the lateral or medial joint compartment (compartmental translation).

For the reasons stated above, it should be kept in mind that a displacement or motion in the degree of freedom being tested is always associated with coupled displacements in other degrees of freedom. This fact should be considered during laxity testing and whenever the terms anterior displacement, posterior displacement, medial opening, and lateral opening are used clinically to describe the test results.

References

1. Abbott LC, Saunders JB, Bost FC, Anderson CE (1944) Injuries of the ligaments of the knee. J Bone Joint Surg [Am] 26: 503-521
2. Abdon P, Asanson M, Turner S (1988) Total meniscectomy in children: A long-term follow-up study. In: Müller W, Hackenbruch W (eds) Surgery and arthroscopy of the knee. Springer, Berlin Heidelberg New York Tokyo, pp 366-368
3. Acufex Microsurgical Inc (1987) The Knee Signature System - KSS. Norwood, USA
4. Adam G, Bohndorf K, Prescher A, Krasny R, Günther RW (1988) Der hyaline Gelenkknorpel in der MR-Tomographie des Kniegelenkes bei 1, 5 T. Fortschr Röntgenstr 148: 648-651
5. Aglietti P, Buzzi R, Bassi PB (1988) Arthroscopic partial meniscectomy in the anterior cruciate deficient knee. Am J Sports Med 16: 597-602
6. Aisen AM, McCune WJ, MacGuire AM, Carson PL, Silver TM, Jafri SZ, Martel W (1984) Sonographic evaluation of the cartilage of the knee. Radiology 153: 781-784
7. Allen PR, Debaham RA, Swan AV (1984) Late degenerative changes after meniscectomy. J Bone Joint Surg [Br] 66: 666-671
8. Allum RL, Jones JR (1987) Acute traumatic haemarthrosis of the knee. J Bone Joint Surg [Br] 69: 160
9. Anderson AF, Lipscomb B (1986) Clinical diagnosis of meniscal tears. Description of a new manipulative test. Am J Sports Med 14: 291-293
10. Anderson AF, Lipscomb B, Liudahl KJ, Addlestone RB (1987) Analysis of the intercondylar notch by computed tomography. Am J Sports Med 15: 547-552
11. Andrew BL (1954) The sensory innervation of the medial ligament of the knee joint. J Physiol 123: 241-250
12. Andrews JR, McLoad WD, Ward T, Howard K (1977) The cutting mechanism. Am J Sports Med 5: 111-121
13. Andrews JR (1985) The classification of the knee ligament instability. Orthop Clin North Am 16: 69-82
14. Appel M, Gradinger R (1989) Die Architektur des Kreuzbandaufbaus. Prakt Sporttrauma Sportmed 5: 12-16
15. Arms SW, Pope MH, Johnson RJ, Fischer RA, Arvidson I, Eriksson E (1984) The biomechanics of anterior cruciate ligament rehabilitation and reconstruction. Am J Sports Med 12: 8-18
16. Arnoczky SP (1983) Anatomy of the anterior cruciate ligament. Clin Orthop 172: 19-25
17. Arnoczky SP, Warren RF (1983) The microvasculature of the meniscus and its response to injury. Am J Sports Med 11: 131-140
18. Arnoczky SP (1985) Blood supply to the anterior cruciate ligament and supporting structures. Orthop Clin North Am 16: 15-28
19. Arnoczky SP (1985) The blood supply of the meniscus and its role in healing and repair. In: Finerman G (ed) Symposium of sports medicine: The knee. Mosby, St. Louis, pp 94-110
20. Arnold JA, Coker TP, Heaton LM, Park JP, Harris WD (1979) Natural history of anterior cruciate ligament tears. Am J Sports Med 7: 305-313
21. Arthornthurasook A, Gaew-Im K (1988) Study of the infrapatellar nerve. Am J Sports Med 16: 57-59
22. Bach BR, Warren RF (1988) Radiographic indicators of anterior cruciate ligament injury. In: Feagin JA (ed) The crucial ligaments. Diagnosis and treatment of ligamentous injuries about the knee. Churchill Livingstone, New York, pp 317-327
23. Bach BR, Warren RF, Wickiewicz TL (1988) The pivot shift phenomenon: Results and description of a modified clinical test for anterior cruciate ligament insufficiency. Am J Sports Med 16: 571-576
24. Bachelin P, Bedat P, Moret O, Fritschy D (1988) Active Lachman test. A radiological control in intercondylar eminence fractures and ACL tears in children. Presented at 3rd Congress of European Society of Knee Surgery and Arthroscopy, Amsterdam
25. Balkfors B (1982) The course of knee-ligament injuries. Acta Orthop Scand (Suppl) 198
26. Bandi W (1981) Die retropatellaren Kniegelenksschäden, 2. Aufl. Huber, Stuttgart
27. Bargar WL, Moreland JR, Markolf KL, Shoemaker SC, Amstutz HC, Grant TT (1980) In vivo stability testing of post-meniscectomy knees. Clin Orthop 150: 247-252
28. Bargar WL, Moreland JR, Markolf KL, Shoemaker SC (1983) The effect of tibia-foot rotatory position on the anterior drawer test. Clin Orthop 173: 200-203
29. Barrack RL, Skinner HB, Buckley SL (1989) Proprioception in the anterior cruciate deficient knee. Am J Sports Med 17: 1-6
30. Barton TM, Torg JS, Das M (1984) Posterior cruciate ligament insufficiency. A review to the literature. Sports Med 1: 419-430
31. Barucha E (1960) Unsere Erfahrungen über den Wert des Rauberschen Röntgenzeichens bei der Meniskusdiagnose. Monatsschr Unfallheilkd 63: 370
32. Basmajian JV, Lovejoy H (1971) Functions of the popliteus muscle in man. J Bone Joint Surg [Am] 53: 557-562

33. Baugher WH, Warren RF, Marshall JL, Joseph A (1984) Quadriceps atrophy in the anterior cruciate insufficient knee. Am J Sports Med 12: 192-195

34. Baumgartl F (1964) Das Kniegelenk. Springer, Berlin Heidelberg New York

35. Beaufils P, Ceolin JL, Perreau M (1988) Medial meniscal cysts: A report on 32 cases. Presented at 3rd Congress of European Society of Knee Surgery and Arthroscopy, Amsterdam

36. Behfar AS, Refior HJ (1986) Arthroskopie des kindlichen Kniegelenkes. Z Orthop Grenzgeb 124: 751-754

37. Bellier G, Dupont JY (1988) Lateral discoid meniscus in children: Pathology and treatment. Presented at 3rd Congress of European Society of Knee Surgery and Arthroscopy, Amsterdam

38. Benedetto KP (1984) Die Technik der arthroskopischen Kreuzbandplastik. Chirurg 55: 756-769

39. Benedetto KP (1985) Der Ersatz des vorderen Kreuzbandes mit dem vasculär gestielten zentralen Drittel des Lig. patellae. Unfallchirurg 88: 189-197

40. Benedetto KP, Glötzer W, Künzel KH, Gaber O (1985) Die Gefäßversorgung der Menisken, morphologische Grundlagen für die Refixation. Acta Anat 124: 88-92

41. Benedetto KP (1986) Indikation zur Arthroskopie bei Verletzungen der Kapselbandstrukturen am Kniegelenk. Hefte Unfallheilkd 181: 772-776

42. Benninghoff A, Goerttler K (1981) Lehrbuch der Anatomie des Menschen, Bd I. Urban & Schwarzenberg, München

43. Bertin KC, Marlowe Goble E (1983) Ligament injuries associated with physeal fractures about the knee. Clin Orthop 177: 188-195

44. Bircher E (1921) Die Arthroendoskopie. Zentralbl Chir 48: 1460-1461

45. Bircher E (1933) Über Binnenverletzungen des Kniegelenkes. Langenbecks Arch Klin Chir 177: 290-350

46. Bird MDT, Sweet MBE (1988) Canals in the semilunar meniscus: brief report. J Bone Joint Surg [Br] 70: 839

47. Blaimont P, Klein P, Alameh M, Van Elegem P (1988) The function of hamstrings: A pathogenic hypothesis of femoropatellar osteoarthritis. In: Müller W, Hackenbruch W (eds) Surgery and arthroscopy of the knee. Springer, Berlin Heidelberg New York Tokyo, pp 55-57

48. Blauth W (1961) Die Sudecksche Dystrophie des Kniegelenkes. Arch Orthop Unfallchir 53: 231-249

49. Blauth W, Karpf P (1981) Grundlagen der klinischen Untersuchung des Kniegelenkes. Prakt Orthop 11: 37-53

50. Blauth W, Hassenpflug J (1983) Die Arthrographie bei Strecksteifen des Kniegelenkes. Z Orthop 121: 706-713

51. Blauth W, Helm C (1988) Vordere Kreuzbandrupturen - ein diagnostisches Problem? Unfallchirurg 91: 358-365

52. Blazina ME (1978) Isolated tear of the anterior cruciate ligament. In: Schulitz KP, Krahl H, Stein WH (eds) Late reconstruction of injured ligaments of the knee. Springer, Berlin Heidelberg New York, pp 22-32

53. Bloier B (1987) Ultraschalldiagnostik am Seitenbandapparat des Kniegelenkes bei Varus-Valgus-Streß. In: Stuhler T, Feige A (Hrsg) Ultraschalldiagnostik des Bewegungsapparats. Springer, Berlin Heidelberg New York Tokyo, S 297-302

54. Blumensaat C (1938) Die Lageabweichungen und Verrenkungen der Kniescheibe. Ergeb Chir Orthop 31: 149-223

55. Blumensaat C (1956) Der heutige Stand des Sudeck-Syndroms. Hefte Unfallheilkd 51: 1-225

56. Böhler J (1943) Röntgenologische Darstellung von Kreuzbandverletzungen. Chirurg 16: 136-138

57. Boniface RJ, Fu FH, Ilkhanipour K (1986) Objective anterior cruciate ligament testing. Orthopedics 9: 391-393

58. Bonnarens FO, Drez D (1987) Clinical examination of the knee for anterior cruciate ligament laxity. In: Jackson DW, Drez D (eds) The anterior cruciate deficient knee. Mosby, St. Louis, pp 72-89

59. Bonnel F, Mansat CH, Jaeger JH (1986) The three-dimensional active rotatory stabilization of the knee. Surg Radiol Anat 8: 37-42

60. Bousquet G (1972) Le diagnostic des laxités chronique du genou. Rev Chir Orthop (Suppl) 58

61. Boyd IA, Roberts TDM (1953) Proprioceptive discharges from stretch- receptors in the knee-joint of the cat. J Physiol 122: 38-58

62. Boyd IA (1954) The histological structure of the receptors in the knee- joint of the cat correlated with their physiological response. J Physiol 124: 476-488

63. Bradley GW, Shives TC, Samuelsen KM (1979) Ligament injuries in the knees of children. J Bone Joint Surg [Am] 61: 588-591

64. Bradley J, Fitzpatrick D, Daniel D, Shercliff, O'Connor J (1988) Orientation of the cruciate ligament in the sagittal plane. J Bone Joint Surg [Br] 70: 94-99

65. Brantigan OC, Voshell AF (1941) The mechanics of the ligaments and the menisci of the knee joint. J Bone Joint Surg [Am] 23: 44-66

66. Brantigan OC, Voshell AF (1943) The tibial collateral ligament: its function, its bursae and its relation to the medial meniscus. J Bone Joint Surg [Am] 25: 121-131

67. Braus H, Elze C (1954) Anatomie des Menschen, Bd I. Springer, Berlin Göttingen Heidelberg

68. Brna JA, Hall RF (1984) Acute monoarticular herpetic arthritis. J Bone Joint Surg [Am] 66: 623

69. Brody DM (1980) Running injuries. Clin Symp 32: 1-36

70. Brühlmann-Keller H, Kieser CH, Züllig R (1986) Arthrographie und Arthroskopie in der Meniskusdiagnostik. Unfallchirurg 89: 547-550

71. Brühlmann H (1986) Ökonomie der Meniskusdiagnostik. In: Tiling TH (Hrsg) Arthroskopische Meniskuschirurgie (Fortschritte in der Arthroskopie Bd 2). Enke, Stuttgart, S 28-29

72. Bruns P (1892) Die Luxation des Semilunarknorpels des Kniegelenkes. Bruns Beitr Klin Chir 9: 435-464

73. Bryant JT, Cooke TDV (1988) A biomechanical function of the ACL: Prevention of medial translation of the tibia. In: Feagin JA (ed) The crucial ligaments. Diagnosis and treatment of ligamentous inju-

ries about the knee. Churchill Livingstone, New York, pp 235-242

74. Bunker TD (1983) Ruptured semimembranosus bursa - A complication of arthroscopy. A short case report. Injury 15: 182-183

75. Burman MS (1931) Arthroscopy or the direct visualisation of joints. An experimental cadaver study. J Bone Joint Surg [Am] 13: 669-695

76. Burman MS, Finkelstein H, Mayer I (1934) Arthroscopy of the knee joint. J Bone Joint Surg [Am] 16: 255-268

77. Burri C, Mutschler W (1982) Das Knie - Verletzungen, Verletzungsfolgen, Erkrankungen. Hippokrates, Stuttgart

78. Butler DL, Noyes FR, Grood ES (1980) Ligamentous restraints to anterior- posterior drawer in the human knee. A biomechanical study. J Bone Joint Surg [Am] 62: 259-270

79. Cailliet R (1984) Knee pain and disability, 2nd edn. Davies, Philadelphia

80. Calville MR, Lee CL, Ciullo JV (1986) The Lenox Hill brace. An evaluation of effectiveness in treating knee instability. Am J Sports Med 14: 257-261

81. Casscells SW (1979) The arthroscope in the diagnosis of disorders of the patellofemoral joint. Clin Orthop 144: 45-50

82. Casscells SW, Fellows B, Axe MJ (1983) Another young athlete with intermittent claudication. Am J Sports Med 11: 180-182

83. Castaing J, Burdin PH, Mougin M (1972) Les conditions de la stabilité passive du genou. Rev Chir Orthop (Suppl) 58: 34-48

84. Casteleyn PP, Handelberg F, Opdecam P (1988) Traumatic haemarthrosis of the knee. J Bone Joint Surg [Br] 70: 404-406

85. Cavlak Y, Heufers D (1979) Die beidseitige Ruptur der Quadricepssehne, ein seltenes Krankheitsbild. Aktuell Traumatol 7: 373-375

86. Cerabona F, Sherman MF, Bonamo JR, Sklar J (1988) Patterns of meniscal injury with acute anterior cruciate ligament tears. Am J Sports Med 16: 603-609

87. Cerulli G, Ceccarini A, Alberti P, Caraffa A (1985) Study of the mechano-receptors of the human menisci. Presented at 4th Congress of the Society of knee, Salzburg

88. Cerulli G, Ceccarini A, Alberti PF, Caraffa A, Caraffa G (1988) Mechanoreceptors of some anatomical structures of the human knee. In: Müller W, Hackenbruch W (eds) Surgery and arthroscopy of the knee. Springer, Berlin Heidelberg New York Tokyo, pp 50-54

89. Cerulli G, Caraffa A, Bensi G, Buompadre V (1988) Biochemical neuromorphological and mechanical studies on ACL. Presented at 3rd Congress of European Society of Knee Surgery and Arthroscopy, Amsterdam

90. Chapman JA (1985) Popliteal artery damage in closed injuries of the knee. J Bone Joint Surg [Br] 67: 420-423

91. Chassaing V, Parier J (1988) Arthroskopie des Kniegelenkes - Diagnostik und operative Therapie. Deutscher Ärzteverlag, Köln

92. Childress HM (1957) Diagnosis of posterior lesions of the medial meniscus. Description of a new test. Am J Surg 93: 782-784

93. Christopher GW, Jurik JA, Janecki CJ, Haake PW, Riley GJ, Chessin GN (1982) Meningococcae arthritis, bacteriaemia and osteomyelitis following arthroscopy. Report of a case. Clin Orthop 171: 127-130

94. Clark FJ, Burgess PR (1975) Slowly adapting receptors in cat knee joint: Can they signal joint angles? J Neurophysiol 38: 1448-1463

95. Cohn AK, Mains DB (1979) Popliteal hiatus of the lateral meniscus. Am J Sports Med 4: 222-226

96. Contzen H (1975) Diagnostik beim instabilen Kniegelenk. Hefte Unfallheilkd 125: 80

97. Cooper DE, Delee JC, Ramamurthy S (1989) Reflex sympathetic dystrophy of the knee. J Bone Joint Surg [Am] 71: 365-369

98. Cotta H, Puhl W, Niethard FU (1982) Der Einfluß des Hämarthros auf den Knorpel der Gelenke. Unfallchirurgie 8: 145-151

99. Crawford E, Dewer M, Aichroth PM (1987) The Westminster cruciometer for measurement anterior cruciate instability. J Bone Joint Surg [Br] 69: 159

100. Cross MJ, Powell JF (1984) Long-term follow-up of posterior cruciate ligament rupture: A study of 116 cases. Am J Sports Med 12: 292-297

101. Cross MJ, Schmidt DR, Mackie IG (1987) A no-touch test for the anterior cruciate ligament. J Bone Joint Surg [Br] 69: 300

102. Cross MJ, Roger GJ, Bokor D, Sorrenti S (1989) Dynamic cruciate tester as a diagnostic tool for the assessment of laxity of the anterior cruciate ligament. J Bone Joint Surg [Br] 71: 162

103. Crowninshield R, Pope MH, Johnson RJ (1976) An analytical model of the knee. J Biomech 9: 397-405

104. Crowninshield R, Pope MH, Johnson R, Miller R (1976) The impedance of human knee. J Biomech 9: 529-535

105. Czerniecki JM, Lippert F, Olerud JE (1988) A biomechanical evaluation of tibiofemoral rotation in anterior cruciate deficient knees during walking and running. Am J Sports Med 16: 327-331

106. Daffner RH, Tabas JH (1987) Trauma oblique radiographs of the knee. J Bone Joint Surg [Am] 69: 568-572

107. Dahners L (1989) Factors influencing ligament healing. Presented at 1st International Symposium on Sporttraumatology „The knee of sportsmen", Bopfingen 9.-10.6.1989

108. Dandy DJ (1981) Arthroscopic surgery of the knee. Churchill Livingstone, Edinburgh

109. Dandy DJ, Pusey RJ (1982) The long-term results of unrepaired tears of the posterior ligament. J Bone Joint Surg [Br] 64: 92-941

110. Dandy DJ, Griffiths D (1989) Lateral release for recurrent dislocation of the patella. J Bone Joint Surg [Br] 71: 121-125

111. Daniel DM, Malcom LL, Losse G, Stone ML, Burks R, Morgan J (1983) The active anterior drawer test. Annual meeting of the AAOS, Anaheim, California

112. Daniel DM, Stone ML, Sachs R, Malcom LL, Losse G, Burks R, Barnett P (1984) Instrumented measure-

ment of acute ACL disruption. Annual meeting of the AAOS, Atlanta, Georgia

113. Daniel DM, Malcom LL, Losse G, Stone ML, Sachs R, Burks R (1985) Instrumented measurement of anterior laxity of the knee. J Bone Joint Surg [Am] 67: 720-726

114. Daniel DM, Stone ML, Sachs R, Malcom LL (1985) Instrumented measurement of the anterior knee laxity in patients with acute anterior cruciate ligament disruption. Am J Sports Med 13: 401-407

115. Daniel DM, Biden EN (1987) The language of knee motion. In: Jackson DW, Drez D (eds) The anterior cruciate deficient knee. Mosby, St. Louis Washington Toronto, pp 1-16

116. Daniel DM, Stone ML (1988) Diagnosis of knee ligament injury: Tests and measurements of joint laxity. In: Feagin JA (ed) The crucial ligaments. Diagnosis and treatment of ligamentous injuries about the knee. Churchill Livingstone, New York, pp 287-300

117. Daniel DM, Stone ML, Barnett P, Sachs R (1988) Use of the quadriceps active test to diagnose posterior cruciate-ligament disruption and measure posterior laxity of the knee. J Bone Joint Surg [Am] 70: 386-391

118. Davies GJ, Malone T, Bassett FH (1980) Knee examination. Phys Ther 60: 1565-1574

119. Dehaven KE (1982) Principles of triangulation for arthroscopic surgery. In: Metcalf R (ed) Symposium on Arthroscopic Knee Surgery. Orthop Clin North Am 13/2: 329-336

120. Dejour H, Walch G (1987) Die chronischen hinteren Instabilitäten. Orthopäde 16: 149-156

121. Dejour H, Chambat P, Walch G, Ranger R (1988) The diagnostic and prognostic value of the „active radiologic Lachman". In: Müller W, Hackenbruch W (eds) Surgery and arthroscopy of the knee. Springer, Berlin Heidelberg New York Tokyo, p 84

122. Delee JC, Curtis R (1983) Anterior cruciate ligament insufficiency in children. Clin Orthop 172: 112-118

123. Delee JC (1985) Complications of arthroscopy and arthroscopic surgery. Results of a national survery. Arthroscopy 1: 214-220

124. Denti M, Bonizzoni C, Ramondetta V, Peretti G (1988) Magnetic resonance imaging of the knee: normal and pathological imaging and correlations with arthroscopy. In: Müller W, Hackenbruch W (eds) Surgery and arthroscopy of the knee. Springer, Berlin Heidelberg New York Tokyo, pp 649-654

125. Dexel M, Langlotz M (1979) Radiologische Diagnostik der chronischen Knieinstabilitäten. In: Morscher E (Hrsg) Funktionelle Diagnostik in der Orthopädie, Enke, Stuttgart

126. Dexel M (1979) Die Klassifikation der chronischen Knieinstabilitäten. In: Morscher E (Hrsg) Funktionelle Diagnostik in der Orthopädie, Enke, Stuttgart

127. Dexel M, Langlotz M (1980) Radiologische Diagnostik der Rotationsinstabilitäten am Kniegelenk. Orthop Prax 10: 336-342

128. Dexel M, Suezawa Y, Rodriguez M (1982) Diagnostik der frischen Bandverletzung am Kniegelenk des Erwachsenen. Orthop Prax 12: 26-32

129. Dick W, Glinz W, Henche HR, Ruckstuhl J, Wruhs O, Zollinger H (1978) Komplikationen der Arthroskopie. Arch Trauma Surg 92: 69-73

130. Dickhaut SC, Delee JC (1982) The discoid lateralmeniscus syndrome. J Bone Joint Surg [Am] 64: 1068-1073

131. Dihlmann W (1987) Gelenke - Wirbelverbindungen, 3rd edn. Thieme, Stuttgart New York

132. Dingerkus MD, Jochum M, Fritz H, Bernett P (1987) Möglichkeiten der biochemischen Differenzierung von Reizergüssen am Kniegelenk. Sportverletzung Sportschaden 2: 86-90

133. Donaldson WF, Warren RF, Wickiewicz T (1985) A comparison of acute anterior cruciate ligament examinations. Initial versus examination under anesthesia. Am J Sports Med 13: 5-10

134. Driessen JJ, van der Werken C, Nicolai JPA, Crul JF (1983) Clinical effects of regional intravenous guanethidine (Ismelin) in reflex sympathetic dystrophy. Acta Anaesthesiol Scand 27: 505-509

135. Dubs L (1984) Bandlaxizität und Sport - ein ätiologischer Beitrag zum femoropatellären Schmerzsyndrom. Orthopäde 13: 46-51

136. Dubs L, Gschwend N (1988) General joint laxity. Arch Orthop Trauma Surg 107: 65-72

137. Dühmke E, Gremmel H (1976) Röntgendarstellung des verletzten Kniegelenkes. Chir Prax 20: 105-124

138. Dupont JY (1988) The jerk test in external rotation in anterior cruciate ligament-deficient knees. In: Müller W, Hackenbruch W (eds) Surgery and arthroscopy of the knee. Springer, Berlin Heidelberg New York Tokyo, pp 71-81

139. Dupont JY, Bellier G, Rodriguez F, Texier G, Houles JP (1988) The behaviour of the remaining patella tendon after harvesting of anterior cruciate ligament reconstruction. An ultrasonographic study. Application to the treatment of patellar tendonitis. Presented at 3rd Congress of European Society of Knee Surgery and Arthroscopy, Amsterdam

140. Dustmann HO, Puhl W, Schulitz KP (1971) Knorpelveränderungen beim Hämarthros unter besonderer Berücksichtigung der Ruhigstellung. Arch Orthop Unfallchir 71: 148-159

141. Dye SF (1988) An evolutionary perspective. In: Feagin JA (ed) The crucial ligaments. Diagnosis and treatment of ligamentous injuries about the knee. Churchill Livingstone, New York, pp 161-172

142. Eady JL, Cardenas CD, Sopa D (1982) Avulsion of the femoral attachment of the anterior cruciate ligament in a seven-year-old child. J Bone Joint Surg [Am] 64: 1376-1378

143. Edholm P, Lindahl O, Lindholm B, Myrnerts R, Ollson KE, Wennberg E (1976) Knee instability. An orthoradiographic study. Acta Orthop Scand 47: 658-663

144. Edixhoven PH (1983) Measurement of the drawer sign of the knee in patients. Acta Orthop Scand 54: 951-959

145. Eichhorn J, Weber A (1987) Die sonographische Darstellung des Laufs der Patella im Gleitlager. In: Stuhler T, Feige A (Hrsg) Ultraschalldiagnostik des Bewegungsapparats. Springer Berlin Heidelberg New York Tokyo, S 282-291

146. Eichhorn J, Strobel M (1988) Problemsituationen bei der Arthroskopie. In: Chassaing V, Parier J (Hrsg) Arthroskopie des Kniegelenkes - Diagnostik und operative Therapie. Deutscher Ärzteverlag, Köln, S 143-145

147. Eichhorn J, Strobel M (1988) Erweiterte Indikationen zur Arthroskopie. In: Chassaing V, Parier J (Hrsg) Arthroskopie des Kniegelenkes - Diagnostik und operative Therapie. Deutscher Ärzteverlag, Köln, S 151-155

148. Eiskjar S, Larsen ST, Schmidt MB (1988) The significance of hemarthrosis of the knee in children. Arch Orthop Trauma Surg 107: 96-98

149. Ellison AE (1985) Embrology, anatomy and function of the anterior cruciate ligament. Orthop Clin North Am 16: 3-14

150. Erlemann R, Pollmann H, Reiser M, Almeida P, Peters PE (1987) Stadieneinteilung der hämophilen Osteoarthropathie mit dem Pettersson-Score. Fortschr Röntgenstr 147: 521-526

151. Evans PJ, Bell GD, Frank C (1989) Prospective evaluation of the McMurray test. J Bone Joint Surg [Br] 71: 350

152. Fabbriciani C, Oransky M (1988) Anatomy of the popliteus muscle and posterolateral structures. In: Müller W, Hackenbruch W (eds) Surgery and arthroscopy of the knee. Springer, Berlin Heidelberg New York Tokyo, pp 58-60

153. Fahrer H, Rentsch HU, Gerber NJ, Beyeler C, Hess CW, Grünig B (1988) Knee effusion and reflex inhibition of the quadriceps. J Bone Joint Surg [Br] 70: 635-638

154. Faro Medical Technologies Inc., 2875 Sabourin, Quebec H4S 1M9, Canada

155. Farquharson MA, Osborne AH (1983) Partial rupture of the anterior cruciate ligament of the knee. J Bone Joint Surg [Br] 65: 32-34

156. Feagin JA, Curl WC (1976) Isolated tear of the anterior cruciate ligament: 5 years follow-up study. Am J Sports Med 4: 95-100

157. Feagin JA, Cabaud HE, Curl WL (1982) The anterior cruciate ligament. Clin Orthop 164: 54-58

158. Feagin JA (1985) Mechanism of injury and pathology of the anterior ligament injuries. Orthop Clin North Am 16: 41-45

159. Feagin JA (1988) Principles of diagnosis and treatment. In: Feagin JA (ed) The crucial ligaments. Diagnosis and treatment of ligamentous injuries about the knee. Churchill Livingstone, New York, pp 3-136

160. Felsenreich F (1935) Radiologische Darstellung pathologischer Beweglichkeit des Kniegelenkes nach Kreuzbandverletzungen. Zentralbl Chir 6: 320

161. Ferretti A, Ippolito E, Mariani P, Puddu G (1983) Jumper's knee. Am J Sports Med 11: 58-62

162. Feretti A (1986) Epidemiology of jumper's knee. Sports Med 3: 289-295

163. Ferguson AB, McMaster JH (1973) Isolated posteromedial capsular lesion of the knee. J Bone Joint Surg [Am] 55: 1316

164. Fetto JF, Marshall JL (1979) Injury to the anterior cruciate ligament producing the pivot-shift sign. J Bone Joint Surg [Am] 61: 710-714

165. Fetto JF, Marshall JL (1980) The natural history and diagnosis of anterior cruciate ligament insufficiency. Clin Orthop 147: 29-38

166. Ficat RP, Philippe J, Hungerford DS (1979) Chondromalacia patellae. A system of classification. Clin Orthop 144: 55-62

167. Fick R (1904) Handbuch der Anatomie und Mechanik der Gelenke unter Berücksichtigung der bewegenden Muskeln, Teil I: Anatomie der Gelenke. Fischer, Jena, S 341-394

168. Fick R (1911) Handbuch der Anatomie und Mechanik der Gelenke unter Berücksichtigung der bewegenden Muskeln, Teil II: Spezielle Gelenk- und Muskelmechanik. Fischer, Jena, S 521-593

169. Finochietto R (1930) El signo del salto. Press Med Argent

170. Finochietto R (1935) Semilunar cartilages of the knee. The „Jump Sign". J Bone Joint Surg [Am] 17: 916

171. Finsterbush A, Friedman B (1975) The effect of sensory denervation on rabbit's knee joints. J Bone Joint Surg [Am] 57: 949-955

172. Finsterbush A, Frankl U, Mann G (1989) Fat pad adhesion to partially torn anterior cruciate ligament: A cause of knee locking. Am J Sports Med 17: 92-95

173. Fischer LP, Guyot J, Gonon GP, Carret JP, Dahan P (1978) The role of the muscles and ligaments in the stabilisation of the knee joint. Anat Clin 1: 43-54

174. Fischer RA, Arms SW, Johnson RJ, Pope MH (1985) The functional relationship of the posterior ligament to the medial collateral ligament of the human knee. Am J Sports Med 13: 390-397

175. Fischer V, Matzen K, Bruns H (1976) Arthroseauslösende Faktoren der Meniskektomie. Z Orthop 114: 735-737

176. Floyd A, Phillips P, Khan MRH, Webb JN, McInnes A, Hughes SPF (1987) Recurrent dislocation of the patella. J Bone Joint Surg [Br] 69: 790-793

177. Forgon M, Szentpetery J (1961) Über angeborene Kniegelenksverrenkungen. Arch Orthop Unfallchir 52: 599-606

178. Fowler PJ (1980) Classification and early diagnosis of the knee joint instability. Clin Orthop 147: 15-21

179. Fowler PJ, Messieh S (1989) Isolated posterior cruciate ligament injuries in athletes. J Bone Joint Surg [Br] 71: 350

180. Franke K (1981) Klassifikation der chronischen Kapselbandinstabilitäten des Kniegelenkes, Teil I: Anatomie und Diagnostik. Beitr Orthop Trauma 28: 125-140

181. Frankel VH, Burstein AH, Brooks DB (1971) Biomechanics of internal derangement of the knee. J Bone Joint Surg [Am] 53: 945-962

182. Freeman MAR, Wyke B (1966) Articular contributions to the limb muscle reflexes. Br J Surg 53: 61-69

183. Freeman MAR, Wyke B (1967) The innervation of the knee joint. An anatomical and histological study of the cat. J Anat 101: 505-532

184. Freising S (1986) Irritation des Nervus saphenus als Ursache von Schmerzen im Kniegelenk. Unfallchirurg 89: 321-325

185. Friederich N, O'Brien W, Müller W, Henning C, Jackson R (1988) Functional anatomy of the cruciate

ligaments and their substitutes, part II: The posterior cruciate ligament. Presented at 3rd Congress of European Society of Knee Surgery and Arthroscopy, Amsterdam

186. Frik K (1932) Röntgenuntersuchungen am Kniegelenk. Fortschr Röntgenstr 46: 155

187. Fritschy D (1988) Jumper's knee and ultrasonography. Am J Sports Med 16: 637–640

188. Fujimoto A, Mori Y, Kuroki Y, Yamamoto R, Hino H, Okumo H (1988) The natural history of anterior knee pain in japanese adolescents. In: Müller W, Hackenbruch W (eds) Surgery and arthroscopy of the knee. Springer, Berlin Heidelberg New York Tokyo, pp 447–451

189. Fukubayashi T, Torzilli PA, Shermann MF, Warren RF (1982) An in vitro biomechanical evaluation of the anterior-posterior motion of the knee. J Bone Joint Surg [Am] 64: 258–264

190. Fullerton LR, Andrews JR (1984) Mechanical block to extension following augmentation of the anterior cruciate ligament. Am J Sports Med 12: 166–168

191. Furman W, Marshall JL, Girgis FG (1976) The anterior cruciate ligament. J Bone Joint Surg [Am] 58: 179–185

192. Gäde EA (1980) Ein Meßgerät zur objektiven Feststellung der Instabilität des Kniegelenkes. Orthop Prax 10: 850–853

193. Gainor BJ (1984) Installation of continous tube irrigation in the septic knee at arthoscopy. Clin Orthop 183: 96–98

194. Gallimore GW, Harms SE (1986) Knee injuries: High-resolution MR imaging. Radiology 160: 457–461

195. Galway R, Beaupre A, McIntosh DL (1972) Pivot-Shift - A clinical sign of symptomatic anterior cruciate insufficiency. J Bone Joint Surg [Br] 54: 763–764

196. Galway R, McIntosh DL (1980) The lateral pivot-shift: A symptom and sign of anterior cruciate ligament insufficiency. Clin Orthop 147: 45–50

197. Gamble JG, Edwards CC, Max SR (1984) Enzymatic adaptation in ligaments during immobilization. Am J Sports Med 12: 221–228

198. Gamble JG (1986) Symptomatic dorsal defect of the patella in a runner. Am J Sports Med 14: 425–427

199. Gardner E (1944) The distribution and termination of nerves in the knee joint of the cat. J Comp Neurol 80: 11–32

200. Gardner E (1948) The innervation of the knee joint. Anat Rec 101: 109–130

201. Gasco J, Del Pino JM, Gomar-Sancho F (1987) Double patella. J Bone Joint Surg [Br] 69: 602–603

202. Gaudernak T (1982) Der posttraumatische Hämarthros des Kniegelenkes - arthroskopische Abklärung der Ursachen. Unfallchirurgie 8: 159–169

203. Gaudernak T, Heine H, Arbogast R (1983) Elektronenmikroskopische Befunde an makroskopischen intakten Kreuzbändern beim Hämarthros. Unfallheilkunde 86: 170–172

204. Geisl H (1983) Beidseitige, simultane, spontane und subkutane Quadricepssehnenruptur. Aktuel Traumatol 13: 201–204

205. Gerngross H, Sohn CH, Griesbeck F (1986) Meniskussonographie und Arthroskopie - Experimentelle Untersuchungen am Leichenknie. Vortrag 50. Jahrestagung der Deutschen Gesellschaft für Unfallheilkunde, Berlin

206. Gerngross H (1987) Persönliche Mitteilung

207. Gillquist J, Hagberg G (1978) Findings at arthroscopy and arthrography in knee injuries. Acta Orthop Scand 49: 398–402

208. Gillquist J, Hamberg P, Lysholm J (1982) Endoscopic partial and total meniscectomy. A comparative study with a short term follow up. Acta Orthop Scand 53: 975–979

209. Girgis FG, Marshall JL, Al Monajem H (1975) The cruciate ligaments of the knee joint. Clin Orthop 106: 216–231

210. Glancy WG, Keene JS, Goletz TH (1984) Symptomatic dislocation of the anterior horn of the medial meniscus. Am J Sports Med 12: 57–64

211. Glashow JL, Katz R, Schneider M, Scott WN (1989) Double-blind assessment of the value of magnetic resonance imaging in the diagnosis of anterior cruciate and meniscal lesions. J Bone Joint Surg [Am] 71: 113–119

212. Glinz W (1980) Diagnostische Arthroskopie und arthroskopische Operationen am Kniegelenk. Huber, Bern Stuttgart Wien

213. Glinz W (1986) Arthroskopische Meniskusresektion: Resultate 1–7 Jahre nach der Operation. In: Tiling T (Hrsg) Arthroskopische Meniskuschirurgie. Enke, Stuttgart (Fortschritte in der Arthroskopie, Bd 2), S 61–71

214. Gobelet C (1984) Algoneurodystrophie. Sandorama 5: 4–11

215. Goldfuss AJ, Morehouse CA, Leveau BF (1973) Effect of muscular tension on knee stability. Med Sci Sports 5: 267–271

216. Gollehon DL, Torzilli P, Warren RF (1987) The role of the posterolateral and cruciate ligaments in the stability of the human knee. J Bone Joint Surg [Am] 69: 233–242

217. Goodfellow J, Hungerford DS, Zindel M (1976) Patellofemoral joint mechanics and pathology. J Bone Joint Surg [Br] 58: 287–291

218. Graf B (1987) Isometric placement of substitute for the anterior cruciate ligament. In: Jackson DW, Drez D (eds) The anterior cruciate deficient knee. Mosby, St. Louis, pp 102–113

219. Grana WA, Connor S, Hollingsworth S (1982) Partial arthroscopic meniscectomy: a preliminary report. Clin Orthop 164: 78–83

220. Grana WA, Hinkley B, Hollingsworth S (1984) Arthroscopic evaluation and treatment of patellar malalignment. Clin Orthop 186: 122–128

221. Grana WA, Muse G (1988) The effect of exercise on laxity in the anterior cruciate ligament deficient knee. Am J Sports Med 16: 586–588

222. Grigg P, Hoffman AH, Fogarty KE (1982) Properties of Golgi-Mazzoni afferents in the cat knee joint capsule, as revealed by mechanical studies of isolated joint capsule. J Neurophysiol 47: 31–40

223. Grood ES, Hefzy MS, Lindenfeld TL, Noyes FR (1988) Isometric points of the posterior cruciate liga-

ment. In: Müller W, Hackenbruch W (eds) Surgery and arthroscopy of the knee. Springer, Berlin Heidelberg New York Tokyo, pp 252–253

224. Grood ES, Noyes FR (1988) Diagnosis of knee ligament injuries: Biomechanical precepts. In: Feagin JA (ed) The crucial ligaments. Diagnosis and treatment of ligamentous injuries about the knee. Churchill Livingstone, New York, pp 245–260

225. Grood ES, Stowers SF, Noyes FR (1988) Limits of movement in the human knee. Effect of sectioning the posterior cruciate ligament and posterolateral structures. J Bone Joint Surg [Am] 70: 88–97

226. Grood ES, Hefzy MS, Lindenfield TN (1989) Factors affecting the region of most isometric femoral attachments, part I: The posterior cruciate ligament. Am J Sports Med 17: 197–207

227. Grosch H (1975) Die Röntgendiagnostik von Seitenbandschäden am Kniegelenk. Radiol Diagn (Berl) 16: 869–873

228. Gross U (1982) Posttraumatische Gelenksteife (pathomorphologische Gesichtspunkte). Unfallchirurgie 8: 251–260

229. Grüber J, Wolter D, Lierse W (1986) Der vordere' Kreuzbandreflex (LCA-Reflex). Unfallchirurg 89: 551–554

230. Grüber J, Wolter D, Lierse W (1988) In vivo study on the proprioceptive function of the knee ligaments. Presented at 3rd Congress of European Society of Knee Surgery and Arthroscopy, Amsterdam

231. Grünwald J, Bauer G, Wruhs O (1987) Tödliche Komplikation bei Arthroskopie im gasförmigen Medium. Unfallchirurg 90: 97

232. Gurtler RA, Stine R, Torg JS (1987) Lachman test evaluated – quantification of a clinical observation. Clin Orthop 216: 141–150

233. Gylys-Morin VM, Hajek PC, Sartoris DJ, Resnick D (1987) Articular cartilage defects: Detectability in cadaver knees with MR. AJR 148: 1153–1157

234. Hackenbruch W, Henche HR (1981) Diagnostik und Therapie von Kapselbandläsionen am Kniegelenk. Eular, Bern

235. Hackenbruch W, Müller W (1987) Untersuchung des Kniegelenkes. Orthopäde 16: 100–112

236. Hackethal KH (1958) Das Sudecksche Syndrom. Hüthig, Heidelberg

237. Hadied AM (1984) An unusual complication of arthroscopy: a fistula between the knee and the praepatellar bursa. J Bone Joint Surg [Am] 66: 624

238. Hafner K, Meuli HC (1975) Röntgenuntersuchung in der Orthopädie. Huber, Bern

239. Hallen LG, Lindahl O (1965) The lateral stability of the knee joint. Acta Orthop Scand 36: 179–191

240. Hallen LG, Lindahl O (1965) Rotation in the knee joint in experimental injury to the ligaments. Acta Orthop Scand 36: 400–407

241. Haller W, Gradinger R, Reiser M (1986) Ergebnisse der magnetischen Resonanz (MR)-Tomographie bei der Nachuntersuchung von Kreuzbandtransplantaten. Unfallchirurg 89: 375–379

242. Haller W, Gradinger R, Lehner K (1989) Die Aussagekraft der MR- Tomographie bei Kreuzbandverletzungen. Prakt Sporttrauma Sportmed 5: 42–46

243. Hallisey MJ, Doherty N, Bennett WF, Fulkerson JP (1987) Anatomy of the junction of the vastus lateralis tendon and the patella. J Bone Joint Surg [Am] 69: 545–549

244. Halperin N, Handel D, Fisher S, Agasi M, Copeliovitch L (1983) Anterior cruciate ligament insufficiency syndrome. Clin Orthop 179: 179–184

245. Halperin N, Oren Y, Hendel D, Nathan N (1987) Semimembranosus tenosynovitis: operative results. Arch Orthop Trauma Surg 106: 281–284

246. Hamberg P, Gillquist J, Lysholm J (1984) A comparison between arthroscopic meniscectomy and modified open meniscectomy. J Bone Joint Surg [Br] 66: 189–192

247. Hang Y (1983) Biomechanics of the knee joint in normal and pathological gait. An electrogoniometric study. J Form Med Assoc 82: 169–189

248. Hanks GA, Joyner DM, Kalenak A (1981) Anterolateral rotatory instability of the knee. Am J Sports Med 9: 225–232

249. Hansphal RS, Older MW, Cardoso TP (1984) The medial shelf: an anatomical, clinical and pathological study. J Bone Joint Surg [Br] 66: 280

250. Harding ML, Steingold RF, Howard L, Aitken W, Stephen RO (1987) Measurement of the knee laxity. J Bone Joint Surg [Br] 69: 159

251. Harms SE, Muschler G (1986) Three-dimensional MR imaging of the knee using surface coils. J Comput Assist Tomogr 10: 773–777

252. Harner CD, Fu FH, Mason GC, Wissinger HA, Rabin BS (1989) Cidexinduced synovitis. Am J Sports Med 17: 96–102

253. Hartung F (1955) Über Ganglienbildung am medialen Kniegelenksmeniskus. Arch Orthop Unfallchir 47: 149

254. Hassenpflug J, Blauth W, Rose D (1985) Zum Spannungsverhalten von Transplantaten zum Ersatz des vorderen Kreuzbandes – zugleich ein Beitrag zur Kritik an der „Over-the-top"-Technik. Unfallchirurg 85: 151–158

255. Hassler H, Jakob RP (1981) Ein Beitrag zur Ursache der anterolateralen Instabilität des Kniegelenkes. Eine Studie an 20 Leichenknien unter besonderer Berücksichtigung des Tractus iliotibialis. Arch Orthop Trauma Surg 98: 45–50

256. Haupt PR (1981) Isolierter Riß des vorderen Kreuzbandes. Arthroskopischer Nachweis. Chir Prax 28: 305–309

257. Haupt PR, Büsing CM, Duspiva W (1986) Isolierte Ruptur des vorderen Kreuzbandes. Unfallchirurg 89: 280–283

258. Hawe W, Dörr A, Bernett P (1989) Sonographische Befunde am verletzten hinteren Kreuzband. Prakt Sporttrauma Sportmed 5: 28–31

259. Hawkins RJ, Bell RH, Anisette G (1986) Acute patellar dislocations. Am J Sports Med 14: 117–120

260. Heckman JD, Alkire CC (1984) Distal patellar pole fractures. Am J Sports Med 12: 424–428

261. Hefzy MS, Grood ES, Noyes F (1989) Factors affecting the region of most isometric femoral attachments, part II: The anterior cruciate ligament. Am J Sports Med 17: 208–216

262. Hegglin R, Siegenthaler W (Hrsg) (1980) Differentialdiagnose innerer Krankheiten, 14. Aufl. Thieme, Stuttgart New York

263. Hehne HJ, Riede UN, Hausschild G, Schlageter M (1981) Tibio-femorale Kontaktflächenmessung nach experimentellen partiellen und subtotalen Meniskektomien. Z Orthop 119: 54–59

264. Hehne HJ (1983) Das Patellofemoralgelenk. Enke, Stuttgart

265. Heijboer MP, Post PJM, van Oostayen JA, Lameris JS (1988) Ultrasonography in patellar tendinitis. Presented at 3rd Congress of European Society of Knee Surgery and Arthroscopy, Amsterdam

266. Hejgaard N, Sandberg H, Hede A, Jacobsen K (1984) The course of differently treated isolated ruptures of the anterior cruciate ligament as observed by prospective stress radiography. Clin Orthop 182: 236–241

267. Helfet AJ (1982) Disorders of the knee, 2nd edn. Lippincott, Philadephia

268. Heller L, Langman J (1964) The meniscofemoral ligaments of the human knee. J Bone Joint Surg [Br] 46: 307–313

269. Helzel MV, Schindler G, Gay B (1987) Sonographische Messung der Gelenkknorpeldicke über den tragenden Femurkondylenanteilen. Vergleich zur Arthrographie und Pneumarthrocomputertomographie. In: Stuhler T, Feige A (Hrsg) Ultraschalldiagnostik des Bewegungsapparats. Springer, Berlin Heidelberg New York Tokyo, S 276–281

270. Hempfling H (1985) Systematik der Plicae am oberen Recessus. In: Hofer H (Hrsg) Fortschritte in der Arthroskopie. Enke, Stuttgart

271. Hempfling H (1987) Farbatlas der Arthroskopie großer Gelenke. Fischer, Stuttgart

272. Henche HR (1974) Indikation, Technik und Resultate der Arthroskopie nach Traumatisierung des Kniegelenkes. Orthopäde 3: 178–183

273. Henche HR, Holder J (1988) Die Arthroskopie des Kniegelenkes. 2. Aufl. Springer, Berlin Heidelberg New York Tokyo

274. Henderson CE, Hopson CN (1982) Pneumoscrotum as a complication of arthroscopy. J Bone Joint Surg [Am] 64: 1238–1240

275. Henning CE, Lynch MA, Glick KR (1985) An in vivo strain gage study of elongation of the anterior cruciate ligament. Am J Sports Med 13: 22–26

276. Hepp WR (1983) Radiologie des Femoro-Patellargelenkes. Enke, Stuttgart

277. Hermann G, Berson BL (1984) Discoid medial meniscus: Two cases of tears presenting as locked knee due to athletic trauma. Am J Sports Med 12: 74–76

278. Hertel P, Schweiberer L (1975) Biomechanik und Pathophysiologie des Kniebandapparates. Hefte Unfallheilkd 125: 1–16

279. Hertel P (1980) Verletzung und Spannung von Kniebändern. Hefte Unfallheilkd 124: 1–91

280. Hertel P, Schweiberer L (1980) Die Akutarthroskopie des Kniegelenkes als diagnostischer und therapeutischer Eingriff. Unfallheilkunde 83: 233–240

281. Hey-Groves E (1919) The crucial ligaments of the knee-joint: their function, rupture and the operative treatment of the same. Br J Surg 7: 505–515

282. Hierholzer G, Ludolph E (1977) Diagnostik von Bandverletzungen am Kniegelenk. Langenbecks Arch Chir 345: 445–449

283. Highgenboten CL (1982) Arthroscopic synovectomy. In: Metcalf R (ed) Symposium on Arthroscopic Knee Surgery. Orthop Clin North Am 13/2: 399–406

284. Highgenboten CL, Jackson A (1988) The reliability of the genucom knee analysis system. In: Müller W, Hackenbruch W (eds) Surgery and arthroscopy of the knee. Springer, Berlin Heidelberg New York Tokyo, pp 107–110

285. Hipp E, Karpf PM, Mang W (1979) Akute Sportverletzungen des Kniegelenkes. Unfallheilkunde 82: 143–154

286. Hohlbach G, Kiffner E, Liepe B (1981) Bilaterale, simultane, spontane und subkutane Quadrizepssehnenruptur. Aktuel Traumatol 11: 234–237

287. Holz U, Weller S (1975) Entstehung und Diagnostik der frischen Bandverletzung. Hefte Unfallheilkd 125: 17–25

288. Holz U, Wentzensen A (1980) Einteilung und klinische Diagnostik der Kapselbandverletzungen am Kniegelenk. Unfallchirurgie 6: 86–93

289. Hönigschmied J (1893) Leichenexperimente über die Zerreißung der Bänder im Kniegelenk. Dtsch Z Chir 36: 587–620

290. Hooper GJ (1986) Radiological assessment of anterior cruciate ligament deficiency. J Bone Joint Surg [Br] 68: 292–296

291. Hördegen KM (1970) Technik und Indikation gehaltener Röntgenaufnahmen. Röntgenpraxis 23: 221–236

292. Hsieh HH, Walker PS (1976) Stabilizing mechanism of the loaded and unloaded knee joint. J Bone Joint Surg [Am] 58: 87–83

293. Hughston JC (1968) Subluxation of the patella. J Bone Joint Surg [Am] 50: 1003–1025

294. Hughston JC (1969) The posterior cruciate ligament in knee joint stability. J Bone Joint Surg [Am] 51: 1045–1046

295. Hughston JC, Eilers AF (1973) The role of the posterior oblique ligament in repairs of acute medial (collateral) ligament tears of the knee. J Bone Joint Surg [Am] 55: 923–940

296. Hughston JC, Andrews JR, Cross MJ, Moschi A (1976) Classification of knee ligament instabilities. Part I: The medial compartement and cruciate ligaments. Part II: The lateral compartement. J Bone Joint Surg [Am] 58: 159–179

297. Hughston JC, Norwood LA (1980) The posterolateral drawer test and external recurvatum test for posterolateral rotatory instability of the knee. Clin Orthop 147: 82–87

298. Hughston JC, Deese M (1988) Medial subluxation of the patella as a complication of lateral retinacular release. Am J Sports Med 16: 383–388

299. Hughston JC (1988) The absent posterior drawer test in some acute posterior cruciate ligament tears of the knee. Am J Sports Med 16: 39–43

300. Imai N, Tomatsu T, Okamoto H, Nakamura Y (1989) Clinical and roentgenological studies on malalignment disorders of the patello-femoral joint. Part III: Lesions of the patella cartilage and subchondral

bone associated with patello-femoral malalignment. Jpn Orthop Assoc 63: 1–17

301. Insall J, Goldberg V, Salvati E (1972) Recurrent dislocation and the high riding patella. Clin Orthop 88: 67–69

302. Irvine GB, Dias JJ, Finlay DBL (1987) Segond fractures of the lateral tibial condyle. J Bone Joint Surg [Br] 69: 613–614

303. Iversen BF, Stürup J, Jacobson K (1988) Stress radiographic comparison of drawer symptoms measured in 90° versus 15° of knee flexion (the Lachman position). In: Müller W, Hackenbruch W (eds) Surgery and arthroscopy of the knee. Springer, Berlin Heidelberg New York Tokyo, pp 91–92

304. Jackson RW, Marans HJ, Glossop N, Willowdale M (1987) Anterior cruciate ligament insufficiency – a three-dimensional motion analysis. Am J Sports Med 15: 388

305. Jackson DW, Jennings LD, Maywood RM, Berger PE (1988) Magnetic resonance imaging of the knee. Am J Sports Med 16: 29–38

306. Jackson RW (1988) The torn ACL: Natural history of untreated lesions and rationale for selective treatment. In: Feagin JA (ed) The crucial ligaments. Diagnosis and treatment of ligamentous injuries about the knee. Churchill Livingstone, New York, pp 341–348

307. Jacobsen K (1976) Landmarks of the knee joint of the lateral radiograph during rotation. RÖFO 125: 399–344

308. Jacobsen K (1976) Stress radiographical measurement of the anteroposterior, medial and lateral instability of the knee joint. Acta Orthop Scand 47: 335–344

309. Jacobsen K (1977) Radiologic technique for measuring instability of the knee joint. Acta Radiol Diagn (Stockh) 18: 113–125

310. Jacobsen K (1978) Demonstration of rotatory instability in injured knees by stress radiography. Acta Orthop Scand 49: 195–204

311. Jacobsen K (1981) Gonylaxometry – stress radiographic measurement of passive stability in the knee joints of normal subjects and patients with ligament injuries. Acta Orthop Scand (Suppl) 194: 1–261

312. Jäger M, Hayd J, Kuzmany J (1973) Klinische und röntgenologische Untersuchungen zur Frage der Sportfähigkeit nach operierten Kniebandschäden. Sportarzt Sportmed 24: 60–63

313. Jäger M, Wirth CJ (1978) Kapselbandläsionen – Biomechanik, Diagnostik, Therapie. Thieme, Stuttgart New York

314. Jäger M, Wirth CJ (1978) Die veraltete anteromediale Kniegelenksinstabilität. Unfallheilkunde 81: 172–177

315. Jäger R, Hassenpflug J (1981) Über die Mechanik des Pivot-shift Zeichens. In: Jäger M, Hackenbroch MH, Refior HJ (Hrsg) Kapselbandläsionen des Kniegelenkes. Thieme, Stuttgart New York, S 104–108

316. Jakob RP, Segesser B (1980) Quadriceps-Dehnungsübungen – ein neues Konzept der Tendinosen des Streckapparates am Kniegelenk (Jumper's knee). Orthopäde 9: 201–206

317. Jakob RP, Hassler H, Staeubli HU (1981) Observations on rotatory instability of the lateral compartement of the knee – experimental studies on the functional anatomy and the pathomechanism of the true and reversed pivot-shift sign. Acta Orthop Scand (Suppl) 191: 1–30

318. Jakob RP (1987) Indikation, Behandlung und Evaluation bei chronischer vorderer Kreuzband-Instabilität. Orthopäde 16: 130–139

319. Jakob RP, Stäubli HU, Deland JT (1987) Grading the pivot shift. J Bone Joint Surg [Br] 69: 294–299

320. Jakob RP, Stäubli HU, Deland J (1988) Grading the pivot shift: an objective system with treatment implications. In: Müller W, Hackenbruch W (eds) Surgery and arthroscopy of the knee. Springer, Berlin Heidelberg New York Tokyo, pp 69–70

321. James SL (1978) Surgical anatomy of the knee. In: Schultz KP, Krahl H, Stein WH (eds) Late reconstructions of injured ligament of the knee. Springer, Berlin Heidelberg New York, pp 3–18

322. Janik B (1955) Kreuzbandverletzungen des Kniegelenkes. De Gruyter, Berlin

323. Jend HH, Schöttle H, Bahnsen J, Crone-Münzebrock W (1986) Achsenanalyse bei Patienten mit Patellaluxation. Unfallchirurgie 12: 263–270

324. Jensen KU, Strich W, Hille E (1989) Dynamische Veränderungen des Patellagleitweges unter isolierter M. vastus medialis Stimulation. Arthroskopie 2: 8–15

325. Johnson LL (1986) Diagnostic and surgical arthroscopy, 3rd edn. Mosby, St. Louis

326. Jonasch E (1958) Untersuchungen über die Form der Eminentia intercondyloidea tibiae im Röntgenbild. RÖFO 89: 81–85

327. Jonasch E (1958) Zerreißung des äußeren und inneren Knieseitenbandes. Hefte Unfallheilkd 59: 1–88

328. Jonasch E (1960) Zur Differentialdiagnose der medialen Meniskuszysten des Kniegelenkes. Arch Orthop Unfallchir 52: 338–340

329. Jonasch E (1964) Das Kniegelenk. De Gruyter, Berlin

330. Jones D, Tanzer T, Mowbray AS, Galway HR (1983) Studies of dynamic ligamentous instability of the knee by elektrogoniometric means. Prosthet Orthot Int 7: 165–173

331. Jonsson T, Peterson L (1982) Objective registration of the anterior stability of the knee. Int J Sports Med [Abstract Service: XXII. Weltkongreß für Sportmedizin Wien vom 28.6.–4.7.1982]

332. Jonsson T, Althoff B, Peterson L, Renström P (1982) Clinical diagnosis of ruptures of the anterior cruciate ligament. Comparative study of the Lachman test and the anterior drawer sign. Am J Sports Med 10: 100–102

333. Jorgensen U, Sonneholm S, Lauridsen F, Rosenklint A (1987) Long-term follow-up of the meniscectomy in athletes. J Bone Joint Surg [Br] 69: 80–83

334. Jung T, Rodriguez M, Augustiny N, Friedrich N, Schulthess G (1988) 1.5 T-MRI, Arthrographie und Arthroskopie in der Evaluation von Knieläsionen. Fortschr Röntgenstr 148: 390–393

335. Jurist KA, Otis JC (1985) Anteroposterior tibiofemoral displacements during isometric extension ef-

forts. The role of external load and knee flexion angle. Am J Sports Med 13: 254–258

336. Kaelin A, Hulin PH, Carlioz H (1986) Congenital aplasia of the cruciate ligaments. J Bone Joint Surg [Br] 68: 827–828

337. Kalenak A, Morehouse CA (1975) Knee stability and knee ligament injuries. JAMA 234: 1143–1145

338. Kamprad F, Hasert V (1972) Traumatische Kreuzbandveränderungen und ihre Darstellung im Röntgenbild. Beitr Orthop 19: 419–425

339. Kannus P, Järvinen M (1988) Knee ligament injuries in adolescents. J Bone Joint Surg [Br] 70: 772–776

340. Kannus P, Järvinen M, Paakkala T (1988) A radiological scoring scale for evaluation of posttraumatic osteoarthritis after knee ligament injuries. Int Orthop 12: 291–297

341. Kapandji IA (1970) The physiology of joints, vol II. Churchill Livingstone, Edinburgh

342. Kaplan EB (1958) The iliotibial tract. J Bone Joint Surg [Am] 40: 817–832

343. Kaplan EB (1961) The fabellofibular and short lateral ligaments of the knee joint. J Bone Joint Surg [Am] 43: 169–179

344. Karpf PM (1977) Anatomische Grundlagen als Voraussetzungen für die Diagnose der Knieverletzungen beim Skifahren. Fortschr Med 95: 191–194

345. Karpf PM, Mang W, Hackenbruch W (1980) Hypermobilität des Kniegelenkes nach dorsalen Kapselbandläsionen. Orthop Prax 10: 154–158

346. Kärrholm J, Selvik G, Elmquist LG, Hansson LI (1988) Instability of the anterior cruciate deficient knee. In: Müller W, Hackenbruch W (eds) Surgery and arthroscopy of the knee. Springer, Berlin Heidelberg New York Tokyo, pp 104–106

347. Kärrholm J, Selvik G, Elmquist LG, Hansson LI, Jonsson H (1988) Three-dimensional instability of the anterior cruciate deficient knee. J Bone Joint Surg [Br] 70: 777–783

348. Kastert J (1953) Die Verwachsung des Kniegelenkfettkörpers als eigenständiges Krankheitsbild. Chirurg 24: 390–394

349. Katz JW, Fingeroth RJ (1986) The diagnostic accuracy of ruptures of the anterior cruciate ligament comparing the Lachman test, the anterior drawer sign and the pivot shift test in acute and chronic knee injuries. Am J Sports Med 14: 88–91

350. Katz MM, Hungerford DS (1987) Reflex sympathetic dystrophy affecting the knee. J Bone Joint Surg [Br] 69: 797–803

351. Kean DM, Preston BJ, Roebuck EJ, McKim TH, Hawkes RC, Holland GN, Phil M, Moore WS (1983) Nuclear magnetic resonance imaging of the knee: examples of normal anatomy and pathology. Br J Radiol 56: 355–364

352. Keene GCR, Paterson RS (1987) Anterior cruciate instability: meniscal and chondral damage. J Bone Joint Surg [Br] 69: 162

353. Kelly DW, Carter VS, Jobe FW, Kerlan RK (1984) Patellar and quadriceps tendon ruptures - jumper's knee. Am J Sports Med 12: 375–380

354. Kennedy JC, Fowler JP (1971) Medial and lateral instability of the knee - an anatomical and clinical study using stress machines. J Bone Joint Surg [Am] 53: 1257–1270

355. Kennedy JC, Weinberg MW, Wilson AS (1974) The anatomy and function of the anterior cruciate ligament. J Bone Joint Surg [Am] 56: 223–235

356. Kennedy JC (1978) Classification of knee joint instability resulting from ligamentous damage. In: Schulitz KP, Krahl H, Stein WH (eds) Late reconstruction of injured ligaments of the knee. Springer, Berlin Heidelberg New York, pp 19–21

357. Kennedy JC (1978) Anterior subluxation of the lateral tibial plateau In: Schulitz KP, Krahl H, Stein WH (eds) Late reconstruction of injured ligaments of the knee. Springer, Berlin Heidelberg New York, pp 94–97

358. Kennedy JC (1979) The injured adolescent knee. Williams & Wilkins, Baltimore

359. Kerlan RK, Glousman RE (1988) Tibial collateral ligament bursitis. Am J Sports Med 16: 344–346

360. Khasigian HA, Evanski PM, Waugh TR (1978) Body type and rotational laxity of the knee. Clin Orthop 130: 228–232

361. Kirchmayr L (1920) Das Röntgenbild als diagnostisches Hilfsmittel bei der Zerreißung der Kniegelenksbänder. RÖFO 27: 425–426

362. Klein J, Tiling TH, Röddecker K (1986) Vergleichende Untersuchung der arthroskopischen Meniskektomie unter Wasser und unter Gas. In: Tiling T (Hrsg) Arthroskopische Meniskuschirurgie. Enke, Stuttgart (Fortschritte in der Arthroskopie, Bd 2) S 50–53

363. Klein KK (1962) An instrument for testing the medial and lateral ligament stability of the knee. Am J Surg 104: 768–772

364. Klein W, Huth F (1980) Arthroskopie und Histologie von Kniegelenkserkrankungen. Schattauer, Stuttgart New York

365. Klein W (1983) The medial shelf of the knee. A follow-up study. Arch Orthop Trauma Surg 102: 67–72

366. Klein W, Schulitz KP (1983) Arthroscopic meniscectomy: Technique, problems, complications and follow-up results. Arch Orthop Trauma Surg 101: 231–237

367. Kliemann L (1952) Die spontane Abbildung des wirklichen Kniegelenksspaltes. RÖFO 76: 602–606

368. Knopp W, Muhr G, Hesoun H, Neumann K (1986) Konservative oder operative Therapie nach Patellaluxation. Unfallchirurg 89: 463–472

369. Koenig F (1889) Lehrbuch der speciellen Chirurgie, 5. Aufl, Bd III. Hirschwald, Berlin

370. Kohn D, Brückl R, Lobbenhofer P (1985) Kurze technische Mitteilung: Videotechnik und Sterilität bei der Arthroskopie. Z Orthop 123: 897–898

371. König H, Sauter R, Schmitt R (1986) Kernspintomographische Diagnostik von Gelenkveränderungen. Fortschr Röntgenstr 145: 43–48

372. König H, Skalej M, Höntzsch, Aicher K (1988) Kernspintomographie von Knorpel-Knochen-Transplantaten im Kniegelenk: Transplantat-Morphologie und Versuch einer quantitativen Beurteilung der Knorpelschäden. Fortschr Röntgenstr 148: 176–182

373. Krahl H (1980) Jumper's knee - Ätiologie, Differentialdiagnose und therapeutische Möglichkeiten. Orthopäde 9: 193–197

374. Krause W (1874) Histologische Notizen. Centralblatt medicinische Wissenschaften 12: 401–403

375. Kreusch-Brinker R, Friedebold G (1987) Indikationen, Technik und Gefahren der intraartikulären Injektionsbehandlung am Knie. Unfallchirurgie 13: 241–248

376. Krömer K (1942) Der verletzte Meniskus. Maudrich, Wien

377. Kujala UM, Kvist M, Heinonen O (1985) Osgood-Schlatter's disease in adolescent athletes. Am J Sports Med 13: 236–241

378. Kujala UM, Kvist M, Österman K (1986) Knee injuries in athletes. Sports Med 3: 447–460

379. Kunitsch G, Oestern HJ, Meyer G (1983) Die Wertigkeit der Kniearthrographie. Röntgenblätter 33: 48–56

380. Lambiris E, Stoboy H (1981) Thermographie bei Osteosynthesen und Totalendoprothesen des Kniegelenkes mit und ohne Infektion. Z Orthop 119: 521–524

381. Langlotz M, Dexel M (1980) Wie zuverlässig ist die intraoperative Untersuchung des medialen Meniskushinterhorns? Diskrepanz zwischen Arthrographie und Arthrotomie. Z Orthop 118: 868–873

382. Larson RL (1983) Physical examination in the diagnosis of rotatory instability. Clin Orthop 172: 38–44

383. Last RJ (1948) Some anatomical details of the knee joint. J Bone Joint Surg [Br] 30: 383–688

384. Last RJ (1950) The popliteus muscle and the lateral meniscus. J Bone Joint Surg [Br] 32: 93–99

385. Latosiewicz R, Popko J, Wasilewski A, Puchalski Z (1986) Gonylaxometrische Untersuchung der Kniestabilität - Technik und Anwendung. Beitr Orthop Traumatol 33: 420–424

386. Lemaire M (1967) Ruptures anciennes du ligament croisé antérior du genou. J Chir (Paris) 93: 311–320

387. Lemaire M, Miremad C (1983) Anteromedial instability of the knee. Physiology, clinical features and radiological diagnosis. Rev Chir Orthop 69: 3–16

388. Lenggenhager K (1940) Über Genese, Symptomatologie und Therapie des Schubladensymptoms des Kniegelenkes. Zentralbl Chir 67: 1810–1825

389. Lerat JL, Moyen B, Dupre La Tour L, Mainetti E, Lalain JJ, Brunet-Gued E (1988) Measure of laxities by stress radiography and by KT 1000 arthrometer. In: Müller W, Hackenbruch W (eds) Surgery and arthroscopy of the knee. Springer, Berlin Heidelberg New York Tokyo, pp 85–90

390. Leven H (1977) Determination of the sagittal instability of the knee joint. Acta Radiol Diagn (Stockh) 18: 689–697

391. Leven H (1978) Radiologic determination of rotational instability of the knee joint. Acta Radiol Diagn (Stockh) 19: 599–608

392. Levy IM, Torzilli PA, Gould JD, Warren RF (1989) The effect of lateral meniscectomy on the motion of the knee. J Bone Joint Surg [Am] 71: 401–406

393. Lewis SL, Pozo JL, Muirhead-Allwood WFG (1989) Coronal fractures of the lateral femoral condyle. J Bone Joint Surg [Br] 71: 118–120

394. Lindenbaum BL (1981) Complications of knee joint arthroscopy. Clin Orthop 160: 158

395. Lindgren PG, Rauschning W (1979) Clinical and arthrographic studies on the valve mechanism in communicating popliteal cysts. Arch Orthop Trauma Surg 95: 245–250

396. Lingg G, Hering L (1984) Computertomographie und pathogenes Potential der Plica parapatellaris medialis. RÖFO 140: 561–566

396a. Liorzu G (1990) Le genou ligamentaire. Springer, Berlin Heidelberg New York

397. Lipscomb B, Anderson AF (1986) Tears of the anterior cruciate ligament in adolescents. J Bone Joint Surg [Am] 68: 19–28

398. Lobenhoffer P, Posel P, Witt S, Piehler J, Wirth CJ (1987) Distal femoral fixation of the iliotibial tract. Arch Orthop Trauma Surg 106: 285–290

399. Locker B, Beguin J, Vielpeau C, Loyau G (1988) Pigmented villonodular synovitis of the knee: Advantages of arthroscopy. In: Müller W, Hackenbruch W (eds) Surgery and arthroscopy of the knee. Springer, Berlin Heidelberg New York Tokyo, pp 661–665

400. Löhnert J, Raunest J (1985) Arthroskopische Chirurgie des Kniegelenkes. Regensberg & Biermann, Münster

401. Löhnert J, Raunest J (1988) Zur Ätiologie und Pathogenese der Baker- Zyste. Aktuel Chir 23: 21–26

402. Loos WC, Fox JM, Blazina ME, Del Pizzo W, Friedman MJ (1981) Acute posterior cruciate ligament injuries. Am J Sports Med 9: 86–92

403. Losee RE, Johnson TR, Southwick W (1978) Anterior subluxation of the lateral tibial plateau. J Bone Joint Surg [Am] 60: 1915–1030

404. Losee RE (1983) Concepts of the pivot-shift. Clin Orthop 172: 45–51

405. Losee RE (1985) Diagnosis of chronic injury to the anterior cruciate ligament. Orthop Clin North Am 16: 83–97

406. Losee RE (1988) The pivot shift. In: Feagin JA (ed) The crucial ligaments. Diagnosis and treatment of ligamentous injuries about the knee. Churchill Livingstone, New York, pp 301–315

407. Lowe PJ, Saunders GAB (1977) Knee analyser: an objective method of evaluating mediolateral stability of the knee. Med Biol Eng Comput 15: 548–552

408. Lucie HS, Wiedel JD, Messner DG (1984) The acute pivot shift: clinical correlation. Am J Sports Med 12: 189–191

409. Ludolph E, Hierholzer G (1980) Anatomie und Biomechanik des Kapselbandapparates am Kniegelenk. Unfallchirurgie 6: 79–85

410. Lukoschek M, Burr DB, Boyd RD, Schaffler MB, Radin EL (1988) Arthrotomie - präarthrotischer Faktor? Aktuel Traumatol 18: 163–167

411. Lysens RJ, Renson LM, Ostyn MS, Stalpaert G (1983) Intermittent claudication in young athletes: Popliteal artery entrapment syndrome. Am J Sports Med 11: 177–179

412. Lyu SR, Wu JJ (1989) Snapping syndrome caused by the semitendinosus tendon. J Bone Joint Surg [Am] 71: 303–305

413. MacDonald DA, Hutton JF, Kelly IG (1989) Maximal isometric patellofemoral contact force in patients with anterior knee pain. J Bone Joint Surg [Br] 71: 296–299

414. Macnicol MF (1986) The problem knee. Heinemann, London

415. Maddox PA, Garth WP (1986) Tendinitis of the patellar ligament and quadriceps (jumper's knee) as an initial presentation of hyperparathyroidism. J Bone Joint Surg [Am] 68: 288–292

416. Mains DB, Andrews JR, Stonecipher T (1977) Medial and anterior-posterior ligament stability of the human knee, measured with a stress apparatus. Am J Sports Med 5: 144–153

417. Manco LG, Kavanaugh JH, Lozman J, Colman ND, Bilfield BS, Fay JJ (1987) Diagnosis of meniscal tears using high-resolution computed tomography. J Bone Joint Surg [Am] 69: 498–502

418. Mandelbaum BR, Finerman GAM, Reicher MA, Hartzman S, Bassett LW, Gold RH, Rauschning W (1986) Magnetic resonance imaging as a tool for evaluation of traumatic knee injuries. Am J Sports Med 14: 361–370

419. Manning MP, Marshall JH (1987) Aneurysm after arthroscopy. J Bone Joint Surg [Br] 69: 151

420. Marcacci M, Gentili R, Felli L (1979) Alcune osservazioni di anatomia funzionale del compartimento posteriore del ginocchio umano (legamento popliteo obliquo). Ital J Sports Traumatol 1: 269–273

421. Markolf KL, Mensch JS, Amstutz HC (1976) Stiffness and laxity of the knee, the contributions of the supporting structures. J Bone Joint Surg [Am] 58: 583–594

422. Markolf KL, Graff-Radford A, Amstutz HC (1978) In vivo knee stability – a quantitative assessment using an clinical testing apparatus. J Bone Joint Surg [Am] 60: 664–674

423. Markolf KL, Girgis FG, Zelko RR (1981) The role of joint load in knee instability. J Bone Joint Surg [Am] 63: 570–585

424. Markolf KL (1984) Measurement of knee stiffness and laxity in patients with documented absence of the anterior cruciate ligament. J Bone Joint Surg [Am] 66: 242–253

425. Markolf KL (1987) Quantitative examination for anterior cruciate laxity. In: Jackson DW, Drez D (eds) The anterior cruciate deficient knee. Mosby, St. Louis, pp 90–101

426. Markolf KL, Amstutz HC (1987) The clinical relevance of instrumented testing for ACL insufficiency. Experience with the UCLA Clinical Knee Testing Apparatus. Clin Orthop 223: 198–207

427. Marshall JL, Girgis FG, Zelko RR (1972) The biceps femoris tendon and its functional significance. J Bone Joint Surg [Am] 54: 1444–1450

428. Marshall JL, Rubin R (1977) Knee ligament injuries – a standardized and therapeutic approach. Orthop Clin North Am 8: 641–668

429. Marshall JL, Fetto JF, Botero PM (1977) Knee ligament injuries: a standardized evaluation method. Clin Orthop 123: 115–129

430. Martens MA, Mulier JC (1981) Anterior subluxation of the lateral tibial plateau. Arch Orthop Trauma Surg 98: 109–111

431. Marymont JV, Lynch MA, Henning CE (1983) Evaluation of meniscus tears of the knee by radionuclide imaging. Am J Sports Med 11: 432–435

432. Mayer L, Burman MS (1939) Arthroscopy in the diagnosis of menisceal lesions of the knee joint. Am J Surg 43: 501–511

433. Mayer PJ, Micheli LJ (1979) Avulsion of the femoral attachment of the posterior cruciate ligament in an eleven-year-old boy. J Bone Joint Surg [Am] 61: 431–432

434. Mayfield GW (1977) Popliteus tendon tenosynovitis. Am J Sports Med 5: 31–36

435. McCoy GF, Hannon DG, Barr RJ, Templeton J (1987) Vascular injury associated with low-velocity dislocations of the knee. J Bone Joint Surg [Br] 69: 285–287

436. McCoy GF, McCrea JD, Beverland DE, Kernohan WG, Mollan RAB (1987) Vibration arthrography as a diagnostic aid in diseases of the knee. J Bone Joint Surg [Br] 69: 288–293

437. McCrea JD, McCoy GF, Kernohan WG, McClelland CJ, Moolan R (1985) Moderne Tendenzen in der Phonoarthrographie. Z Orthop 123: 13–17

438. McCrea JD, McCoy GF, Kernohan WG, McClelland CJ, Moolan R (1985) Vibrationsarthrographie in der Diagnostik von Kniegelenkskrankheiten. Z Orthop 123: 18–22

439. McCullough RW, Gandsman EJ, Litchman HE, Schatz SL (1988) Dynamic bone scintigraphy in osteochondritis dissecans. Int Orthop 12: 317–322

440. McGinty JB, McCarthy JC (1981) Endoscopic lateral release: A preliminary report. Clin Orthop 158: 120–125

441. McGinty JB (1982) Arthroscopic removal of loose bodies. In: Metcalf R (ed) Symposium on Arthroscopic Knee Surgery. Orthop Clin North Am 13/2: 313–328

442. McIntosh DL, Darby TA (1976) Lateral substitution reconstruction. J Bone Joint Surg [Br] 58: 142

443. McLean ID (1989) Isolated intra-articular popliteus tendon rupture. J Bone Joint Surg [Br] 71: 166

444. McLoad WD, Moschi A, Andrews JR, Hughston JC (1977) Tibial plateau topography. Am J Sports Med 5: 13–18

445. McMaster JH, Weinert CR, Scranton P (1974) Diagnosis and management of isolated anterior cruciate ligament tears. J Trauma 14: 230–235

446. McMaster JH (1975) Isolated posterior cruciate ligament injury: literature review and case reports. J Trauma 15: 1025–1029

447. McPhee IB, Fraser JG (1981) Stress radiography in acute ligamentous injuries of the knee. Injury 12: 383–388

448. Menschik A (1974) Mechanik des Kniegelenkes, Teil 1. Z Orthop 112: 481–495

449. Menschik A (1975) Mechanik des Kniegelenkes, Teil 2. Z Orthop 113: 388–400

450. Menschik A (1974) Mechanik des Kniegelenkes, Teil 3. Sailer, Wien

451. Menschik A (1984) Grundsätzliches zur Kinematik und Selbstverwirklichung der unbekannten biologischen Bewegungssysteme unter besonderer Berücksichtigung des Kniegelenkes. Hefte Unfallheilkd 167: 23–47

452. Menschik A (1985) Persönliche Mitteilung

453. Menschik A (1988) The theory of movement and the modern mode of thought in biology. In: Müller W, Hackenbruch W (eds) Surgery and arthroscopy of the knee. Springer, Berlin Heidelberg New York Tokyo, pp 3-11

454. Menschik A (1988) Biometrie. Springer, Berlin Heidelberg New York Tokyo

455. Menschik A (1989) Persönliche Mitteilung

456. Merk H (1986) Einsatzmöglichkeiten der Sonographie am Bewegungsapparat. Beitr Orthop Traumatol 33: 347-354

457. Meyer H (1853) Die Mechanik des Kniegelenks. Müllers Archiv

458. Meyers MH (1975) Isolated avulsion of the tibial attachment of the posterior cruciate ligament of the knee. J Bone Joint Surg [Am] 57: 669-672

459. Minkhoff J, Shermann O, Bonamo J, Goldman A, Schlesinger I, Firooznia H, Rafii M, Golimbu C (1988) MRI: An assessment of its diagnostic capabilities as it pertains to the knee. Presented at 3rd Congress of European Society of Knee Surgery and Arthroscopy, Amsterdam

460. Mirbey J, Besancenot J, Chambers RT, Durey A, Vichard P (1988) Avulsion fractures of the tibial tuberosity in the adolescent athlete. Am J Sports Med 16: 336-340

461. Mohr W (1987) Pathologie des Bandapparates: Sehnen, Sehnenscheiden, Faszien, Schleimbeutel. Springer, Berlin Heidelberg New York Tokyo

462. Molitor PJA, Dandy DJ (1989) Permanent anterior dislocation of the proximal tibiofibular joint. J Bone Joint Surg [Br] 71: 240-241

463. Moller BN, Krebs B, Jurik AG (1986) Patellar height and patellofemoral congruence. Arch Orthop Trauma Surg 104: 380-381

464. Moore TH, Meyers MH (1977) Apparatus to position knees for varus-valgus stress roentgenogramms. J Bone Joint Surg [Am] 59: 984

465. Moraldo M, Schleberger R (1986) Die Behandlung des arthroskopisch gesicherten basisnahen hinteren Längsrisses des Innen- und Außenmeniskus durch Ruhigstellung. In: Tiling T (Hrsg) Arthroskopische Meniskuschirurgie. Enke, Stuttgart, (Fortschritte in der Arthroskopie, Bd 2) S 115-116

466. Muhr G, Wagner M (1981) Kapsel-Band-Verletzungen des Kniegelenkes - Diagnostikfibel. Springer, Berlin Heidelberg New York

467. Müller W (1975) Die Rotationsinstabilität am Kniegelenk. Hefte Unfallheilkd 125: 51-68

468. Müller W (1979) Neuere Aspekte der funktionellen Anatomie des Kniegelenkes. Hefte Unfallheilkd 129: 131-137

469. Müller W (1980) Allgemeine Diagnostik und Soforttherapie bei Bandverletzungen am Kniegelenk. Unfallheilkunde 83: 389-397

470. Müller W (1982) Das Knie - Form, Funktion und ligamentäre Wiederherstellungschirurgie. Springer, Berlin Heidelberg New York Tokyo

471. Müller W (1984) Pathophysiologie des Kniegelenkes. Hefte Unfallheilkd 167: 48-60

472. Müller W, Biedert R, Hefti F, Jakob RP, Munzinger U, Stäubli HU (1988) OAK knee evaluation - A new way to assess knee ligament injuries. Clin Orthop 232: 37-50

473. Munzinger U, Dubs L, Buchmann R (1985) Das femoropatellare Schmerzsyndrom. Orthopäde 14: 247-260

474. Mysnyk C, Wroble RR, Foster T, Albright JP (1986) Prepatellar bursitis in wrestlers. Am J Sports Med 14: 46-54

475. Nagel DA, Burton DS, Manning J (1977) The dashboard knee injury. Clin Orthop 126: 203-208

476. Nakajima N, Kondo M, Kurosawa H, Fukubayashi T (1979) Insufficiency of the anterior cruciate ligament. Review of 118 cases. Arch Orthop Trauma 95: 233-240

477. Nakamura T, Kurosawa H, Kawahara H, Watari K, Miyashita H (1986) Muscle fibre atrophy in the quadriceps in knee-joint disorders. Arch Orthop Trauma Surg 105: 163-169

478. Naver L, Aalberg JR (1985) Avulsion of the popliteus tendon. Am J Sports Med 13: 423-424

479. Nicholas JA (1973) The five-one-reconstruction for anteromedial instability for the knee. J Bone Joint Surg [Am] 55: 899-922

480. Nicholas JA (1978) Report of the commitee on research and education. Am J Sports Med 6: 295-306

481. Niederdöckl U, Höllwarth M (1982) Zur Problematik des unklaren Hämarthros des Kniegelenkes im Kindesalter. Unfallchirurgie 8: 155-158

482. Nielsen S, Ovesen J, Rasmussen O (1985) The posterior cruciate ligament and rotatory knee instability. Arch Orthop Trauma Surg 104: 53-56

483. Nielsen S, Helmig P (1986) The static stabilizing function of the popliteus tendon in the knee. Arch Orthop Trauma Surg 104: 357-362

484. Nielsen S, Helmig P (1986) Posterior instability of the knee joint - an experimental study. Arch Orthop Trauma Surg 105: 121-125

485. Noesberger B (1975) Untersuchung des Kniegelenkes. Hefte Unfallheilkd 125: 86-95

486. Noesberger B (1981) Grundlagen der Diagnostik frischer und veralteter Kapselbandläsionen des Kniegelenkes. In: Jäger M, Hackenbroch MH, Refior HJ (Hrsg) Kapselbandläsionen des Kniegelenkes. Thieme, Stuttgart New York, S 78-87

487. Norwood LA, Cross MJ (1977) The intercondylarshelf and the anterior cruciate ligament. Am J Sports Med 5: 171-176

488. Norwood LA, Cross MJ (1979) Anterior cruciate ligament, functional anatomy of its bundles in rotatory instabilities. Am J Sports Med 7: 23-26

489. Nottage WM, Sprague NF, Auerbach BJ, Shahriaree H (1983) The medial patellar plica syndrome. Am J Sports Med 11: 211-214

490. Noyes FR, Grood ES, Butler DL, Raterman L (1980) Knee ligament test. What do they really mean? Phys Ther 60: 1578-1581

491. Noyes FR, Mooar PA, Matthews DS (1983) The symptomatic anterior cruciate deficient knee. Part I: The long-term functional disability in athletically active individuals. J Bone Joint Surg [Am] 65: 154-162

492. Noyes FR (1985) The variable functional disability of the anterior cruciate ligament - deficient knee. Orthop Clin North Am 16: 47-67

493. Noyes F, Grood E, Stowers S (1985) A biomechanical analysis of knee ligament injuries producing posterolateral subluxation. Presentation at the 4th Congress of Society of knee, Salzburg 12.-17.5.1985

494. Noyes FR, Grood ES (1988) Diagnosis of knee ligament injuries: Clinical concepts. In: Feagin JA (ed) The crucial ligaments. Diagnosis and treatment of ligamentous injuries about the knee. Churchill Livingstone, New York, pp 261–285

495. Noyes FR, Grood ES, Torzilli PA (1989) The definitions of terms for motion and position of the knee and injuries of the ligaments. J Bone Joint Surg [Am] 71: 465–472

496. Nyga W (1970) Röntgendarstellung von Kreuzbandverletzungen des Kniegelenkes. Z Orthop Grenzgeb 107: 340–344

497. O'Brien W, Friederich N, Müller W, Henning C, Jackson R (1988) Functional anatomy of the cruciate ligaments and their substitutes. Part I: The anterior cruciate ligament. Presented at 3rd Congress of European Society of Knee Surgery and Arthroscopy, Amsterdam

498. O'Connor B, McConnaughey S (1978) The structure and innervation of cat knee menisci and their relation to a „sensory hypothesis" of meniscal function. Am J Anat 153: 431–442

499. O'Connor's textbook of arthroscopic surgery. (1984) Shahriaree H (ed) Lippincott, Philadelphia

500. Odensten M, Gillquist J (1985) Functional anatomy of the anterior cruciate ligament and a rationale for reconstruction. J Bone Joint Surg [Am] 67: 257–262

501. Odensten M, Lysholm J, Gillquist J (1985) The course of partial anterior cruciate ligament ruptures. Am J Sports Med 13: 183–186

502. O'Donoghue DH (1950) Surgical treatment of fresh injuries to the major ligaments of the knee. J Bone Joint Surg [Am] 32: 721–738

503. O'Donoghue DH (1961) Injury to the ligaments of the knee. Am J Orthop 3: 46–52

504. Ogata K, McCarthy JA, Dunlap J, Manske PR (1988) Pathomechanics of posterior sag of the tibia in posterior cruciate deficient knees. Am J Sports Med 16: 630–636

505. Ogilvie-Harris DJ, Jackson RW (1984) The arthroscopic treatment of chondromalazia patellae. J Bone Joint Surg [Am] 66: 660–665

506. Ogilvie-Harris DJ, Roscoe M (1987) Reflex sympathetic dystrophy of the knee. J Bone Joint Surg [Br] 69: 804–806

507. Oliver JH, Coughlin LP (1987) Objective knee evaluation using the genucom knee analysis system. Am J Sports Med 15: 571–578

508. Osternig LR, Bates BT, James SL, Larson RL (1978) Rotary mechanics after pes anserinus transplant. Am J Sports Med 6: 173–179

509. Otto R, Menninger H (1977) Die Diagnose von Weichteilprozessen der Knieregion mit Hilfe der Xerographie. Röntgenblätter 30: 79–83

510. Paar O, Fürbringer W, Bernett P (1984) Verletzungen des Innenmeniskus- Hinterhorns und des hinteren Schrägbandes. Chirurg 55: 49–52

511. Paar O, Reiser M, Bernett P (1985) Stellenwert der Arthrographie in der Diagnostik unklarer Kniebeschwerden - Erfahrungen zur Läsion der Meniskusansatzzone. Unfallchirurg 88: 452–456

512. Pagenstecher A (1903) Die isolierte Zerreißung der Kreuzbänder des Kniegelenkes. Dtsch Med Wochenschr 47: 872–875

513. Palmer I (1938) On the injuries to the ligaments of the knee joint: A clinical study. Acta Chir Scand (Suppl) 53: 1–283

514. Palmer I (1958) Pathophysiology of the medial ligament of the knee joint. Acta Chir Scand 115: 312–318

515. Parolie JM, Bergfeld JA (1986) Long-term results of nonoperative treatment of isolated posterior cruciate ligament injuries in the athlete. Am J Sports Med 14: 35–38

516. Pässler H, Henkemeyer H, Burri C (1972) Funktionelle Behandlung nach Bandnaht und -plastik am Kniegelenk. Langenbecks Arch Chir Suppl Chir Forum: 51–53

517. Pässler H, März S (1986) Der radiologische Lachman-Test - eine einfache und sichere Methode zum Nachweis von Kreuzbandschäden. Unfallchirurgie 12: 295–300

518. Pässler H (1989) Persönliche Mitteilung

518a. Pässler H, Michel D (1990) Persönliche Mitteilung

519. Patel D (1981) Proximal approaches of arthroscopic surgery of the knee. Am J Sports Med 9: 296–303

520. Patel D (1982) Superior lateral approach to the arthroscopic meniscectomy. In: Metcalf R (ed) Symposium on Arthroscopic Knee Surgery. Orthop Clin North Am 13/2: 299–306

521. Paulos LE, Rosenberg TD, Drawbert, Manning J, Abbott P (1987) Infrapatellar contracture syndrome. Am J Sports Med 15: 331–341

522. Pavlow H, Hirschy JC, Torg JS (1979) Computed tomography of the cruciate ligaments. Radiology 132: 389–393

523. Peterson L, Pitman MI, Gold J (1984) The active pivot shift: the role of the popliteus muscle. Am J Sports Med 12: 313–317

524. Pfeil E (1981) Das Femoropatellargelenk. Barth, Leipzig

525. Pförringer W (1982) Hämarthros und Kreuzbänder - biomechanische Untersuchungen. Unfallchirurgie 8: 353–367

526. Pförringer W (1982) Hämarthros und Kreuzbänder - morphologische Untersuchungen. Unfallchirurgie 8: 368–378

527. Poigenfürst J (1960) Technik und Bedeutung gehaltener Röntgenbilder. Chir Prax 4: 467–488

528. Poigenfürst J (1973) Gehaltene Röntgenaufnahmen. Orthop Prax 3: 45–63

529. Polly DW, Callaghan JJ, Sikes RA, McCabe JM, McMahon K, Savory CG (1988) The accuracy of selective magnetic imaging compared with the findings of arthroscopy of the knee. J Bone Joint Surg [Am] 70: 192–198

530. Pope MH, Crowninshield R, Miller R, Johnson R (1976) The static and dynamic behavior of the human knee in vivo. J Biomech 9: 449–452

531. Pope MH, Johnson RJ, Brown DW, Tighe C (1979) The role of the musculature in injuries of the medial

collateral ligament. J Bone Joint Surg [Am] 61: 398–402

532. Pun WK, Chow SP, Chan KC, Ip FK, Leong JCY (1988) Effusions in the knee in elderly patients who were operated on for fracture of the hip. J Bone Joint Surg [Am] 70: 117–118

533. Quellet R, Levesque HP, Laurin CA (1969) The ligamentous stability of the knee. Can Med Assoc J 100: 45–50

534. Rauber A (1944) Ein wenig bekanntes Röntgensymptom bei älteren Meniskusaffektionen. Z Orthop 37: 1–4

535. Rauschning W, Lindgren PG (1979) The clinical significance of the valve mechanism in communicating popliteal cysts. Arch Orthop Trauma Surg 95: 251–256

536. Ravelli A (1949) Zum Röntgenbild des menschlichen Kniegelenkes. RÖFO 71: 614–619

537. Ray JM, Clancy WG, Lemon RA (1988) Semimembranosus tendinitis: An overlooked cause of medial knee pain. Am J Sports Med 16: 347–351

538. Rehm KE, Schultheis KH, Ecke H (1986) Technik und Indikation der arthroskopischen Kreuzbandplastik. Hefte Unfallheilkd 181: 805–809

539. Reichelt A (1983) Die klinische Diagnostik des retropatellaren Knorpelschadens. In: Küsswetter W, Reichelt A (Hrsg) Der retropatellare Knorpelschaden. Thieme, Stuttgart New York

539a. Reicher MA, Hartzmann S, Duckwiler GR, Bassett LW, Anderson LJ, Gold RH (1986) Menical injuries: Detection using MR imaging. Radiology 166: 753–757

540. Reider B, Clancy W, Langer LO (1984) Diagnosis of cruciate ligament injury using single contrast arthrography. Am J Sports Med 12: 451–454

541. Reiser M, Rupp N, Karpf PM (1980) Die Darstellung der Kreuzbänder durch die xeroradiographische Tomographie. RÖFO 132: 316–319

542. Reiser M, Rupp N, Karpf PM, Feuerbach ST, Paar O (1982) Erfahrungen mit der CT-Arthrographie der Kreuzbänder des Kniegelenkes. RÖFÖ 137: 372–379

543. Reiser M, Rupp N, Pfänder K, Schepp S, Lukas P (1986) Die Darstellung von Kreuzbandläsionen durch die MR-Tomographie. RÖFO 145: 193–198

544. Reiser M, Lehner K, Zacher J, Rupp N, Heizer K, Weigert F (1986) MR- Tomographie bei Gelenkerkrankungen. Darstellung der normalen und verdickten Synovialmembran. Röntgenpraxis 39: 300–305

545. Reiser M, Bongartz G, Erlemann R, Strobel M, Pauly T, Gebert K, Stoeber U, Peters PE (1988) Magnetic resonance in cartilaginous lesions of the knee with three-dimensional gradient-echo imaging. Skeletal Radiol 17: 465–471

545a. Reiser M (1989) Persönliche Mitteilung

546. Renström P, Arms SW, Stanwyck TS, Johnson RJ, Pope MH (1986) Strain within the anterior cruciate ligament during hamstring and quadriceps activity. Am J Sports Med 14: 83–87

547. Resnik D, Niwayama G (eds) (1988) Diagnosis of bone and joint disorders. Saunders, Philadelphia London Toronto

548. Richter H (1948) Muskulär bedingte Knieschmerzen. Chirurg 19: 451–458

549. Ricklin P (1976) Spätergebnisse nach Meniskektomie. Hefte Unfallheilkd 129: 51–58

550. Ricklin P, Rüttimann A, Del Buono MS (1980) Die Meniskusläsion. Thieme, Stuttgart New York

551. Rippstein J (1983) Prospekt Firma F Scholz X-ray Corp Needham Heights, MA (USA)

552. Ritchey SJ (1960) Ligamentous disruption of the knee. A review with analysis of 28 cases. US Armed Forces Med J 11: 167–176

553. Ritter U (1952) Zur Klinik und Röntgendiagnose der Meniskusverkalkungen. Chirurg 23: 22–27

554. Robert (1855) Untersuchungen über Anatomie und Mechanik des Kniegelenkes. Rickersche Buchhandlung, Giessen

555. Rodriguez M, Suezawa Y, Jacob HAC (1981) Experimentelle Untersuchungen zur Diagnose des Kapselbandapparates. In: Jäger M, Hackenbroch MH, Refior HJ (Hrsg) Kapselbandläsionen des Kniegelenkes. Thieme, Stuttgart New York, S 93–97

556. Röhr E (1988) Kniegelenksonographie. Thieme, Stuttgart New York

557. Rombold C (1936) Osteochondritis dissecans of the patella. A case report. J Bone Joint Surg [Am] 18: 230–231

558. Rosenberg TD, Rasmussen GL (1984) The function of the anterior cruciate ligament during anterior drawer and Lachman's testing. Am J Sports Med 12: 318–322

559. Rosenberg TD, Paulos LE, Parker RD, Coward DB, Scott SM (1988) The forty- five-degree posteroanterior flexion weight-bearing radiograph of the knee. J Bone Joint Surg [Am] 70: 1479–1483

560. Ross KR, Glasgow MMS (1984) The suprapatellar plica. J Bone Joint Surg [Br] 66: 280

561. Ross RF (1932) A quantitative study of rotation of the knee joint in man. Anat Rec 52: 209–223

562. Rovere GD, Nichols AW (1985) Frequency, associated factors and treatment of breaststroker's knee in competitive swimmers. Am J Sports Med 13: 99–104

563. Ruetsch H, Morscher E (1977) Measurement of the rotatory stability of the knee joint. In: Chapchal G (ed) Injuries of the ligaments and their repair. Thieme, Stuttgart New York, S 116–122

564. Sandberg R, Balkfors B (1988) Reconstruction of the anterior cruciate ligament. A 5-year follow-up. Acta Orthop Scand 59: 288–293

565. Sandholzer K, Häfele H (1988) Röntgenologisches Zeichen der vorderen Kreuzbandinsuffizienz. Sportverl Sportschaden 4: 106–111

566. Sandow MJ, Goodfellow JW (1985) The natural history of the anterior knee pain in adolescents. J Bone Joint Surg [Br] 67: 36–38

567. Sarkar K, Buckley C, Uhthoff (1986) Liposarcoma simulating a baker's cyst: a case study. Arch Orthop Trauma Surg 105: 316–319

568. Satku K, Chew CN, Seow H (1984) Posterior cruciate ligament injuries. Acta Orthop Scand 55: 26–29

569. Schabus R, Wagner M (1984) Chirurgische Anatomie des Kniegelenkes. Hefte Unfallheilkd 167: 10–22

570. Schaer H (1938) Der Meniskusschaden. Thieme, Leipzig

571. Scharf W, Schabus R, Wagner M (1981) Das laterale Kapselzeichen. Unfallheilkunde 84: 518–523

572. Scharf W, Weinstabl R, Orthner E (1985) Anatomische Unterscheidung und klinische Bedeutung zweier verschiedener Anteile des M. vastus medialis. Acta Anat 123: 108-111

573. Scharf W, Weinstabl R, Firbas W (1986) Anatomische Untersuchungen am Streckapparat des Kniegelenkes und ihre klinische Relevanz. Unfallchirurg 89: 456-462

574. Scheuba G (1978) Die gehaltene Aufnahme. Telos, Griesheim

575. Schlepckow P, Ernst HU (1988) Congenital absence of cruciate ligaments: clinical, radiological and arthroscopic aspects. In: Müller W, Hackenbruch W (eds) Surgery and arthroscopy of the knee. Springer, Berlin Heidelberg New York Tokyo, pp 116-120

576. Schlüter K, Becker R (1954) Fehlform des äußeren Meniskus als Ursache des schnappenden Kniegelenkes. Chirurg 25: 499-505

577. Schmid A, Schmid F (1988) Objektivierbarkeit des Lachman-Testes durch Arthro-Sonographie. Unfallchirurg 91: 70-76

578. Schmidt M, Thiel HJ, Lohkamp F, Bisping B (1982) Diagnostischer Aussagewert der Arthrographie des Kniegelenkes. Schnetztor, Konstanz

579. Schmitt O, Mittelmaier H (1978) The biomechanical significance of the vastus medialis and lateralis muscles. Arch Orthop Trauma Surg 91: 291-295

580. Schuler M, Naegele M, Lienemann A, Münch O, Siuda S, Hahn D, Lissner J (1987) Die Wertigkeit der hochauflösenden CT und der Kernspintomographie im Vergleich zu den Standardverfahren bei der Diagnostik von Meniskusläsionen. Fortschr Röntgenstr 146: 391-397

581. Schulitz KP, Hille E, Kochs W (1983) The importance of the mediopatellar synovial plica for the chondromalazia patellae. Arch Orthop Trauma Surg 102: 37-44

582. Schulitz KP, Klein W, Hille E (1985) Meniskektomie – totale, partielle, offene oder geschlossene Operation? Z Orthop 123: 837-840

583. Schultz RA, Müller DC, Kerr CS, Micheli L (1984) Mechanoreceptors in human cruciate ligaments. An histological study. J Bone Joint Surg [Am] 66: 1072-1076

584. Schutzer SF, Gossling HR (1984) The treatment of reflex sympathetic dystrophy syndrome. J Bone Joint Surg [Am] 66: 625-629

585. Schutte MJ, Dabezies EJ, Zimny ML, Happel LT (1987) Neural anatomy of the human anterior cruciate ligament. J Bone Joint Surg [Am] 69: 243-247

586. Schwarz C, Blazina ME, Sisto DJ, Hirsh LC (1988) The results of operative treatment of osteochondritis dissecans of the patella. Am J Sports Med 16: 522-529

587. Sciuk J (1989) Persönliche Mitteilung

588. Segond P (1879) Recherches cliniques et expérimentales sur les épanchements sanguins du genou par entorse. Prog Med 7: 297-299, 319-321, 340-341, 379-381, 400-401, 419-421

589. Seybold K (1988) Szintigraphische Infektdiagnostik mit monoklonalen Antigranulozyten-Antikörpern. Nuklearmedizin 2: 101-108

590. Shelbourne DK, Benedict F, McCarroll JR, Rettig AC (1989) Dynamic posterior shift test. An adjuvant in evaluation of posterior tibial subluxation. Am J Sports Med 17: 275-277

591. Sherman OH, Fox JM, Snyder SJ, Del Pizzo W, Friedman MC, Ferkel RD, Lawley MJ (1986) Arthroscopy - „No-problem surgery". J Bone Joint Surg [Am] 68: 256-265

592. Shibata T, Shiraoka K, Takubo N (1986) Comparison between arthroscopic and open synovectomy for the knee in rheumatoid arthritis. Arch Orthop Trauma Surg 105: 257-262

593. Shino K, Ohta N, Horibe S, Ono K (1984) In vivo measurement of a-p instability in the ACL-disrupted knees and in the postoperative knees. Trans Orthop Res Soc 9: 394-396

594. Shino K, Horibe S, Ono K (1987) The voluntarily evoked posterolateral drawer sign in the knee with posterolateral instability. Clin Orthop 215: 179-186

595. Shino K, Inoue M, Horibe S, Nakamura H, Ono K (1987) Measurement of anterior instability of the knee. J Bone Joint Surg [Br] 69: 608-613

596. Shoemaker SC, Markolf KL (1982) In vivo rotatory knee stability. J Bone Joint Surg [Am] 64: 208-216

597. Shoemaker SC, Markolf KL (1986) The role of the meniscus in the anteriorposterior stability of the loaded anterior cruciate deficient knee. J Bone Joint Surg [Am] 68: 71-78

598. Siebert W, Kohn D, Siebert B, Wirth CJ (1988) Was kann die Infrarot- Thermographie bei der Diagnostik und Therapiekontrolle am Kniegelenk leisten? Orthop Prax 18: 321-323

599. Siebert W, Kohn D, Münch EO, Wirth CJ (1988) Was kann die Thermographie bei der Diagnose der Chondropathia patellae leisten? Orthop Prax 18: 143-144

600. Silva I, Siler DM (1988) Tears of the meniscus as revealed by magnetic resonance imaging. J Bone Joint Surg [Am] 70: 199-202

601. Simonsen O, Jensen J, Mouritsen P, Lauritzen J (1984) The accuracy of clinical examination of injury in the knee joint. Injury 16: 96-101

602. Skalej M, Klose U, Küper K (1988) Optimierte Untersuchungstechnik von Meniskopathien durch kernspintomographisches 3 D-imaging bei 1, 5 Tesla. Fortschr Röntgenstr 148: 183-188

603. Skoff H (1985) Verletzungen des vorderen Kreuzbandes: ein offenes Kapitel? Orthopäde 14: 64-68

604. Skoglund S (1973) Joint receptors and kinaesthesis. In: Iggo A (ed) Somatosensory system, vol 2. Springer, Berlin Heidelberg New York, pp 111-136

605. Slocum DB, Larson RL (1966) Rotatory instability of the knee. J Bone Joint Surg [Am] 48: 1221

606. Slocum DB, Larson RL (1968) Rotatory instability of the knee. J Bone Joint Surg [Am] 50: 211-225

607. Slocum DB, James SL, Larson RL, Singer KM (1976) Clinical test for anterolateral instability of the knee. Clin Orthop 118: 63-69

608. Small NC (1986) Complications in arthroscopy: The knee and other joints. Arthroscopy 2: 253-258

609. Small NC (1988) Complications in arthroscopic surgery performed by experienced arthroscopists. Arthroscopy 4: 215-221

610. Smillie IS (1985) Kniegelenksverletzungen. Enke, Stuttgart

611. Sodem SA (1985) Computerized Accurate Ligament Tester C.A.L.T. Sodemsystems, Genf

612. Sommerlath KG, Gillquist J (1988) Evaluation of sagittal knee instability with two measuring devices. Communication at 3rd Congress of European Society of Knee Surgery and Arthroscopy, Amsterdam

613. Sonnenschein A (1952) Biologie, Pathologie und Therapie der Gelenke dargestellt am Kniegelenk. Schwabe, Basel

614. Soudry M, Lanir A, Angel D, Roffman M, Kaplan N, Mendes DG (1986) Anatomy of the normal knee as seen by magnetic resonance imaging. J Bone Joint Surg [Br] 68: 117–120

615. Souryal TO, Moore HA, Evans JP (1988) Bilaterality in anterior cruciate ligament injuries: Associated intercondylar notch stenosis. Am J Sports Med 16: 449–454

616. Southmayd W, Quigley TB (1982) The forgotten popliteus muscle. Clin Orthop 164: 9–12

617. Sprague NF (1981) Arthroscopic debridement for degenerative knee joint disease. Clin Orthop 160: 118–123

618. Sprague RB, Tipton CM, Flatt AE, Asprey GM (1966) Evaluation of a photographic method for measuring leg abduction and adduction. J Am Phys Ther Assoc 46: 1068–1078

619. Sprague RB, Asprey GM (1965) Photographic method for measuring knee stability: a preliminary report. J Am Phys Ther Assoc 45: 1055–1058

620. Stankovic P, Zürcher K, Stuhler TH, Heise A (1979) Zur Röntgendiagnostik von Kapselbandschäden am Kniegelenk. Chirurg 50: 658–660

621. Stäubli HU, Jakob RP, Noesberger B (1981) Experimentelle Grundlagen zur Diagnostik der posterolateralen Knierotationsinstabilität. In: Jäger M, Hackenbroch MH, Refior HJ (Hrsg) Kapselbandläsionen des Kniegelenkes. Thieme, Stuttgart New York, S 109–116

622. Stäubli HU, Jakob RP, Noesberger B (1988) Translation and rotation in knee instability : a prospective stress radiographic analysis with the knee in extension. In: Müller W, Hackenbruch W (eds) Surgery and arthroscopy of the knee. Springer, Berlin Heidelberg New York Tokyo, pp 82–83

623. Stedtfeld HW, Strobel M (1983) Ein neues Haltegerät zur Anfertigung gehaltener Röntgenaufnahmen des Kniegelenkes. Unfallheilkunde 86: 230–235

624. Stedtfeld HW, Strobel M (1983) Zur Wahl gehaltener Ausmeßverfahren für gehaltene Röntgenaufnahmen des Kniegelenkes. Unfallheilkunde 86: 463–471

625. Stedtfeld HW, Strobel M (1984) Beitrag zur Frage der posteromedialen Instabilität des Kniegelenkes. Unfallheilkunde 87: 290–297

626. Steinbrück K (1987) Epidemiologie von Sportverletzungen - 15-Jahres- Analyse einer sportorthopädischen Ambulanz. Sportverl Sportschaden 1: 2–12

627. Steinbrück K, Wiehmann JC (1988) Untersuchung des Kniegelenks - Wertigkeit klinischer Befunde unter arthroscopischer Kontrolle. Z Orthop 126: 289–295

628. Steiner ME, Grana WA, Chillag K, Schelberg-Karnes E (1986) The effect of exercise on anterior-posterior knee laxity. Am J Sports Med 14: 24–29

629. Steinmann B, Gitzelmann R (1984) Vererbte Krankheiten mit Bandlaxität. Orthopäde 13: 9–18

630. Stickland A (1984) Examination of the knee joint. Phys Ther 70: 144–150

631. Stoltze D, Harms J, Böttger E, Heckl RW (1982) Der Knieschmerz als Erstsymptom bei retroperitonealen Raumforderungen. Z Orthop 120: 10–13

632. Strobel M, Stedtfeld HW (1986) Die gehaltene Röntgenuntersuchung des Kniegelenkes - eine Bestandsaufnahme. Unfallchirurg 89: 272–279

633. Strobel M, Stedtfeld HW, Stenzel H (1986) Die mikroprozessorgestützte dreidimensionale Darstellung von Kapselbandinstabilitäten des Kniegelenkes. Hefte Unfallheilkd 181: 144–150

634. Strobel M, Stedtfeld HW, Neumann HS (1988) Ein aktiver klinischer Test zur Differenzierung einer hinteren Schublade bei sagittaler Instabilität. Chir Prax 38: 227–234

635. Strobel M, Eichhorn J (1988) Komplikationen bei der Arthroskopie. In: Chassaing V, Parier J (Hrsg) Arthroskopie des Kniegelenkes - Diagnostik und operative Therapie. Deutscher Ärzteverlag, Köln

636. Strobel M, Stedtfeld HW, Stenzel H (1987) Pathomechanik der anteromedialen Rotationsinstabilität des Kniegelenkes in ihren verschiedenen Verletzungsgraden. Hefte Unfallheilkd 189: 119–128

637. Strobel M, Eichhorn J, Schießler W (1989) Arthroskopische Untersuchung des Kniegelenkes. Deutscher Ärzteverlag, Köln

638. Stuhler TH (1978) Funktionelle Stenose: Pathogenetisches Prinzip des Ganglions. Arch Orthop Trauma Surg 93: 43–48

639. Suezawa J, Rodriguez M, Jakob HAC, Dexel M (1981) Schonende Streßaufnahmen bei frischen Knietraumen. Orthop Prax 11: 909–913

640. Sutker AN, Barber FA, Jackson DW, Pagliano JW (1985) Iliotibial band syndrome in distance runners. Sports Med 2: 447–451

641. Swiontkowski MF, Schlehr F, Sanders R, Limbird TA, Pou A, Collins JC (1988) Direct, real time measurement of meniscal blood flow. Am J Sports Med 16: 429–433

642. Sylvin LE (1975) A more exact measurement of the sagittal stability of the knee joint. Acta Orthop Scand 46: 1008–1011

643. Takagi K (1933) Practical experiences using Takagi's arthroscope. J Jap Orthop Assoc 8: 132

644. Takagi K (1939) The arthroscope. J Jap Orthop Assoc 14: 359–441

645. Tamea CD, Henning CE (1981) Pathomechanics of the pivot-shift maneuver. An instant center analysis. Am J Sports Med 9: 31–37

646. Tegner Y, Lysholm J, Gillquist J (1988) Evaluation of knee ligament injuries. In: Müller W, Hackenbruch W (eds) Surgery and arthroscopy of the knee. Springer, Berlin Heidelberg New York Tokyo, pp 123–129

647. Teichert G (1955) Beitrag zur Röntgenbildanalyse des Kniegelenkes. Röntgenblätter 8: 4–8

648. Teitge RA (1988) Stress x-rays for patellofemoral instability. Communication at 3rd Congress of Europe-

an Society of Knee Surgery and Arthroscopy, Amsterdam

649. Tegner Y, Lysholm J, Lysholm M, Gillquist J (1986) A performance test to monitor rehabilitation and evaluate anterior cruciate ligament injuries. Am J Sports Med 14: 156-159

650. Terry GC (1985) Associated joint pathology in the anterior cruciate ligament - deficient knee. Orthop Clin North Am 16: 29-39

651. Terry GC, Hughston JC, Norwood LA (1986) The anatomy of the iliopatellar band and the iliotibial tract. Am J Sports Med 14: 39-45

652. Thomas NP, Jackson AM, Aichroth PM (1985) Congenital absence of the anterior cruciate ligament. J Bone Joint Surg [Br] 67: 572-575

653. Thurner J, Marcacci M, Felli L (1981) Kinästhesie. Z Orthop 119: 301-305

654. Tibone JE, Antich TJ, Perry J, Moynes D (1988) Functional analysis of untreated and reconstructed posterior cruciate ligament. Am J Sports Med 16: 217-223

655. Tiling T, Nasse GV, Sattel W, Schmid A (1984) Der arthroskopische Befund beim Hämarthros bei frischer und alter vorderer Kreuzbandruptur. Langenbecks Arch Chir 364: 329-330

656. Tiling T (1986) Operative Arthroskopie beim Hämarthros des Kniegelenkes. Hefte Unfallheilkd 181: 782-784

657. Tiling T, Röddecker K (1986) Knieinstabilität und Meniskusschaden. In: Tiling T (Hrsg) Arthroskopische Meniskuschirurgie. Enke, Stuttgart (Fortschritte in der Arthroskopie, Bd 2) S 101-107

658. Tillmann B, Blauth M, Schleicher A (1981) Zugverspannungen der Patella In: Jäger M, Hackenbroch MH, Refior HJ (Hrsg) Kapselbandläsionen des Kniegelenkes. Thieme, Stuttgart New York, S 68-73

659. Tittel K, Kotter M, Schauwecker F (1984) Zur Messung von Kniegelenksinstabilitäten in sagittaler Richtung. Unfallchirurg 10: 316-321

660. Toft J (1985) Die arthroskopische vordere Kreuzbandplastik mit Dacron und Lyodura in „over-the-top"-Technik. In: Hofer H (Hrsg) Fortschritte in der Arthroskopie. Enke, Stuttgart, S 167-171

661. Torg JS, Conrad W, Kalen V (1976) Clinical diagnosis of anterior cruciate ligament instability in the athletes. Am J Sports Med 4: 84-91

662. Torzilli P, Greenberg RL, Insall J (1981) An in vivo biomechanical evaluation of anterior-posterior motion of the knee - roentgenographic measurement technique, stress machine and stable population. J Bone Joint Surg [Am] 63: 960-968

663. Townsend MA, Izak M, Jackson RW (1977) Total motion knee goniometry. J Biomech 10: 183-193

664. Tretter H (1928) Beiträge zur Biomechanik des Kniegelenkes. Dtsch Z Chir 212: 93-100

665. Trickey EL (1968) Rupture of the posterior cruciate ligament of the knee. J Bone Joint Surg [Br] 50: 334

666. Trickey EL (1978) Instability of the knee joint. J Bone Joint Surg [Br] 60: 4-5

667. Trickey EL (1980) Injuries of the posterior cruciate ligament. Clin Orthop 147: 76-81

668. Trillat A (1962) Lésions traumatique du ménisque interne du genu. Classement anatomique et diagnostic clinique. Rev Chir Orthop 48: 551-563

669. Trillat A (1978) Posterolateral instability. In: Schulitz KP, Krahl H, Stein WH (eds) Late reconstructions of injured ligaments of the knees. Springer, Berlin Heidelberg New York, pp 99-103

670. Tudisco C, Conteduca F, Puddu G (1988) Synovial hemangioma of the meniscal wall simulating a meniscal cyst. Am J Sports Med 16: 191-192

671. Turner DA, Prodromos CC, Petasnick JP, Clark JW (1985) Acute injury of the ligaments of the knee: magnetic resonance evaluation. Radiology 154: 717-722

672. Turner PG, Grinshaw PN (1987) Measurement of the instability of unstable knees. J Bone Joint Surg [Br] 69: 160

673. Valentin B (1961) Die erste Beschreibung der Kniegelenksmeniskusläsion. Arch Orthop Unfallchir 52: 666-670

674. Van Dijk R (1983) The behaviour of the cruciate ligaments of the human knee. Universität Nijmegen, Niederlande

675. Vanni M (1986) Die normale Anatomie der Kniescheibe im hohen Lebensalter. Z Orthop Grenzgeb 124: 201-204

676. Vaubel J (1938) Die Endoskopie des Kniegelenkes. Zentralbl Rheumaforsch 1: 210-213

677. Volkov VS (1971) Apparatus for determing rupture of the anterior cruciate ligament. Vestn Khir 106: 135-137

678. Vollbrecht (1898) Über umschriebene Binnenverletzungen des Kniegelenkes. Bruns Beitr Klin Chir 21: 216-283

679. Vollmar J, Benz K (1960) Der Knieanprall und seine Verletzungen bei Auto- und Motorradfahrern. Arch Orthop Unfallchir 52: 438-459

680. Wagner M, Schabus R (1980) Anatomie des Kniegelenkes. Hollinek, Wien

681. Wagner M, Schabus R (1981) Das laterale Pivot-shift Phänomen. Untersuchungen am Leichenknie nach artifiziellen Kapselbandläsionen. In: Jäger M, Hakkenbruch MH, Refior HJ (Hrsg) Kapselbandläsionen des Kniegelenkes. Thieme, Stuttgart New York, S 98-103

682. Waldrop JI, Broussard TS (1984) Disruption of the anterior cruciate ligament in a three-year-old child. J Bone Joint Surg [Am] 66: 1113-1114

683. Walker DM, Kennedy JC (1980) Occult knee ligament injuries associated with femoral shaft fractures. Am J Sports Med 8: 172-174

684. Walsh ME, Bennet GC, Gaballa M (1988) McMurray's test and joint laxity in the normal child. J Bone Joint Surg [Br] 70: 857

685. Wang JB, Walker PS (1974) Rotatory laxity of the human knee joint. J Bone Joint Surg [Am] 56: 161-170

686. Wang JB, Rubin RM, Marshall JL (1975) A mechanism of isolated anterior cruciate ligament rupture. J Bone Joint Surg [Am] 57: 411-413

687. Wang JK, Johnson KA, Ilstrup DM (1985) Sympathetic blocks for reflex sympathetic dystrophy. Pain 23: 13-17

688. Warren LF, Marshall JL, Girgis FG (1974) The prime static stabilizer of the medial side of the knee. J Bone Joint Surg [Am] 56: 665-674

689. Warren LF, Marshall JL (1979) The supporting structures and layers on the medial side of the knee. J Bone Joint Surg [Am] 61: 56-62

690. Warren LF (1985) Initial evaluation and management of acute anterior cruciate ligament ruptures. In: Finerman G (ed) American Academy of Orthopedic Surgeons. Symposium on Sportsmedicine, The knee. Mosby, St. Louis, pp 212-221

691. Watanabe M, Takeda S (1953) On the popularization of arthroscopy. J Jap Orthop Assoc 27: 258

692. Watanabe M (1954) The development and present status of the arthroscope. J Jap Med Instr 25: 11

693. Watanabe M, Takeda S, Ikeuchi H (1957) Atlas of arthroscopy. Igaku Shoin, Tokyo

694. Weatherwax JR (1981) Anterior drawer sign. Clin Orthop 154: 318-319

695. Weber M (1983) Das Pterygium. Enke, Stuttgart

696. Weber W, Weber E (1836) Mechanik der menschlichen Gehwerkzeuge. Dieterichsche Buchhandlung, Göttingen

697. Weh L (1988) Die überdehnte Kniescheibensehne beim Patellaspitzensyndrom. Sportverl Sportschaden 2: 26-34

698. Weh L (1989) Ursachen des „vorderen Knieschmerzes". Arthroskopie 2: 2-7

699. Weller S, Köhnlein E (1962) Die Traumatologie des Kniegelenkes. Thieme, Stuttgart

700. Wentzlik G (1952) Mechanisierung der „gehaltenen Aufnahme" nach Böhler unter Berücksichtigung der Strahlenschutzvorschriften. Teil 1: gehaltene Aufnahme des Kniegelenkes. Röntgenblätter 5: 162-168

701. White BF, Brown DW, Hundal M, Johnson RJ, Pope MH (1979) Knee impedance testing machine. Med Instrum 13: 227-231

702. White BF, Brown DG, Johnson RJ, Pope MH (1979) In vivo laxity testing of the knee. Anterior displacement test. Trans Orthop Res Soc 4: 255

703. Wiberg G (1941) Roentgenographic and anatomical studies on the femoropatellar joint. With special reference to chondromalacia patellae. Acta Orthop Scand 12: 319-323

704. Wilcke KH (1933) Endoskopie des Kniegelenkes an der Leiche. Bruns Beitr Klin Chir 169: 75-83

705. Winkel D, Vleeming A, Fisher S, Mejer OG, Vroege C (1985) Nichtoperative Orthopädie der Weichteile des Bewegungsapparates, Teil 2: Diagnostik. Fischer, Stuttgart

706. Winkel D, Hirschfeld P (1988) Orthopädische Medizin, Bd 2: Das Knie, 2. Aufl. Perimed, Erlangen

707. Wirth CJ, Artmann M (1974) Verhalten der Roll-Gleitbewegung des belasteten Kniegelenkes bei Verlust und Ersatz des vorderen Kreuzbandes. Arch Orthop Unfallchir 78: 356-361

708. Wirth CJ, Artmann M (1975) Diagnostische Probleme bei frischen und veralteten Kreuzbandverletzungen des Kniegelenkes. Arch Orthop Unfallchir 81: 333-340

709. Wirth CJ, Küsswetter W (1978) Die isolierte Ruptur des vorderen Kreuzbandes. Arch Orthop Unfallchir 91: 239-242

710. Wirth CJ, Jäger M (1981) Röntgenologische Diagnostik der Kapselbandläsionen. Röntgenpraxis 34: 399-409

711. Wirth CJ, Häfner H (1981) Biomechanische Aspekte und klinische Wertigkeit des Lachman-Testes bei der Diagnostik von Kreuzbandverletzungen. Orthop Prax 11: 904-908

712. Wirth CJ, Jäger M, Kolb M (1984) Die komplexe vordere Knie-Instabilität. Thieme, Stuttgart New York

713. Wirth CJ, Kolb M (1985) Hämarthros und „isolierte" vordere Kreuzbandläsion. Unfallchirurg 88: 419-423

714. Wirth CJ, Rodriguez M, Milachowski KA (1988) Meniskusnaht - Meniskusrefixation. Thieme, Stuttgart New York

715. Witt AN, Jäger M, Refior HJ, Wirth CJ (1977) Das instabile Kniegelenk - Grundlagenforschung, Diagnose, Therapie. Arch Orthop Unfallchir 88: 49-63

716. Wojtys E, Wilson M, Buckwalter K, Braunstein E, Martell W (1987) Magnetic resonance imaging of the hyaline cartilage and intraarticular pathology. Am J Sports Med 15: 455-463

717. Woods GW, Stanley RF, Tullos HS (1979) Lateral capsular sign: x-ray clue to a significant knee instability. Am J Sports Med 7: 27-33

718. Worth RM, Kettelkamp DB, Defalque RJ, Duane KU (1984) Saphenous nerve entrapment. Am J Sports Med 12: 80-81

719. Yasuda K, Majima T (1988) Intra-articular ganglion blocking extension of the knee. J Bone Joint Surg [Br] 70: 837

720. Youmans WT (1978) The so called „isolated" anterior cruciate ligament tear or anterior cruciate ligament syndrome: a report of 32 cases with some observation on treatment and its effect on result. Am J Sports Med 6: 26-30

721. Zarins B, Rowe CR, Harris BA, Watkins MP (1983) Rotational motion of the knee. Am J Sports Med 11: 152-156

722. Zelko RR (1982) The Lachman sign vs the anterior drawer sign in the diagnosis of acute tears of the anterior cruciate ligament. Orthop Trans 6: 45-49

723. Zimny ML, Schutte M, Dabezies E (1986) Mechanoreceptors in the human anterior cruciate ligament. Anat Rec 214: 204-209

724. Zippel H (1973) Meniskusverletzungen und Meniskusschäden. Barth, Leipzig

Subject Index

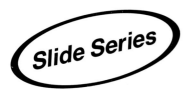

A. Gächter, F. K. Freuler, Basle

Arthroscopic Findings in the Knee Joint

Arthroskopische Befunde am Kniegelenk
Arthroscopie diagnostique du genou

1988. II, 56 pp. 250 slides (125 b/w) with legends in English, German and French. Supplied in a ringbinder. DM 378,– ISBN 3-540-92593-7

The usefulness of arthroscopic examinations is not limited to revealing lesions of the meniscus; far more, the strength of this method lies in the possibilities it offers for identification of complex lesions as well. Arthroscopy also allows the testing of function with the benefit of intra-articular vision; the implications of the injuries and the exact treatment procedures to be followed – operative or conservative – can thus be established. For correct identification of injuries, clinical knowledge needs to be supplemented by familiarity with the visual findings. Recognition is dependent upon knowledge; and it is for this reason that this slide series has been created, in which each arthroscopic image is paired with an explanatory line drawing.

The slides were selected from the 8000 arthroscopic examinations carried out at the University Orthopedic Hospital in Basle. Emphasis is placed on presenting clear and unambiguous images of important findings of types that are seen daily in arthroscopy.

Springer-Verlag
Berlin Heidelberg
New York London
Paris Tokyo Hong Kong

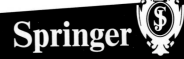

Springer

H.-R. Henche, Rheinfelden; **J. Holder,** Frankfurt

Arthroscopy of the Knee Joint

Diagnosis and Operation Techniques

With Forewords by R. W. Jackson and E. Morscher

Drawings by F. Freuler and M. Jauch

Translated from the German by D. Le Vay

2nd, rev. and enlarged ed. 1988. XI, 190 pp. 225 figs., mostly in color. Hardcover DM 268,– ISBN 3-540-18218-7

Rapid developments in this successful diagnostic and operative technique have called for a new edition of **Arthroscopy of the Knee Joint.** This second edition has been completely revised and retains very little material from the first edition. The diagnostic section has been considerably expanded and elucidated and the operative section adapted to modern technology.

The first part of the book presents the external conditions and prerequisites for diagnostic arthroscopy. The endoscopic anatomy and pathology of the knee joint are covered in detail. Particular emphasis is placed on practical hints for accurate arthroscopic procedures.

The second part then discusses operative techniques. The reader discovers step-by-step how and which pathological findings should, in the authors' opinion, be treated. Here, too, the problems and possible complications of arthroscopic surgery relevant to the individual techniques are dealt with in detail.

Equipped with this book, the reader will be thoroughly informed on all current arthroscopic methods and possibilities.

Prices are subject to change without notice.

Springer-Verlag
Berlin Heidelberg
New York London
Paris Tokyo Hong Kong

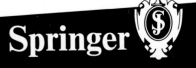